G000153890

P 37 tine ?

PERIODONTICS IN PRACTICE

PERIODONTICS IN PRACTICE
Science with humanity

Trevor LP Watts BDS, MDS, PhD, FDSRCPS
Senior Lecturer and Honorary Consultant in
Periodontology at Guy's, King's College and
St Thomas' Dental Institute, London, UK

MARTIN DUNITZ

© Martin Dunitz Ltd 2000

Although every effort has been made to ensure that all owners of copyright material
have been acknowledged in this publication, we would be glad to acknowledge in
subsequent reprints or editions any omissions brought to our attention.

First published in the United Kingdom in 2000
by Martin Dunitz Ltd, The Livery House,
7–9 Pratt Street, London NW1 0AE
Tel. 207 482 2202

All rights reserved. No part of this publication may be reproduced, stored in a
retrieval system, or transmitted, in any form or by any means, electronic, mechanical,
photocopying, recording, or otherwise, without the prior permission of the publisher
or in accordance with the provisions of the Copyright Act 1988 or under the terms of
any licence permitting limited copying issued by the Copyright Licensing Agency,
90 Tottenham Court Road, London W1P 0LP.

The Author has asserted his right under the Copyright, Designs and Patents Act 1988
to be identified as the Author of this Work.

Although every effort has been made to ensure that drug doses and other information
are presented accurately in this publication, the ultimate responsibility rests with the
prescriber. Neither the publishers nor the authors can be held responsible for errors or
for any consequences arising from the use of information contained herein. For
detailed prescribing information or instructions on the use of any product or procedure discussed herein, please consult the prescribing information or instructional
material issued by the manufacturer.

A CIP catalogue record for this book is available from the British Library.

ISBN 1–85317–830–6

Distributed in the United States and Canada by:
Thieme New York
333 7th Avenue
New York, NY 10001
USA
Tel. 212 760 0888

Composition by Scribe Design, Gillingham, Kent
Printed and bound in Singapore by Kyodo Printing Pte Ltd

CONTENTS

RELATED DENTAL SUBJECTS

CASE MANAGEMENT AND DECISION MAKING

PREFACE

There are several excellent books on periodontology in print on both sides of the Atlantic Ocean. Like many teachers, I had intended not to write a book, but when the publishers kindly approached me with the suggestion, I thought hard. We live at a time when the evidential basis of medicine is rightly the centre of attention, and truth is what we seek to approach.

For over 10 years I have provided abstracts of current research papers from the scientific literature for the *British Dental Journal*. These have related to all aspects of dentistry, with a clinical orientation. In this book, I have given similar brief summaries of over 140 of the many papers that have helped to form modern periodontology. These are a personal selection, naturally, but many are classic studies and others are chosen to illustrate specific points. I hope that my approach will be helpful to dentists and students at the level of interpreting the research literature.

However, there is another aspect of periodontology that concerns me as a teacher, and that is the way in which we apply science to our patients. Applying science to human patients is a skill that does not always come naturally to scientists, and I have tried to balance this educational need with a critical approach to the interpretation of periodontal research. For 20 years I have developed a tutorial course for first-year Master's degree students in my subject. About 70 of them have interacted with me and I thank them for it. This has given the overall framework to the book. These bones have been clothed in flesh with regard to the needs of the 2000 or more dental undergraduates whom I have been privileged to serve over 25 years. In addition, many practising dentists have asked my advice on a wide range of topics. As a teacher, I have been helped by all these experiences to perceive issues where there is a need for careful explanation.

When I was a student in the 1960s, I counted some 23 different subjects in my dental surgery course. A few years after qualifying, when I returned to university to teach and research periodontology, a similar pleasing diversity was apparent within this dental subject. Now, over 25 years after entering the speciality, I can truthfully say that my subject is fascinating and has never bored me. Not only does it involve the function of an anatomically unique part of the human body, but periodontal diseases also have their own unique pathological and immunological characteristics in an environment boasting some 300 known species of microorganism. Treatment is frequently dependent upon altering human behaviour and may also involve a wide variety of non-surgical and surgical techniques, with many interesting pharmacological and regenerative adjuncts. There is a strong basis of good epidemiological work, and a large number of clinical trials.

The book is aimed primarily at practising dentists, and is meant to complement an education in clinical periodontology by raising questions and providing answers to some of them. With the information explosion, we all need to be researchers in one form or another. Although I have designed the book to unwrap gradually the subject of periodontology, I do not intend to bore readers with more than brief accounts of subjects under the headings of anatomy, bacteriology and pathology, which they will have encountered elsewhere.

One final note: because this book encompasses a practising lifetime, some of the earlier photography shows ungloved fingers in the patients' mouths, which was common practice at the time. Naturally, I have adhered to gloved practice since it became the norm in dentistry, and I fully support all accepted infection control procedures.

ACKNOWLEDGEMENTS

First, I am deeply grateful to Elizabeth, my wife of over 30 years. Her love, gentleness and sensitivity, both as a wife and mother and in her long-standing work of personal counselling, have provided my most consistent and challenging role-model.

I would like to thank many colleagues and students who have contributed over the years to the development of this work. They have all helped me to learn. Out of those who have occupied the official relationship of a teacher to me, I would like especially to thank Professors Phil Holloway and Harold Jones most warmly for their kindness in years past when I studied, taught and researched at the University of Manchester.

As a result of two mergers, the institution that I entered next as the Royal Dental School has become part of Guy's, King's College and St Thomas' Dental Institute, or GKT Dental Institute for short. Most of my time is spent on Floor 21 at Guy's Hospital, and sincere thanks are due to many very kind and helpful colleagues throughout the Institute and elsewhere in the hospital. I feel privileged to be part of this large but very friendly and supportive establishment, and would like to thank the Dean of the Dental Institute, Professor Frank Ashley, for his personal encouragement and friendship over many years.

My abstracting work for the *British Dental Journal* has benefited from the encouragement of the immediate past editor, Dame Margaret Seward, and the current editor, Mike Grace, to both of whom I give sincere thanks. Without this work, I would not have thought of one of the prime features of the present book.

I am indebted to several generous colleagues who have permitted me to publish their photographs, as well as to the *British Medical Journal* for allowing me to reproduce figures from one of my papers. This courtesy is acknowledged in the text. Photographs have been provided by Mr Malcolm Lawrence, Mr Guy Palmer, Dr Paul Palmer, Professor Richard Palmer, Dr Ravi Saravanamuttu and Mr Brian Smith. Colleagues who have kindly read portions of the manuscript and offered advice include Professor David Gibbons, Dr Mark Ide, Professor Richard Palmer, Mr Brian Smith, Professor William Wade and Dr Ron Wilson. The responsibility for any errors and significant omissions in the final text is the author's alone.

I would also like to thank Messrs Hu-Friedy and their Authorised Consultant, Mr Peter Oxley, for the generous donation of Gracey pattern curettes that appear in the relevant photographs.

My thanks are also due to Mr Robert Peden and Miss Catherine Stuart at Martin Dunitz Ltd. If it had not been for Mr Peden's initial contact, this book would not have been written, and both he and Miss Stuart have given me kind support and encouragement in the work.

CONVENTIONS AND ABBREVIATIONS

TOOTH NOTATION

Where teeth are referred to by a number, this is according to the FDI (International Dental Federation) two-digit system. The first digit indicates quadrant: in the permanent dentition, upper right is 1, upper left is 2, lower left is 3 and lower right is 4, to indicate deciduous teeth, the respective quadrants are numbered 5, 6, 7 and 8. The second digit indicates the tooth: permanent teeth are numbered from the central incisor (1) to the third molar (8). Thus the permanent lower-left second premolar is tooth 35, for instance, and the deciduous upper-right first molar is tooth 54.

PROBING CHARTS

In the interests of clarity, I have used a simple chart of probing depths most of the time, so that conditions for the whole tooth or a group of teeth may be compared easily in sequential recordings (see Chapter 30 for comment). Where a figure is the same as in the previous chart, it is black; where it is reduced (better), it is red; and where it is increased (worse), it is blue. As with caries charts, lingual and palatal records are in the line closer to the tooth number in the quadrant, and buccal records are in the further line.

ABBREVIATIONS

Some of the abbreviations given below are widely used in medical practice; others are found less frequently outside periodontology circles. They are generally indicated with their first usage in the text.

Aa	*Actinobacillus actinomycetemcomitans*
AIDS	acquired immune deficiency syndrome
ANUG	acute necrotizing ulcerative gingivitis
BOP	bleeding on probing
CAL	clinical attachment level or loss (used by some authors to denote PAL)
CEJ	cementoenamel junction
CPITN	Community Periodontal Index of Treatment Need
EMD	enamel matrix derivative
GI	Gingival Index (of Löe and Silness)
GJP	generalized juvenile periodontitis
GTR	guided tissue regeneration
HIV	human immunodeficiency virus
IDDM	insulin-dependent diabetes mellitus
Ig	immunoglobulin (specified further, e.g. IgM, IgA, IgG4)
IL-	interleukin (specified further, e.g. IL-6, IL-1β)
LJP	localized juvenile periodontitis
MAb	monoclonal antibody
NIDDM	non-insulin-dependent diabetes mellitus
NSPH	non-specific plaque hypothesis
NUP	necrotizing ulcerative periodontitis
OHI	oral hygiene instruction
PAL	probing attachment level or loss (see also CAL)
PD	probing depth
Pg	*Porphyromonas gingivalis*
PI	Periodontal Index (of Russell)
RPP	rapidly progressive periodontitis
SAFT	self-achieved furcation tunnel
SPH	specific plaque hypothesis
VPI	Virginia Polytechnic Institute

1 THE HUMAN ENVIRONMENT OF THE PERIODONTIUM

- What are the prime influences on the periodontium, for better or worse?
- Why is behaviour so significant in periodontics?
- Why is communication so important in periodontics?
- What periodontal objectives do patients have?

Periodontology is a term derived from three Greek words: περι (peri, meaning 'around'), οδους (odous – 'tooth'), and λογος (logos – 'discourse'). It is the science of the supporting tissues of the tooth. Many factors have a bearing on the state of these tissues. The clinical practice of periodontology (periodontics) starts and finishes with the patient. The clinician needs to bring together several diverse

Table 1,1: *The periodontium and its environment*

The scene
- Periodontal tissue structure
- Active tissue turnover

Principal protagonists
- Microbial plaque with threat of damage
- Active host defence

Host behaviour
- Positive host behaviour, e.g. plaque control
- Negative host behaviour, e.g. tobacco smoking

Influences on host behaviour
- Positive, e.g. dental team giving effective oral hygiene education, and press articles and advertisements that reinforce this
- Negative, e.g. poor attempts at oral hygiene education, and press or advertising misinformation

---

areas of scientific understanding (Table 1,1) and apply them to a real human being with a specified periodontal condition.

CHANGING ANATOMICAL STRUCTURE

First, there is the structure of the periodontium and adjacent tissues, and its relation to function. It would be quite wrong to view this structure as something static, as mere scenery for the other actors such as bacteria and host response. The scene is undergoing continual revision, as actors come and go, with a continuous turnover of cells and cellular products, such as the collagen fibres that hold the body together. The high turnover rates of the junctional epithelium and periodontal ligament collagen are of significance in both the initial development of disease and some of its later effects, such as drifting of individual teeth.

DYNAMIC DEFENCES

There is an equivalent mistaken view of the periodontal host defences. These are not only reactive, but proactive. The defence is active even in the absence of an enemy, as demonstrated by the continual flow of neutrophils into the healthy gingival crevice. These are randomly moving cells that search for intruders, such as bacteria, and are well-equipped to destroy them. The whole complex system of inflammation is available to protect the human body against the threat of microbial invasion. This system is currently viewed as responsible for much of the damage caused in periodontal diseases. It is even possible to view tooth loss from periodontitis as a protective event: the human body is relieved of the bacterial threat in the well-organized plaque.

COMPLEX MICROBIAL HABITAT

It is well established that a large number of microbial species may be found adjacent to the periodontal tissues. If they are allowed to remain undisturbed, they form the complex biofilm called bacterial plaque. This has a life of its own and has clearly been shown to be the cause of several widespread periodontal diseases. However, some investigators have gone to considerable lengths to show that not all bacteria are equally important, and that certain specific organisms may be particularly damaging.

SIGNIFICANT BEHAVIOURAL CONTEXT

Although human beings have varying individual susceptibility to destructive periodontal diseases, many may prevent or control such diseases by controlling the bacterial plaque. In recent years it has become apparent that other behavioural factors, such as tobacco addiction, may predispose to periodontitis, exacerbate it and reduce the effects of treatment. To treat the patient effectively usually involves modifying the behavioural factor, and there may be more than one treatment option for the same problem. The patient must be involved in making the most appropriate choice, with advice and discussion of potential risks, benefits and treatment outcomes.

EVIDENCE AND ITS INTERPRETATION

There is a considerable body of periodontal research literature, and many basic periodontal truths are established. The clinician needs to know how and where to find evidence of these truths in support of advice that may be given to the patient.

However, the professional is not the only contender for the patient's ear. Skilful advertising and publicity seek to exploit human insecurities and fears, and make money out of them. Journalists may also unintentionally misinform the public with attention-seeking articles and create unnecessary conflict between clinicians and their patients.

Another group of well-intentioned people advocates the treatment methods of various alternative medicine philosophies. Unfortunately, these have little or no basis in science. There are also less scrupulous individuals who try to create a gullible and loyal market for quackery.

Consequently, there may be a tension between the clinician and patient that needs to be resolved. No-one likes to be told that they are wrong, but some patients may even apologetically blame themselves for the state of their periodontium. However, there are also individuals who seek aggressively to dictate the course of their treatment and manipulate the clinician. Both extremes may result from anxiety, which guides so much of human behaviour.

TREATMENT INVOLVES TRUST

It is important to establish a basic relationship of trust with the patient from the start. This may include gently reasoning with some patients that they are not to blame for their disease, and that going to the dentist regularly might not have prevented it. Above all else, it is important to establish common goals and shared motives for treatment. This does not preclude either clinician or patient having other individual goals and motives.

In the complex arena of the professional relationship, trust is the first stage in establishing truth – about the patient's condition, about the knowledge relating to it and about the appropriate course of action for both clinician and patient. The clinician has a dual responsibility: to know the evidence or where to find it, and to communicate it to the patient with clarity.

this is the 'Plaque-infected dentitions' study referred to in Chapter 21 (Abstract 21,1).

THE DENTIST–PATIENT RELATIONSHIP APPLIED TO PERIODONTOLOGY

It has been said that periodontology is the foundation of good dentistry. This is true in more than one sense. Not only do the teeth need to be well supported by the periodontium, but the dentist who can lead a patient through the explanation, advice and execution of a periodontal treatment plan, including complicated behaviour changes in oral hygiene, is rightly to be viewed as a support to the patient.

Dentists may have a number of conflicts about giving information and advice. It is important to start where the patient is, which means being ready to listen. At the outset, the patient should be made to feel in control. This may be done quite simply, by the dentist giving the patient the right to interrupt with a comment or question at any time. Some dentists feel uncomfortable at the thought of a question that they may not be able to answer, but we all have to admit to gaps in our knowledge.

In all aspects of dentistry, communication is important. The patient is a partner in treatment, and entitled to a discussion of the options. Refusal of treatment is one of those options and so is a second opinion. There is no worse basis for treatment than a patient who reluctantly agrees to persuasion from the dentist, or the converse. Both situations are potentially explosive. Faced with an adverse outcome, each may try to blame it on the other.

There is an additional reason why communication is of special importance in periodontics. There is a need not only for patient cooperation, but also for substantial and permanent behaviour change in most cases. Although cooperation is needed for orthodontics or removal of impacted teeth, there is a perceived endpoint that does not apply to periodontal treatment. In other words, many periodontal outcomes are open to subsequent reversal by the patient. A classic example of

THE OBJECTIVES OF PATIENTS WITH PERIODONTAL PROBLEMS

Patients may arrive at the dentist with a variety of personal complaints arising from their periodontal condition. A common complaint is that the gums bleed; less frequently, teeth may feel loose; sometimes halitosis is a problem perceived by the patient or mentioned by a close friend or relative. Teeth may have moved because of periodontitis, or the gums may have receded. On occasions, tooth loss or movement may make problems for mastication or speech.

Patients often perceive these complaints as threats to their social or physical well-being. Their overall aim in consulting a dentist may be to correct any problems that they feel are likely to cause embarrassment or discomfort. Four objectives may be listed that cover most patients with periodontal problems (Table 1,2).

Table 1,2: *Periodontally-associated patient objectives*

Social relations
- Appearance and arrangement of teeth (aesthetics or beauty)
- Avoidance of oral malodour
- Avoidance of other embarrassment, e.g. from loose prostheses

Self-image
- Tooth retention
- Avoidance of prostheses

Comfort
- Satisfactory masticatory function
- Avoidance of uncomfortable conditions such as:
  Dentine hypersensitivity
  Periodontal abscesses
  Dental hypermobility

Speech
- Maintenance of usual speech behaviour
- Avoidance of distorted speech patterns

First, there is the question of how patients think others perceive them. We may call this the social objective and, in addition to visual appearance, it can include matters like halitosis.

Secondly, how do patients perceive themselves? In the minds of many, loss of teeth is viewed as an unwelcome sign of advancing age. Others may view it as an unwelcome surgical intervention, to be followed by the equally unwelcome prospect of removable partial dentures.

A third objective is comfort: in mastication, which may also manifest itself as a desire to retain all teeth, or at least to replace missing ones with fixed bridgework and implants, if necessary and affordable; and in avoiding discomfort related to periodontal pathology.

The fourth objective is to retain normal speech. Movement, especially of upper incisors, may cause some patients undesired alterations that are potentially embarrassing. The replacement of teeth with any form of prosthesis also may affect speech in some people.

Patients may have any or all of these objectives. Because of the limitations of treatment, certain objectives are not realistic for some individual patients. There may be a conflict between the aesthetic and tooth retention objectives in some patients with advanced disease. These patients may have to choose between retention of teeth in unsatisfactory positions and loss of these teeth followed by their aesthetic replacement with a prosthesis. An example of management of a patient who was unable to fulfil the objective of tooth retention is given in Case History 1 (Figs 1,1–1,5).

CASE HISTORY 1: a suspicious and depressed patient (Figs 1,1–1,5)

A 39-year-old single white female was referred for periodontal assessment. Throughout the procedure she asked questions and made written notes about the conversation. It emerged that she had seen several dentists who had said different things and treated her in different ways for the same aggressive periodontal problem. Several teeth had recurring abscesses. Teeth were beginning to drift because of advanced disease, but she did not want to lose any, and hoped that somehow she would be able to keep her teeth if only she could find the right treatment. She also had severe personal problems and smoked 20 cigarettes per day.

DIAGNOSIS

Advanced chronic adult periodontitis, possibly an early-onset form of periodontitis at a previous stage, but now exacerbated by tobacco smoking. Prognosis for several teeth was very poor. Plaque control was also poor, despite some knowledge and previous instruction.

MANAGEMENT

An initial treatment phase of oral hygiene education, root planing and scaling was important in demonstrating to the patient that she was unable to maintain good plaque control. Although advised, she was not able to quit smoking, but did succeed in reducing the quantity. As treatment progressed, she appreciated the need for some extractions and aesthetic partial dentures. She had a supportive general dental practitioner who was willing to provide gradual transition to complete dentures, and was given hygienist maintenance support at 4-month intervals.

COMMENT

An insecure patient with low self-image. Listening and discussion were important throughout treatment. At one point she was almost suicidal. She needed kindness and help to reconstruct her life, and had to accept the likelihood of eventual loss of her teeth, which initially she resisted strongly. The main lines of periodontal counselling were: that plaque was not controlled, but she still had

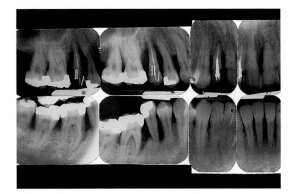

Fig. 1,1

Radiographs of right side of patient in Case History 1 at initial examination.

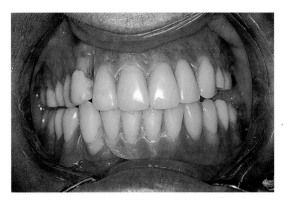

Fig. 1,3

Case history 1: 10 years later almost complete dentures are worn, retained by the two right canine teeth.

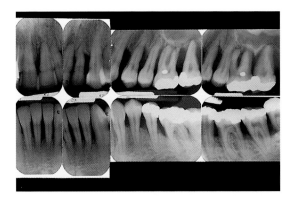

Fig. 1,2

Radiographs of left side of patient in Case History 1 at initial examination.

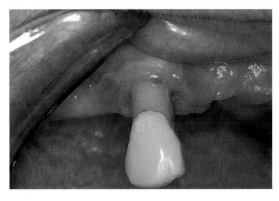

Fig. 1,4

Case history 1: tooth 13, probing depth (PD) 1–3 mm.

alternative options; that dentures could be a positive option to improve her life; and that she could retain control of decisions to lose individual teeth and to add teeth to the dentures. Once trust had become apparent, over a period of 10 years all but two teeth were lost and replaced with dentures. The patient's personal characteristics were greatly improved once the initial severe depressive state was resolved. It is possible that sympathetic management of her periodontal problems contributed to overcoming depression. Hope played a considerable part in a satisfactory outcome, although false hopes were rightly lost.

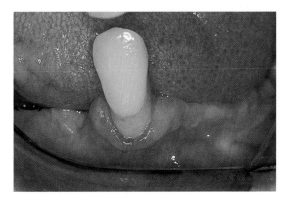

Fig. 1,5

Case history 1: tooth 43, PD 1–3 mm.

HYGIENISTS AND OTHER MEMBERS OF THE TEAM

Management of periodontal treatment inevitably involves delegation by the dentist of important parts of treatment to other personnel. Hygienists have a leading role in this work, but so may nurses (dental health education), and receptionists may be asked for advice; and they all may be considered more approachable than the dentist by some patients.

The ground rules are simple: nothing must conflict with the dentist's management of the patient, and openness must be the norm. As a result, time must be made for all personnel to come together so that advice guidelines can be established. Once this has been done, regular meetings for a few minutes every 2-3 months can deal with new questions that patients have asked. In all cases of doubt, the staff must, of course, refer queries to the dentist at the next convenient opportunity.

The hygienist has a special position by reason of intimate involvement with the progress of treatment. A detailed set of guidelines should be established for hygiene personnel, and a clear treatment plan for each patient. It may be useful to have a checklist covering all likely procedures, including which teeth need special attention and for what reason.

An essential aspect of team management is the interest shown by the dentist in each person's work. This should include joint review of patients by dentist and hygienist. In every way, the dentist, as an authority figure, should ensure that patients view any attending staff as carrying the same authority within their spheres of practice. It is central to patient welfare that no conflict should exist, or be perceived to exist, within the team.

CONCLUSION

The periodontal environment is extensive: not only does it include the microflora adjacent to the tissues and the host response, but also the patient's behaviour and a wide variety of influences on it. If the members of the dental team are aware of this complicated background, it will help them to anticipate and deal with their patients' problems.

2 THE AMAZING MAZE OF PERIODONTAL RESEARCH

- Why worry about research?
- What sorts of research are relevant to periodontics?
- How is research done?
- Why may some research findings be difficult to apply?

Research is the foundation for all our knowledge, yet for many people the papers published in research journals are quite incomprehensible. A few clinicians view researchers with contempt as people shut away in their academic ivory towers and divorced from reality. This is interesting because the object of most researchers is to achieve a better understanding of reality than others before them. There are also a paranoid few who view research as a closed shop with a hidden agenda, full of conspiracies and ready to persecute its opponents. Actually, researchers are likely to disagree over a wide range of matters, and should not be seen as having a common agenda.

At the other extreme, a few view research with awe, a perspective derived from respect of their teachers in dental school and knowledge of the mysterious laboratories in which some research is performed, and they may feel that researchers are beyond the criticism of ordinary mortals. However, research has always benefited from thoughtful criticism, whatever the source. The greatest researchers are often the most humble, and they are well aware of their capacity for error.

Somewhere in the middle there is a valiant and perhaps increasing band of people who appreciate the value of research but have difficulty understanding it because they have not participated in it. It is probably still true to say that many clinicians simply ignore most research for most of the time. This may be

partly from feelings that much research is irrelevant to clinical practice, and partly because they just do not know where to start looking.

CLINICIANS NEED TO UNDERSTAND RESEARCH

In today's evidence-based clinical world, however, there is an increasing need to understand the foundations of periodontology. Manufacturers seek to introduce the clinician to new and expensive technologies for periodontal treatment and diagnosis. Clinicians then may seek to persuade patients to pay for these services, and patients naturally will want to know the potential benefit.

To form a professional judgement and to inform and advise patients correctly, the clinician needs knowledge not only of the new technology in question, but also of the whole

Table 2,1: *Some types of periodontal research study*

Theoretical	In vitro
• Review	• Microbiological
• Statistical	• Histological
• Modelling	• Immunological
	• Biochemical
	• Genetic
	• Cell culture
In vivo (animal)	**In vivo (human)**
• Analogical	• Observational
• Therapeutic	• Investigative
• Toxicological	• Clinical trials
	• Cohort studies

background of periodontal research, of the ways in which a new technology has arisen, the ways in which it has been tested and the actual clinical benefits that have been shown. Is the new technology a real advance in practice?

THE PANORAMA OF PERIODONTAL RESEARCH

A simple classification of research studies is given in Table 2,1. Theoretical studies employ existing data to see whether further useful conclusions are forthcoming. New research models may be developed from an assessment of past research, and because of the complexity of measuring periodontal disease, there is also a strong tradition of statistical research.

Studies *in vitro* (Latin: in glass – i.e. originally in test tubes and other glass apparatus) are carried out in the laboratory and may involve a wide range of different investigations. Studies *in vivo* (in a live subject) may be performed in animals when there is an important reason for not doing them in human subjects.

Finally, there is a huge variety of studies in human beings, varying from painstaking epidemiological observation to complex clinical trials of treatment procedures. This list is not intended to be exhaustive, and various aspects of research may be combined with each other.

THE PROCESS OF EXPERIMENTAL RESEARCH (Table 2,2)

All types of experimental research have a basis in theory. Ideas are tested to see whether they are correct. The ideas or hypotheses come from observing natural events, or from careful examination of previous observations and experiments in a particular field of interest.

It is therefore customary for experimental researchers to begin by reviewing the particular published literature that summarizes relevant previous work. From this they will identify a suitable hypothesis that needs to be examined. Next, they will devise a suitable experiment to test the hypothesis, and write a

Table 2,2: *Stages of an experimental research study*

Planning
- Literature search and review
- Hypothesis formulation
- Protocol writing

Provision and approval
- Funding and resource allocation
- Ethical approval

Execution
- Recruitment of volunteer participants (if required)
- Performance of study according to approved protocol
- Analysis of results

Publication
- Writing of paper
- Submission to journal
- Peer review
- Possible adjustment or rewriting of paper, or further experimental work
- Acceptance and publication
- Response of other researchers

protocol indicating how the experiment is to be performed.

At this stage, the implications of the research are examined. Funding this will need to be approved by the appropriate authority – perhaps a university department head or other budget-holder – or, in the case of large sums, by an independent grant-awarding body that will seek specialist advice.

Ethical implications also are examined. In the UK, all research with animals is subject to the most rigorous control by the Home Office. For studies in human beings, there are ethics committees and institutional review boards which have to be satisfied that the study is both scientifically appropriate and unlikely to harm participants. The participants must be clearly informed about the study and give their consent to take part. They have the right to withdraw their cooperation at any stage and for any reason.

The next stage is that the research study is actually performed. This may take a few weeks for some types of laboratory study, or a few years for some clinical studies of treatment in human beings.

The finished account of research is then written as a paper. The first part is the introduction or literature review, which leads up to the aim of the study. This is followed in turn with details of the methods and materials employed, the results of the research and a discussion that links these findings to the literature review and explains what conclusions may be drawn.

At this point the researchers send their paper to a journal publisher for possible publication. The editor seeks expert advice from other scientists (usually, but not always, anonymous) about the scientific merit of the work. This process of peer review is to improve or eliminate, as far as possible, work that is not scientifically sound before it reaches a wider audience. Reviewers make suggestions that lead frequently to a more accurate account and occasionally to further research.

Finally, on publication, the research can be read and evaluated by many others who are familiar with the field of study. This will lead to further discussion of the research, sometimes in public correspondence, particularly if the study is controversial.

It is possible for poor research to be published, but this long and arduous process certainly tends to maintain a higher standard than otherwise. There are other checks on the research community in the shape of regular conferences. At the International Association for Dental Research's annual meeting, and at its divisional meetings all over the world, short accounts of several thousand studies are made public and discussed. As a result, researchers may undertake further experiment to improve their work, or cease a particular line of study if it seems unfruitful or inappropriate.

EXAMPLE OF A THEORETICAL STUDY

One type of theoretical study is when an attempt is made to bring together the results of a number of separate studies concerning the same issue. Abstract 2,1 concerns whether there is any advantage in the use of the antibiotic tetracycline in treating a widespread form of periodontitis. This is called a meta-analysis,

Abstract 2,1 *Quality assessment and meta-analysis of systemic tetracycline use in chronic adult periodontitis*

Hayes C, Antczak-Bouckoms A, Burdick E, *Journal of Clinical Periodontology* 1992; **19**: 164–168

A search on the computer database MEDLINE identified 13 studies (nine randomized controlled trials, four non-randomized studies) that evaluated systemic use of tetracycline alone or as an adjunct to non-surgical therapy of human periodontitis. Two readers who did not know the origin of these studies assessed their methods and results. Quality of all studies was scored for protocol, and for data analysis and presentation. Only two studies gave adequate information for comparison, with respect to periodontal pockets of depth initially 5 mm or more. These studies did not report significant differences between different groups. By considering the likely level of error, the present investigators concluded that there was no evidence for indiscriminate use of tetracycline in adult periodontitis.

Comment: The apparently harsh judgement on quality of these studies really reflected many different approaches that could not be combined easily to give a clear answer to the question.

where an attempt is made to bring together the results of a number of studies in order to approach the objective truth more closely and rule out the effect of occasional misleading studies.

The studies had been designed in many different ways, and most were therefore not suitable for direct comparison. Outcome was expressed in dissimilar ways, but when the investigators compared carefully selected studies they concluded that evidence did not support using the drug in adult periodontitis.

The result of this study did not mean that the drug had no effect; it simply meant that no effect had been shown by the studies identified with a bearing on human adult periodontitis. Positive evidence is required before subjecting patients to a treatment.

The study also shows how important it is for researchers to report their methods and results as fully as possible. When weighing the evidence for and against a particular treatment, the results of different studies need to be translated into a common system. It is a waste of research if this cannot be done. Scientific evidence in one study needs to be confirmed in others before it can be regarded as established.

A STUDY *IN VITRO*

Much experimental research involves extensive laboratory study of specimens removed from living subjects. An interesting study of this type is outlined in Abstract 2,2. The background is that for at least 10 years, researchers had been interested in the potential of tetracycline as an antibiotic for possible use in some sorts of periodontitis. This was reasonable because periodontitis is a result of microbial action, and many periodontal microbes are susceptible to the action of tetracycline. However, experiments suggested that there was a different way in which tetracycline might help periodontal treatment.

Because tetracycline affects bacteria, any effect of the drug on periodontal health might be explained wholly or partly by this antibiotic effect. To show that there was a different effect preventing collagen breakdown, these researchers tested the fluid exudate from the

Abstract 2,2 *Further evidence that tetracyclines inhibit collagenase activity in human crevicular fluid and from other mammalian sources*

Golub LM, Wolff M, Lee HM, et al., *Journal of Periodontal Research* 1985; **20**: 12–23

Gingival crevicular fluid was collected from human periodontal pockets of varying depth and assessed for its ability to break down collagen. This was greater in deeper pockets. Treatment of human subjects with different tetracyclines markedly reduced the activity 1–2 weeks later. Studies of skin and gingiva from diabetic rats (in which there is excessive collagenase activity) and of collagenases from rabbit chondrocytes and rat neutrophils showed that tetracyclines also inhibit these collagen-destroying systems.

Comment: One of several papers by these investigators to confirm this effect.

gingival crevice in people with periodontitis, and in others who received a course of a tetracycline group drug. To show that there was a more general effect, they also demonstrated a reduction in activity of collagenase in other mammalian systems.

This shows how research techniques *in vitro* may contribute to understanding a periodontal matter that could not be studied directly. Tetracyclines are antibiotics. This research shows another mechanism that may be beneficial – an effect on the host, rather than the microorganisms.

ANIMAL STUDIES *IN VIVO*

A detailed ethical treatise on studies in animals and human beings is beyond the scope of this book. However, we may list a few questions that are relevant to this matter and indicate a possible approach.

If we want to help human beings, why can we not study their actual problem rather than an animal model that may not be directly applicable? If a study in human beings is not possible, then we must be reasonably certain that the animal study will give us some answers. Can we justify killing an animal? People do this for both food and clothing. Is it right to use a live animal? People have done this from antiquity, for transport in particular and also for hunting and guarding.

Although many would answer yes to the two previous questions, there are still concerns over the way the animal is treated. Is it treated kindly? People who object to intensive farming may dislike animal laboratories for the same reason.

A researcher will have to find answers to these questions for the sake of conscience. If animals are used, every consideration should be given to their welfare, and their sacrifice should help to answer an important question in the interests of human welfare.

EXAMPLE OF CONFLICTING RESULTS FROM ANIMAL STUDIES

An example of studies on occlusal trauma, a subject that is dealt with more fully in Chapter

Abstract 2,3 *Influence of trauma from occlusion on progression of experimental periodontitis in the beagle dog*

Lindhe J, Svanberg G, *Journal of Clinical Periodontology* 1974; **1**: 3–14

In beagle dogs, experimental periodontitis was induced by a surgical method and maintained with subgingival plaque accumulation on a metal band. Teeth were jiggled by means of a small cap splint with an inclined plane on the experimental tooth, which made it contact prematurely on occluding, and a spring that returned the tooth to its former position when the mouth opened. When compared 180 days later with a control tooth with periodontitis only on the other side of the mouth, occlusal trauma caused increased attachment loss and increased bone loss.

Comment: This was evidence of co-destruction – occlusal trauma approximately doubled attachment loss (which is irreversible, unlike the bone loss caused by trauma).

Abstract 2,4 *Co-destructive factors of marginal periodontitis and repetitive mechanical injury*

Meitner S, *Journal of Dental Research* 1975; (Special Issue C): C78–C85

In squirrel monkeys, experimental periodontitis was induced with plaque accumulation on ligatures, and jiggling was started 10 weeks later by using orthodontic interdental separators to change the position of teeth every 48 h. After 20 weeks of periodontitis, there was increased bone loss from occlusal trauma over and above that caused by periodontitis on control teeth, but only one of four experimental teeth had a recognizable but moderate increase in loss of periodontal attachment.

Comment: The trauma had an effect in the shape of increased bone loss but there was no overall evidence of co-destruction.

25, may be used to show that animal studies do not always give clear evidence. In Abstracts 2,3 and 2,4 an outline is given of two studies of the same question in different animal models. The question is whether moderately jiggling a tooth to and fro over a period of time can exacerbate the loss of attachment which is caused by dental plaque in the disease of periodontitis.

This question cannot be studied ethically in human beings directly because it would involve deliberately causing an irreversible disease. Researchers in Sweden therefore turned to the beagle dog, an animal in which they had previously studied periodontitis; in the USA, other researchers used the squirrel monkey for similar reasons.

However, although the two groups of researchers showed similar effects for other questions regarding occlusal trauma, the results of their models disagreed over this particular issue. Furthermore, repeated studies with modified methods at a later date gave the same disagreement. This means that these results cannot be applied to the human condition of periodontitis, unlike other animal studies that are in agreement. The matter is still an open question.

HUMAN STUDIES

There have been many thousands of periodontal research studies in human beings. As an example, we shall consider one of the most celebrated and quoted papers of all time (Abstract 2,5). The authors are renowned for their work, and the study is part of the evidence that plaque causes gingivitis. It was also the creation of a widely used model – experimental human gingivitis – with which numerous clinical studies have been performed.

Yet there is a problem. At the time the work was done, many clinicians had come to regard gingivitis as a disease caused by bacteria. However, there were other, older ideas, notably that massaging the gingiva was necessary to maintain health. Even today, this disproven concept is espoused by some.

Abstract 2,5 *Experimental gingivitis in man*

Löe H, Theilade E, Jensen SB, *Journal of Periodontology* 1965; **36**: 177–187

Twelve healthy subjects stopped oral hygiene, and plaque accumulated until they had developed clinical gingivitis over a period of 10–21 days. They were then instructed in thorough oral hygiene with brush and woodsticks. In the next 3–10 days the gingivitis resolved while plaque was reduced to a very low level. Microscopic examination of plaque showed changes in its composition as it developed. The authors concluded that removal of plaque resolved gingival inflammation.

Comment: This classic study may be interpreted differently.

The problem is one of interpretation. In this study, plaque control was performed with instruments that could also be considered likely to massage or stimulate the gingiva –

brushes and woodsticks. The authors did point out that the coarse Scandinavian diet of their subjects failed to stop gingivitis, but the oral hygiene methods were considerably more thorough and direct than the movement of loose foodstuffs in the mouth.

To provide clear evidence that plaque causes gingivitis, methods of plaque control are needed that cannot be interpreted as stimulating or massaging the gingiva. This was exactly what happened next. At a symposium 5 years later, Löe described how the use of a chlorhexidine mouthrinse prevented plaque development in healthy mouths, and with it gingivitis (see Abstract 24,2).

CONCLUSION

As will be seen in the rest of this book, ingenious researchers have studied most aspects of periodontology, and much of our knowledge is well established. It is also true that the more we know, the more we realize where we are ignorant.

3 'NORMAL' PERIODONTIUM AND DISEASE

- What is periodontal health?
- What structures are affected by periodontal diseases?
- What are the main dynamic features of periodontal health?
- How may biological misunderstandings affect periodontics?

When we speak of what is normal in the periodontium, we may have a concept of health that is ideal. If that is so, then normal periodontium is rare. In most mouths there are at least traces of gingival inflammation.

Gingivitis is not serious, and some have even questioned whether it should be called a disease. Because it involves a response to external challenge, we may define it as a pathological condition. It may also be a cosmetic inconvenience, and interfere with the performance of good dental treatment.

Periodontitis is more serious, because it can lead to tooth loss and a number of other undesirable events. Both periodontitis and gingivitis result from the presence of bacterial plaque, and we cannot predict when gingivitis may become periodontitis. It is customary, therefore, to teach patients to control plaque and to use the absence of gingivitis as a sign that plaque is controlled.

Only when bacterial plaque has been controlled for a long period do human periodontal tissues manifest the characteristics of 'health' (Figs 3,1–3,2). These are often defined in terms of the anatomical structures: the hard tissues of the tooth, epithelia, soft gingival connective tissue, periodontal ligament and alveolar bone (Fig. 3,3). There are also other important aspects: the condition

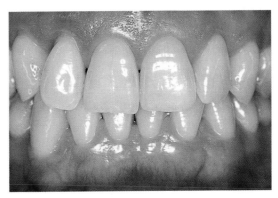

Fig. 3,2

A 34-year-old patient who has been treated for periodontitis, 18 months after active treatment was completed. There was attachment loss on the distal of the upper-right lateral incisor, and this tooth now shows slight distal recession, as a result of successful treatment. It is also slightly mesially rotated, which is a variation on drifting, as a result of the initial disease. In other respects, the gingival tissues may be described as 'normal', and are healthy.

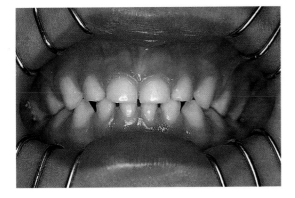

Fig. 3,1

Healthy periodontium in a child aged 3 years. She is the daughter of a periodontist and regular plaque control has been performed daily since the age of 18 months.

13

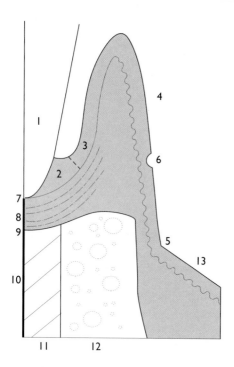

Fig. 3,3

Structure of healthy periodontium that has not experienced attachment loss. 1 = enamel; 2 = junctional epithelium; 3 = oral sulcular epithelium; 4 = oral epithelium; 5 = mucogingival junction; 6 = free gingival groove; 7 = cementoenamel junction; 8 = dentogingival fibres; 9 = dentoperiosteal fibres; 10 = cementum; 11 = periodontal ligament; 12 = alveolar bone; 13 = reflected mucosa.

of the dental pulp, the position of teeth in each dental arch and the relations of the two arches in function.

CEMENTUM

This is a very hard substance with some similarities to bone. It mediates the attachment of the tooth into the gum by means of periodontal ligament fibres that are incorporated into it. Cementum is a living tissue and towards the tooth apex (apically) it has incorporated cementocytes, whereas towards the tooth crown (coronally) these are largely on its surface. Secondary cementum may be laid

down in the apical region of teeth when they erupt further into the mouth as a result of attrition or loss of opposing teeth. The cementum meets the enamel at the cementoenamel or amelocemental junction (CEJ), which is an important clinical landmark.

EPITHELIA

A layer of junctional epithelium is attached to the enamel adjacent to the CEJ. This epithelium merges with the oral sulcular epithelium, which lines the gingival crevice and at the crest of the free gingiva merges into the oral epithelium on the keratinized external aspect of the gingiva. This continues in an apical direction to the mucogingival junction, after which the epithelium becomes the non-keratinized covering of the reflected or buccal sulcus mucosa.

JUNCTIONAL EPITHELIUM

Junctional epithelium has several unique characteristics. It has a large basement membrane area, from which new cells move rapidly to a small surface at the base of the gingival crevice. At the enamel, hemidesmosomes (otherwise related to the basement membrane in basal cells) mediate attachment. Within the epithelium, desmosomes are less frequent than in other epithelia – perhaps about 25% of the level – reflecting the high speed of turnover and greater permeability of this tissue.

ORAL SULCULAR EPITHELIUM

Oral sulcular epithelium, like junctional epithelium, does not usually keratinize. The keratin-rich layer on the surface of many epithelia serves to reduce their permeability, and may be viewed as a protective mechanism. However, it has been shown that very thorough removal of bacteria from the gingival sulcus over a period of time induces a

Abstract 3,1 *The width of radiologically-defined attached gingiva over permanent teeth in children*

Saario M, Ainamo A, Mattila K, et al., *Journal of Clinical Periodontology* 1994; 21: 666–669

In 123 children aged 6, 10 and 12 years, panoramic radiographs were taken with a wire marker over the mucogingival junction. The distance from this to the midpoint of the cementoenamel junction was measured. The attached gingiva over first molars and incisors increased significantly at both time intervals.

Comment: This cross-sectional study compared different children at the three ages. Ideally, the same children should be followed over a 6-year period to show the changes, because otherwise an assumption is needed about the similarity of the three differently aged groups. However, other cross-sectional studies have shown similar results.

Abstract 3,2 *The role of gingival connective tissue in determining epithelial differentiation*

Karring T, Lang NP & Löe H, *Journal of Periodontal Research* 1975; **10**: 1–11

In seven monkeys, 14 epithelium-free grafts of gingival connective tissue were placed in pouches underneath the mucosa apical to the mucogingival junction. For each of these, another graft of connective tissue from alveolar mucosa was also implanted as a control. In 3–4 weeks, the overlying mucosa was removed from all grafts, and healing followed with re-epithelialization from the adjacent non-keratinized mucosa. Subsequent examination showed that the epithelium over the graft areas was in accordance with the graft; new keratinized tissue had developed where this type of connective tissue had been placed, and the controls had not produced this change.

Comment: A clear demonstration that the connective tissue determines the type of epithelium, and can alter cells of another type that grow over it.

form of keratinization. Taking this together with other studies suggesting that the sulcus may disappear after long-term prevention of plaque formation, we may be tempted to ask whether a sulcus is part of 'normal' gingival anatomy, or whether it is part of the response to plaque. However, for all practical purposes, the sulcus may be viewed as 'normal' in the sense that we encounter it in virtually all periodontally healthy patients.

ORAL EPITHELIUM

Oral epithelium is well keratinized and well bound down to the underlying connective tissue. Intersecting rete ridges of this epithelium ensure a much extended basement membrane area, and nutrition of the whole epithelium is maintained by digits of well-vascularized connective tissue between the ridges. Except for where it covers the free gingival margin related to the gingival sulcus, oral epithelium is part of a mucoperiosteum extending to the mucogingival junction. This is called the attached gingiva.

ATTACHED GINGIVA

Attached gingiva serves to anchor the gingiva firmly around the tooth, but has been a source of controversy. Although no-one would think of needlessly discarding it in the course of surgery (see Chapters 19 and 23), studies have suggested that it is not essential to gingival health in the case of individual teeth (see Abstracts 23,1 and 23,2). For instance, a tooth that has no attached gingiva, say, on its buccal surface may still be maintained in a state of health by plaque control with no predisposition to further disease.

Two important facts about attached gingiva are worth remembering. First, it appears to increase with age. There are several studies confirming this finding, and one is summarized in Abstract 3,1. The first such study appeared in 1976, when mucogingival surgery was in a boom period and many children had been provided with extra attached gingiva that was probably unnecessary. The advice nowadays is to wait a few years to see if there

really is a problem. Secondly, if there *is* a clinically justifiable reason for increasing the
attached gingiva in a patient, another timely
study (Abstract 3,2) warns us to choose the
right procedure. The nature of this tissue is
determined by the underlying connective
tissue. To increase attached gingiva, more
connective tissue of the right sort must be
provided, as discussed in Chapter 23.

GINGIVAL SOFT TISSUE

Underneath the epithelium there is a varying
amount of gingival connective tissue, of which
the principal cells are fibroblasts and the main
component is collagen. A good blood supply
carries nutrients and the components of the
host response against disease to where they
are needed. Vessels pass superficially within
the mucoperiosteum of the attached gingiva,
and deeply within the periodontal ligament.
Blood flows in a coronal direction, ensuring
that a surgically raised mucoperiosteal flap
retains its supply and so is able to heal.

The form of the gingival soft tissues is
usually related to the underlying bone.
Recession is often related to the presence of
dehiscences, which are alveolar defects (Fig.
3,4). However, in health the characteristic
gingival papilla that separates each tooth
from the next is adapted to the shape of their
proximal surfaces.

PERIODONTAL LIGAMENT

Separating the cementum from adjacent
alveolar bone, the ligament is a cushion with
several complex features to help teeth
function.

The supporting bundles of collagen fibres are
in several groups. Principal fibres form the
bulk, suspending the tooth in its socket with
a gap of 0.2–0.3 mm. At the alveolar crest,
dentoperiosteal fibres join the periosteum.
Coronally to them, a group of dentogingival
fibres passes into the soft connective tissue of
the gingiva. Proximally, the trans-septal groups
of fibres connect teeth together at this level.

The ligament has a good blood supply
passing up from the apical region of the tooth,
joined by other vessels from the cribriform
alveolar bone of the socket. Like other connective tissues, the ligament also contains the
components of ground substance, particularly
proteoglycans.

Altogether, the ligament functions as a
viscoelastic structure. It deforms when a tooth
is moved by a force (e.g. when teeth occlude)
and allows the tooth subsequently to return to
its former position.

The ligament is essential to the tooth's well-
being. Loss of ligament means loss of flexible
support for the tooth.

ALVEOLAR BONE

In contrast, the alveolar bone is not essential
to the tooth. Perhaps we should view it as a
response to the tooth, because it does not form
if the tooth does not develop, and when teeth
are removed, it tends to atrophy. Where there
are alveolar defects (Fig. 3,4), periodontal
ligament fibres simply pass into soft tissue.
Abstract 3,3 is a case history that illustrates
that bone is not necessary for a tooth to
function satisfactorily.

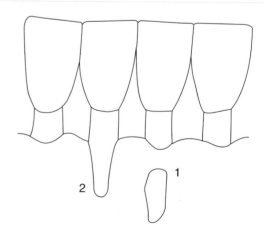

Fig. 3,4

Alveolar defects. A fenestration (1) is a window in the
bone over a tooth, and a dehiscence (2) is a fenestration
that is open at the coronal end.

Abstract 3,3 *A periodontal attachment mechanism without alveolar bone*

Novak MJ, Polson AM, Caton J, et al., *Journal of Periodontology* 1983; **54**: 112–118

This fascinating case history describes the periodontium of a 22-year-old black male whose dentist referred him for specialist assessment because of apparent widespread bone loss on radiographs. However, clinical examination detected no hypermobility of teeth and minimal, if any, attachment loss. Laboratory tests of plaque bacteria and host response indicated a normal patient with clinical gingivitis only. A maxillary third molar, with most proximal bone missing, was removed and its attachment structure and ultrastructure examined. This appeared to have normal fibres inserted into atypical cementum. The authors postulated a developmental defect affecting bone and cementum.

Comment: Bone is not essential to the periodontal ligament attachment, and the soft tissue support in this patient was adequate for normal function.

Abstract 3,4 *The relationship between attachment level loss and alveolar bone loss*

Goodson JM, Haffajee AD & Socransky SS, *Journal of Clinical Periodontology* 1984; **11**: 348–359

In a study of 22 patients with untreated periodontitis for 1 year, clinical measurements were made at monthly intervals and periapical radiographs were taken of 231 sites with pockets $\geq$ 5 mm deep at baseline, 6 months and 1 year. Fourteen (6%) of these sites showed bone loss of $\geq$ 0.5 mm. Following a careful analysis of all data, the authors concluded that significant attachment loss preceded bone loss by 6–8 months.

Comment: The time lapse indicates that bone loss is one of the later changes in the progression of periodontitis.

These facts have important implications for periodontal treatment and diagnosis, and will be discussed in relation to surgery (Chapter 19).

Alveolar bone is also susceptible to forces other than those that make pockets in periodontitis. As we shall see, occlusal forces may affect the bone in the absence of bacterial plaque, and gingival inflammation without attachment loss may lead to loss of bone. However, when the periodontal ligament is reduced in periodontitis, it is usual for adjacent alveolar bone to be reduced also because of the accompanying inflammation. One interesting study suggests that loss of attachment may occur some 6–8 months before bone loss becomes apparent (Abstract 3,4).

COLLAGEN IN THE PERIODONTIUM

Evidence clearly indicates that some cells may have their activities localized to a particular part of the tissues. When we consider the cells that form collagen in the periodontium, for instance, there are at least four distinct regional populations in addition to the subgroups that form the several different types of this molecule.

Both osteoblasts and cementoblasts may form collagen, and there are at least two types of fibroblast according to their anatomical region of activity. Gingival fibroblasts form collagen in the marginal and papillary gingiva, and are distinct from those that work in the periodontal ligament. As will become apparent in our discussion of wound healing (Chapter 20), these matters have a direct bearing on the development of regenerative technologies.

Another point to remember is that as collagen matures, its fibrils contract. There is a continuous turnover of this protein in the tissues and an especially high turnover in the periodontal ligament. We may view this mechanism therefore as a permanent force that holds the tissues firmly together unless collagen processing is disrupted. There is also a contraction in the fibroblast as it moves through the tissues. These forces may have an effect on teeth, although there is still controversy over their role in eruption.

OTHER MATTERS CONCERNING PERIODONTAL HEALTH

The dental pulp is not a part of the perio-dontium, but the condition of each of these two dental organs may affect the other. Communication between the two will be considered in Chapter 27, and there are relevant comments in Chapter 22.

Position of teeth in the arch is of importance to periodontal health in that oral hygiene may be impeded by malposition. Gingival reces-sion may be facilitated where teeth are so out of alignment that they are not covered by bone (Chapter 23).

Arch relations are of significance when opposing teeth contact the gingival tissues and sometimes (but by no means always) damage them in function. This may occur with Angle's class II division II malocclusion in those cases where upper incisors contact lower labial gingiva (Chapter 25). It is also possible where lower incisors contact upper palatal gingiva in a class II malocclusion of either division.

CONCLUSION

This brief description of the components of the periodontium has links to many questions regarding periodontal diseases and their treatment. It is intended to be a relevant rather than exhaustive account of the anatomy and activities of these tissues.

4

THE SPECTRUM OF PERIODONTAL DISEASES

- What are the four basic periodontal lesions?
- What factors produce periodontal diseases?
- Why do teeth move?
- How successful may treatment be?
- Can different types of periodontitis be distinguished?
- When may pain occur in periodontal diseases?

In one sense, all chronic periodontal diseases are similar because inflammatory mechanisms can probably account for them. But why should the inflammation have no sequel at one site, lead to attachment loss in another site a tiny distance away, cause hyperplastic or drug-related enlargement at another site and lead to recession in another?

The response to treatment also varies. Abstract 4,1 describes a famous classic study in periodontal practice. Why should not every periodontal pocket of the same depth respond in the same way to the same treatment? We are not able to answer this question yet, but part of the answer at least lies in the patient.

When patients are studied with regard to host response defects, clear answers do not emerge. It is clear that some with a well-defined clinical disease such as juvenile periodontitis have a defective host response, but not all of them. Even worse, the defect may not be sufficient to explain why the disease occurs in those patients who have both.

Periodontal diseases are multifactorial. They require a battle between the host and the resident bacterial plaque in a setting where damage is possible. This gives at least three groups of determinants for disease – host

defence mechanisms, bacterial mechanisms and host structure.

Furthermore, as we shall see in future chapters, each of these determinants can affect the others, and also themselves (Table 4,1).

Abstract 4,1 *A long-term survey of tooth loss in 600 treated periodontal patients*

Hirschfeld L & Wasserman B, *Journal of Periodontology* 1978; **49**: 225–237

After 15–50+ years (mean 22 years) of post-treatment maintenance, 600 patients were re-examined. Prognosis was originally described as questionable for teeth with furcation involvement, deep ineradicable pocket, severe bone loss or marked mobility with deep pocket. During maintenance, patients varied greatly and were grouped according to response to treatment: 499 well-maintained patients (WM) lost three teeth or fewer; 76 downhill patients (D) lost four to nine teeth; and 25 extreme downhill patients (ED) lost 10–23 teeth. Overall, two out of three questionable teeth were kept; 7% of all teeth were lost for periodontal reasons and 1% for other reasons. During follow-up, WM lost 0.68 teeth per patient, of which 4/5 were predicted as questionable; for D these figures were 5.7 and 4/7; for ED, 13.3 and 3/7. Most teeth were kept with simple thorough traditional periodontal treatment, and 300 patients lost no teeth at all.

Comment: Treatment outcome was less predictable in the ED and D groups, and a few patients lost most teeth. These results also set a high standard for those who endeavour to produce more effective treatment methods.

Table 4,1: *Some interactions between determinants of periodontal diseases*

Active determinant	Determinant acted upon		
	Host structure	Host defence	Bacteria
Host structure	Developmental factors may predispose to disease, e.g. mild hypophosphatasia	Factors affect the micro-circulation, e.g. hormones may increase tissue permeability	Determines basic bacterial environment
Host defence	Produces numerous enzymes, especially collagenase	Interaction occurs within defences, e.g. opsonins from complement enhance neutrophil activity	Initiates a multitude of actions, including phagocytosis, antibodies and other mechanisms
Bacteria	Have potential for considerable damage, with endotoxins, proteases etc.	May interfere directly, e.g. *Actinobacillus actinomycetemcomitans* leucotoxin can kill neutrophils	Have a variety of interactions, some of mutual benefit; others may be inhibitory

INFLAMMATION

To understand how inflammation is manifest in the periodontium, let us consider how the four cardinal signs described by the Roman physician Celsus in the 1st century A.D. may be exhibited or modified.

REDNESS

Redness (Latin: *rubor*) is an early sign in the gingiva, resulting from augmented local blood flow as many resting capillaries open. These vessels have a greatly increased blood pressure and significant quantities of fluid escape, with the active movement of many neutrophils into the tissues.

SWELLING

Swelling (*tumor*) results from the fluid flow, but this oedema is severely modified by the loss of much crevicular fluid as an inflammatory exudate through the junctional and sulcular epithelium.

HEAT

Heat (*calor*) increases, but the temperature rise is modest; the fluid loss and opening the mouth may account for this.

PAIN

Pain (*dolor*) is not commonly reported with periodontal inflammation, except that probing untreated disease may at times cause marked discomfort. The absence of pain under normal circumstances is probably due to the escape of crevicular fluid. When the crevice is probed, however, there may be considerable local pressure in these oedematous tissues.

A further sign of gingival inflammation is bleeding on probing (BOP). Even with light pressure, when the periodontal probe is placed in the crevice it passes into the inflamed tissue. Capillaries and other small vessels are under stress because of high internal pressure, and rupture because of the added force in the tissues. Blood appears at the gingival margin almost immediately in many cases, and in nearly all cases within

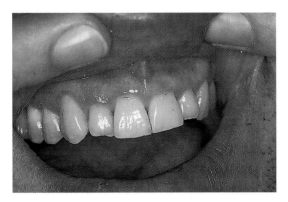

Fig. 4,1

Marked gingivitis on the labial of upper anterior teeth in a patient aged 28 years. Redness and swelling are apparent.

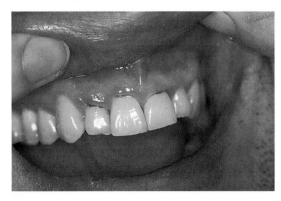

Fig. 4,2

After gentle movement of a probe in the gingival crevice, bleeding is evident.

30 s (Figs 4,1 and 4,2). Occasionally in advanced disease, a small abscess is ruptured by the probe and pus may appear at the margin, with or without blood.

ATTACHMENT LOSS

This constitutes the greatest enigma in periodontitis, and we shall therefore spend some time (Chapters 5, 9 and 10) examining it. For attachment loss to occur, it seems that inflammation is a necessary predisposing factor. However, only a tiny minority of inflamed sites progress to measurable attachment loss on proximal surfaces in the inhabitants of developed countries. This may be related to a degree of plaque control, as we shall see, but it clearly indicates something of considerable interest to us. If we can predict where it will occur, then we will be able to direct attention to those sites.

What is attachment loss? It is the irreversible destruction of the periodontal ligament, commencing at the coronal aspect and progressing in any possible direction but primarily apically. The crucial feature is destruction of collagen without its replacement. If there is adjacent bone, the spread of inflammation will also lead to bone resorption, but this is not the essence of the lesion (Fig. 4,3).

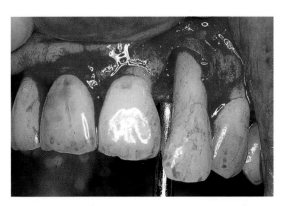

Fig. 4,3

Attachment loss on an upper-left lateral incisor over which a flap of gingiva has been raised during surgery. Bone has also receded from the associated inflammatory tissue that has been removed. The patient was aged 22 years and had localized juvenile periodontitis. This clearly shows the site specificity of such lesions. The tooth has lost much attachment on the mesial and buccal surfaces and has overerupted with a tendency to move distally, where the attachment is largely intact with minimal inflammatory tissue. The adjacent central incisor is unaffected with full periodontal support. This figure was first published in the *British Medical Journal* (Watts TLP, Periodontitis for medical practitioners, 1998; 316: 993–996) and is reproduced by permission of the BMJ.

How is attachment lost? This is not known, but there are several mechanisms for losing collagen. Bacteria and phagocytes can produce collagenase. Tissues contain metallo-proteinases, of which collagenase is a member, and these are normally kept under control by at least three varieties of tissue inhibitors of metalloproteinases (TIMP), which are secreted by many different cells and may be obstructed. Fibroblasts and other cells may destroy too much, or produce too little, collagen. Any or all of these mechanisms may participate and also there may be unknown mechanisms.

If we merely seek a mechanism then we are deluding ourselves because there are abundant mechanisms. The central issue is not how, but where and when the collagen is destroyed.

Why is the ligament so special that it is evidently destroyed only on infrequent occasions and in particular places? Or does the problem perhaps lie in the fact that the usual replacement of collagen does not follow?

Attachment may be lost rapidly or slowly, and is a very selective process. The presumed speed of destruction and the specific sites attacked have been the basis for certain diagnoses. It is not easy to measure true attachment loss because it is always accompa-nied by inflammation (if untreated). We there-fore talk of 'clinical attachment loss', 'clinical attachment level', 'probing attachment loss' or 'probing attachment level', which will be discussed in the next chapter.

GINGIVAL ENLARGEMENT

A large variety of stimuli may lead to gingival enlargement (Table 4,2). The reasons and the appearances may vary. In most cases, plaque-related inflammation is involved, but in a rare few, enlargement may occur without the involvement of plaque.

The appearance may be characteristic (Figs 4,4–4,8). Some lesions may be generalized, or nearly so, as with drug-related enlargement (Figs 4,9–4,12). Some may have an appearance that is hard to explain (Figs 4,13–4,18).

The enlargement may be oedematous, but the response to plaque may also involve hyperplasia. Hormonal effects in pregnancy

Table 4,2: *Causes of gingival enlargement*

Cause	Type	Effect
Common causes		
Plaque	Oedematous	Inflammation
	Fibrous	Hyperplasia
Mouthbreathing/ reduced lip coverage	Fibrous	Excessive collagen formation
Hormones		
Oestrogens	Oedematous	Intensified
Progesterone		inflammation
Systemic drugs		
Phenytoin	Fibrous	Excessive
Cyclosporin		collagen
Calcium channel blockers		formation
Rare causes		
Familial fibromatosis	Fibrous	Excessive collagen formation
Neoplasia		
Leukaemias	Solid	Tissues
Local tumours		enlarged by leukaemic or tumour cells
Sarcoidosis	Solid	Hyperplasia
Wegener's granulomatosis		with elements of
Crohn's disease		the disease in question
Nutritional variation		
Scurvy	Oedematous	Intensified
Vitamin A overdose		inflammation

or puberty allow plaque-related oedema to increase (Fig. 4,19).

In drug-related enlargement, the bulk of the lesions are fibrous in nature because excessive amounts of collagen are deposited in the connective tissues. In the UK probably only a minority of patients on the relevant drugs develop the overgrowth, which often can be reversed with improved plaque control.

Where systemic involvement is suspected, full examination is advisable of all possible

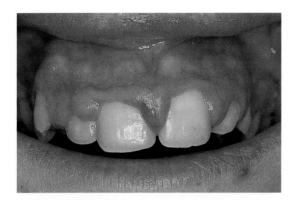

Fig. 4,4

Mouthbreathing-associated gingival enlargement in a 15-year-old male (see Chapter 14).

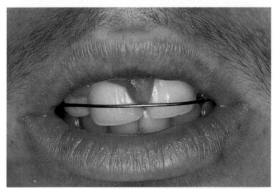

Fig. 4,5

The orthodontic retainer, worn day and night, may have helped to exacerbate the incompetent lips. It is possible that pubertal changes contribute to some cases like this.

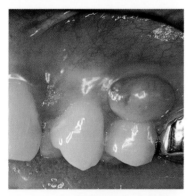

Fig. 4,6

Ossifying fibrous epulis in 23-year-old female, who had never been pregnant.

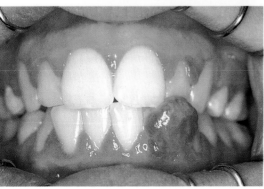

Fig. 4,7

In a pregnancy of seven months, a large epulis (Greek: on the gums) is present, with a 'pregnancy gingivitis' (see Chapter 14).

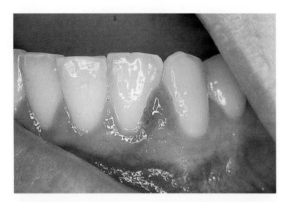

Fig. 4,8

Within a week of parturition, the epulis has separated. There is rarely a need to remove epulides during pregnancy, when haemostasis may pose problems in the gingiva. If necessary, minor surgery may be used later.

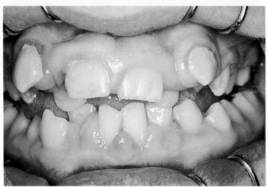

Fig. 4,9

Phenytoin-related enlargement in an 11–year-old epileptic male who was also on diazepam, phenobarbitone and carbamazepine. With a cocktail like that, the patient was often too drowsy to attend to oral hygiene.

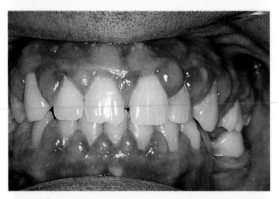

Fig. 4,10

Gingival enlargement in a 52-year-old male treated with nifedipine for angina and hypertension.

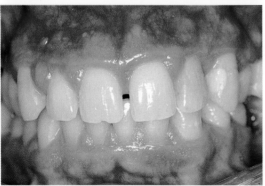

Fig. 4,11

The same patient after 18 months of hygienist treatment and follow-up. Most lesions have regressed to manageable proportions.

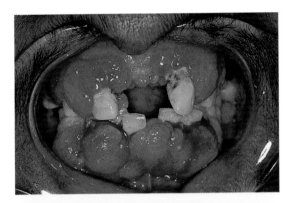

Fig. 4,12

Renal transplant patient aged 56 years, on cyclosporin and nifedipine. The hirsutism (marked hair) of this female is due to cyclosporin. Unfortunately, she also had advanced periodontitis, which led to removal of her teeth. The marked enlargement is partly due to the very large volume of inflamed gingiva that has been affected by the drugs.

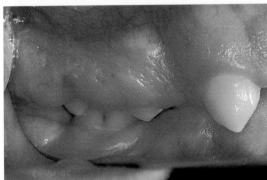

Fig. 4,13

Hereditary gingival fibromatosis in female aged 33 years: right side.

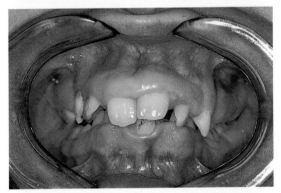

Fig. 4,14

Central view.

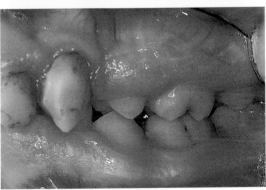

Fig. 4,15

Left side.

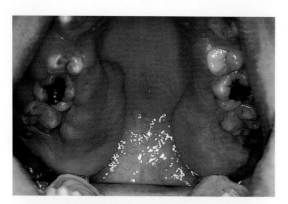

Fig. 4,16

Upper occlusal view.

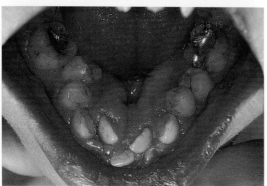

Fig. 4,17

Lower occlusal view.

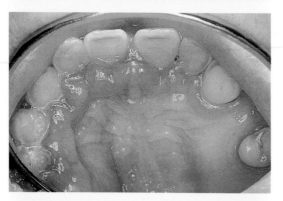

Fig. 4,18

Characteristic gingival enlargement in patient with chronic myeloid leukaemia (See Chapter 14).

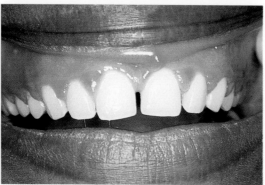

Fig. 4,19

Oedematous gingival enlargement in pregnancy.

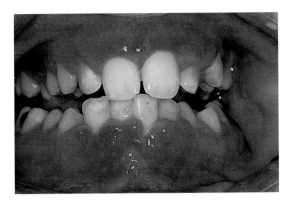

Fig. 4,20

Sarcoidosis in patient in third decade. Biopsy showed areas of sarcoid in the gingiva.

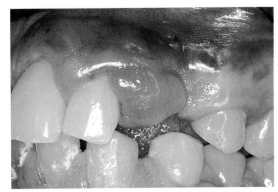

Fig. 4,21

Fibrous epulis in patient with monoclonal gammopathy.

related features accessible in a dental surgery. For instance, if leukaemia is suspected, lymph nodes should be palpated and skin and mucous membranes should be examined for signs of anaemia, jaundice and haemorrhagic effects. Immediate referral should be the response to evidence of such a condition: blood tests may not be conclusive, and marrow tests are the only way to confirm the definite presence of a leukaemia.

Wherever there is doubt over the nature of any enlargement, biopsy is a wise course of action. In some cases, it may confirm the presence of a more widespread disease (Fig. 4,20). In others it will set the mind at rest, as in a patient with a known monoclonal gammopathy where the sudden appearance of a fibrous epulis (Fig. 4,21) raised the question of a myeloma.

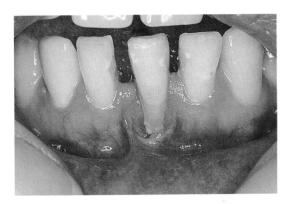

Fig. 4,22

Labial gingival recession over a lower incisor with plaque obviously present.

GINGIVAL RECESSION

This is a common occurrence, and may happen as an isolated event (Fig. 4,22), or as a more generalized phenomenon (Fig. 4,23) with related pathology. It is a frequent sequel to any successful periodontal treatment. Evidence suggests that it results from an inflammatory process, caused either by plaque or mechanical trauma (Abstract 4,2), and it is obvious that there must be some attachment loss for it to occur.

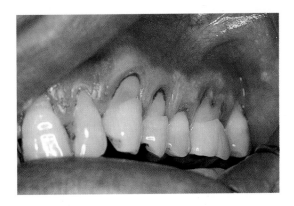

Fig. 4.23

Long-standing recession associated with cervical abrasion cavities and dark calculus deposits on several teeth.

Abstract 4,2 *The possible pathogenesis of gingival recession. A histological study of induced recession in the rat*

Baker DL & Seymour GJ, *Journal of Clinical Periodontology* 1976; **3**: 208–219

After extraction of an upper incisor in each of 20 rats, acrylic resin was placed in the sockets. Following sacrifice 25–40 weeks later, three histological zones were identified in tissue from horizontal sections adjacent to implants. Zone I was identified in thick marginal gingiva, and had normal characteristics. Zone II, in thinner gingiva, showed epithelial hyperplasia with elongated rete ridges and mononuclear cell infiltration in subjacent connective tissue. In zone III, the diverging mesial and distal aspects of the recession were identified. The authors suggest a mechanism for recession, consisting of very localized inflammation under the epithelium, proliferation of the epithelium and remodelling, as a result of which the gingival margin moves apically.

Comment: This provides a unified explanation for all recession in terms of inflammation, whether induced by plaque or by trauma such as vigorous oral hygiene.

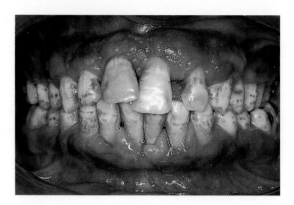

Fig. 4,24

An upper-left central incisor with distal attachment loss has moved mesially, displacing the other in a labial direction.

It is clear that teeth most affected by marked recession often have dehiscences or fenestrations, and are in positions where the gingiva may be thin. Because they may be closely associated with a fraenum, some have suggested that this structure may play a part in the recession (see comment on 'fraenal pull', Chapter 13). However, a fraenum normally contains no muscle fibres and can only produce gingival blanching when the lip is extended to a position that it does not normally reach. It is more likely that the fraenum is only involved fortuitously or by impeding plaque control.

DRIFTING AND OVERERUPTION

Why do teeth move? Normal periodontal support is sufficient to hold them in balance, but when this is disrupted by disease, other factors enter the equation.

In normal dental equilibrium there is balance between occlusal forces and this is probably the most powerful constraint acting on teeth. As orthodontists also remind us, if muscle balance is disturbed between the tongue and cheeks, it may also alter tooth position.

In disease there are two other potential factors. Where neither occlusal force nor muscle balance is greatly involved (Fig. 4,24), a tooth moves away from the greatest attachment loss on its surface. By Newton's first law of motion, for it to move, a force must either push or pull the tooth.

If the tooth is pushed, the obvious candidate is inflammatory oedema in the pocket wall. However, this is subject to the limitation that its pressure is reduced by loss of crevicular fluid.

If the tooth is pulled, the continual rapid turnover of collagen in the periodontal ligament provides a suitable force. As the collagen matures and contracts, there is a greater force on the side of the tooth where least attachment has been lost. The coronal position of the extra force will also account for tilting, where this occurs, because the fulcrum for a tilt will be in the apical region of the tooth.

GINGIVITIS AND ITS VARIATIONS

In gingivitis we are faced with a universal epidemic of inflammation which seems to do little harm as long as it remains limited to the gingival margin.

There are a few acute diseases that affect the gingiva, such as acute necrotizing ulcerative gingivitis and acute herpetic gingivostomatitis, which will be discussed in Chapter 12. Unlike chronic marginal gingivitis, these are provoked lesions with an initiating factor: either infection by an exogenous pathogen or a lowered host resistance, permitting endogenous infection.

A rare lesion that has been given the tentative label of an allergic response is so-called plasma cell gingivitis (Fig. 4,25). This may be observed alone or with angular cheilitis and glossitis. A precipitating allergen has been suggested in some cases where resolution occurred on avoidance of a chewing gum, a dentifrice, a herbal toothpaste or red peppers. However, features of an allergic reaction are not always found.

In the early days of acquired immune deficiency syndrome (AIDS) and human immunodeficiency virus (HIV) studies, some observers suggested that an unusual 'linear gingivitis' was a specific feature. A thin line of erythema of uniform width was described along the marginal gingival tissues. However, further studies have shown that the appearance is not unique and indeed not frequent in this group of patients.

Overall, chronic marginal gingivitis may be regarded as a simple inflammatory response to different stimuli. In most cases, the stimulus will be plaque bacteria or local trauma from oral hygiene and dental procedures.

A TENTATIVE PERIODONTITIS CLASSIFICATION

The basis for modern classification of periodontitis is the work of Page and Schroeder, who listed five distinguishable types in 1982. In Table 4,3 the grouping of diseases is related to the host immune response.

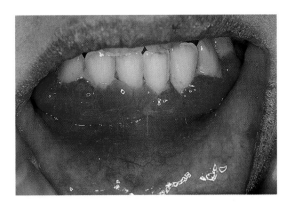

Fig. 4,25

Plasma cell gingivitis in a 16-year-old female patient who chewed gum. There was also a generalized juvenile periodontitis (GJP).

Early-onset periodontitis runs a course that may be defined as aggressive or severe in relation to chronic adult disease. The usual accepted upper age limits for juvenile periodontitis and rapidly progressive periodontitis (RPP) are 25 and 35 years, respectively. It is possible that the former is frequently over long before 25 years, and that the latter may occur after 35 years. The diseases may vary widely in presentation, and the associated

Table 4,3: *A classification of clinical forms of periodontitis*

Type	Features
Early-onset aggressive periodontitis 　Prepubertal periodontitis 　Juvenile periodontitis 　Rapidly progressive periodontitis	Neutrophil and macrophage defects and associated immune dysfunction
Slow progression adult periodontitis 　Chronic marginal periodontitis	No detectable immune defects
Necrotizing periodontitis 　Necrotizing ulcerative periodontitis	Multiple suppression of host response mechanisms

immune disorders may vary from profound and life-threatening in some patients with prepubertal periodontitis to moderate without further consequence in most localized juvenile periodontitis.

Slowly progressing adult periodontitis appears to be a straight battle between a normal host and bacterial plaque.

Necrotizing periodontitis was extremely rare until AIDS caused more cases. It appears to be related to immune suppression involving more than the phagocyte division of the host response. Typically, there is severe invasion of host tissue by bacteria and death of much tissue around the teeth, particularly alveolar bone, which may be sequestrated.

In addition to these basic forms of periodontitis, we may add two others. Post-juvenile periodontitis is the term given to the pattern of localized juvenile periodontitis, affecting incisors and first molars but diagnosed at a much later age than 25 years. This is usually treated as adult periodontitis. There is also frequent reference in the literature to periodontitis that is 'refractory'. This term may be interpreted as 'I tried hard to treat it but it didn't improve.' If one rules out contributing factors to treatment failure, such as inadequate plaque control, refractory periodontitis cases are very few.

PAIN IN THE PERIODONTIUM

Most periodontal diseases are insidious and without pain. The occasional acute disorder (Chapter 12) may be very uncomfortable. Periodontitis may be painful on probing but not otherwise. An endodontic problem may be mistaken for a periodontal disorder.

On rare occasions, however, a patient may present complaining of a diffuse pain on both sides of the mouth and affecting the whole of the periodontal tissues, including the attached gingiva. If no contributing dental factors are apparent, referral to an oral physician is recommended. Sometimes menopausal endocrine changes are responsible.

With cyclosporin-related enlargement, diffuse gingival pain is noted by some patients. It appears to be a genuine drug effect, and not a device of the patient to obtain treatment (some patients think that we are interested in diseases to the exclusion of cosmetic quality of life).

Severe localized pain from attached gingiva is extremely rare. Case History 2 is an account of such an occurrence that had a clear organic cause. In the absence of a true neuralgia, and with anatomically unrelated pain distribution, atypical facial pain is a possible diagnosis but should be made by an oral surgeon or physician.

CASE HISTORY 2: a patient with severe pain in the attached gingiva

A 45-year-old patient was referred for urgent periodontal attention. She had a severe recurring pain in the lower left premolar region of the buccal attached gingiva. The appearance had been diagnosed provisionally as acute necrotizing ulcerative gingivitis, but it had not responded to treatment with metronidazole. Teeth in this region responded to vitality tests and there was no other apparent pathology. The patient arrived accompanied by her husband and one child. She was quite tearful, and her husband was noticeably unsympathetic. She had apparently been complaining of severe pain for several days, and had eaten little food in that time. Examination revealed generalized gingivitis and plaque, and in the painful area there was a small region of attached gingiva with desquamative debris, which the patient had not touched since the pain began. Further questioning revealed that even to touch the area caused a severe prolonged pain. There were no other signs of disease.

DIAGNOSIS

Trigeminal neuralgia. The trigger zone and patient behaviour were characteristic. She was, however, rather young to have the condition, which usually affects people over 50 years of age.

MANAGEMENT

Immediate prescription of carbamazepine, with prompt referral for full neurological examination. Trigeminal neuralgia may be 'idiopathic' or it may have a cause such as tumours. The medication completely relieved the pain, which helped confirm the diagnosis.

COMMENT

When the problem was explained, the husband's behaviour changed. There are few conditions that cause such severe pain – certainly not periodontal diseases. Some patients will not permit examination because they fear it will trigger an attack. This was an extremely rare presentation for the condition.

CONCLUSION

Four principal types of lesion may present in many different ways in the periodontal tissues. According to the host response, three groups of disease may be discerned in periodontitis. Teeth may move as a result of periodontal diseases, but there is rarely any noticeable pain. Many other diseases may be manifest in the periodontal tissues, and the clinician should be aware of this. Such manifestations are often non-specific, but the history and occasional tests may guide towards a diagnosis.

5   ASSESSING PERIODONTAL HEALTH AND DISEASE

- Why is detailed periodontal assessment so important?
- What needs to be examined?
- How do we interpret the findings of a periodontal examination?
- Do clinicians need to use constant force or automated periodontal probes?
- Is the CPITN any use to the clinician?

The context of periodontology is incomplete without reflection on how this complex group of diseases may be measured. People sometimes think of measurement and mathematics as a boring and tedious necessity, something to be left to statisticians. But if we clinicians leave the measurement of disease to such people, we may find ourselves misled by their advice. For instance, if a statistician does not know that two different things – attachment level and more apically placed inflammatory tissue – are measured simultaneously by probing a diseased pocket and that certain often undefined assumptions (such as position of the probe) underlie any use of these data, we may end up with wrong conclusions.

A full periodontal clinical assessment of a patient takes an experienced clinician anything up to 1 h, depending on details of the examination, problems in judging prognosis and uncertainties in planning treatment. It is important that this expensive time should be well used.

Periodontal measurement is about making decisions. These vary from individual treatment decisions on which many patients rely, to decisions about which treatment has shown the best results in a large clinical trial. If measurement can be in numbers, then mathematics may help us to reach good decisions.

At the same time, there is an element of interpretation even where we use numbers. A healthy gingival crevice should not be more than 3 mm, say some. In fact, when treating someone with advanced disease, we may be glad to see some pockets reduce to 5 mm, and the patients may be able to keep them healthy without detectable inflammation.

TYPES OF PERIODONTAL ASSESSMENT

There are two types of periodontal assessment. Both may use similar examination procedures and both are decision-making appointments but they differ in one extremely important point. An 'initial assessment', as its name implies, is when a new patient is examined and the only information available is what is gathered by the clinician, contributed by another dentist or provided by the patient. At a 'reassessment', however, a further potentially valuable piece of information is available: the response of the individual patient to the treatment provided. Without this information, some decisions are hard to make, if indeed they are rationally possible. This will be discussed further in Chapter 30.

Response is judged by the change in the patient's periodontal condition since the previous assessment. There are two contributing factors to take into account: the change in the patient's behaviour and the operator's direct intervention. If the patient is unchanged, there is no basis for success. At its worst, non-compliance with advice may doom a patient to a palliative treatment plan, where support is given but gradual prosthetic transition occurs (see Case History 1, Chapter 1).

Patient behaviour is largely judged by events at the gingival margin, but actions such as smoking cessation also should be praised and encouraged. Because plaque control is of fundamental importance, plaque status should be accurately recorded at every visit.

Most of the operator's direct contribution to treatment response is seen apically to the gingival margin. Reductions in PD and improvements in probing attachment level are a good indication of effective treatment, particularly if crevicular bleeding is reduced.

OBSERVING

The foundation of good periodontal practice is observation. Visual observation may note colour and shape of the tissues, identify positions for probing, read the probe scale and recognize bleeding. The sensation of probing is important when encountering subgingival obstructions such as calculus and identifying the CEJ.

Observation begins when the patient arrives and continues throughout the history-taking and examination. Every patient needs to be made at home in unfamiliar surroundings, so the clinician encourages the patient to ask questions and participate in discussion. Where necessary, direct questions may be used to elicit information about the patient's goals and objectives in periodontal treatment (Chapter 1). The patient's feelings also should be explored as a basis for empathy and understanding. The initial assessment is an encounter of two people who need to work together.

Careful observations, if not recorded at the time, should be written down immediately after the patient leaves. A dictation machine may be used during a busy session as an aide-memoire, although recording the entire visit like a psychiatrist or psychotherapist is likely to prove counter-productive.

PLAQUE

The main aetiological agent for the majority of periodontal diseases is an important diagnos-

tic marker. When some patients visit the dentist they take special precautions to avoid getting blamed and the remaining plaque, therefore, is a clear indication of what they are unable to remove.

There are several ways of assessing plaque. If the teeth are dried with air, a probe may be used to identify deposits. Alternatively, a disclosing solution may be used, with these precautions: lips and anterior restorations are protected with petroleum jelly, and care is taken to keep the fluid off clothing. The patient is asked to rinse *gently*. Vigour may wash the fluid out of some plaque. If there is doubt about whether the colour indicates plaque, a probe will usually show the deposit for what it is.

Because the aim is to remove plaque entirely, the approach of O'Leary and colleagues in 1972 is appropriate. Presence or absence is marked on a chart with four surfaces (mesial, buccal, distal and lingual) shown for each tooth. A score of 10% or below is usually considered satisfactory, but experienced patients often achieve scores below 5%.

The score should be recorded at every visit. Without this information, we do not know how the patient has varied during treatment: plaque control evaluation in terms such as 'good', 'fair' or 'poor' is so vague as to be meaningless for treatment decisions. The O'Leary chart has the added advantage that areas and surfaces are identified for attention on future occasions.

WHAT INDICATES PERIODONTAL HEALTH?

Absence of plaque is a useful goal when we consider control of aetiological factors in periodontal diseases. We need a similar indicator for health in the tissues when treating patients.

The study in Abstract 5,1 is a test of BOP – a gingivitis marker – that shows that its continued absence is a strong indicator of periodontal health. Our goal, therefore, should be to eradicate this phenomenon. On the other hand, the study shows that all is not necessarily lost if some sites bleed, because this is a very poor predictor of breakdown.

Abstract 5,1 *Absence of bleeding on probing. An indicator of periodontal stability*

Lang NP, Adler R, Joss A, et al., *Journal of Clinical Periodontology* 1990; **17**: 714–721

After completion of active treatment, 41 patients attended at 2–6 month intervals over 2.5 years for periodontal maintenance. All supragingival plaque and calculus was removed. Sites that bled on probing were also scaled subgingivally. Recurrence or progression of disease was defined as a probing attachment loss of 2 mm or more. Only 6% of sites that bled actually lost 2 mm, which is a very low positive predictive value. The negative predictive value, of sites that did not bleed as a proportion of sites that did not lose 2 mm attachment, was 98%. It was therefore very likely that a non-bleeding site would remain stable.

Comment: Presence of bleeding did not indicate instability, but its absence did indicate the converse.

Abstract 5,2 *Bleeding/plaque ratio. A possible prognostic indicator for periodontal breakdown*

van der Velden U, Winkel EG, Abbas F, *Journal of Clinical Periodontology* 1985; **12**: 861–866

Seven untreated juvenile periodontitis patients (susceptible group: mean age 15.5 years) were compared with seven patients (insusceptible: mean age 58 years) with much plaque and no evidence of attachment loss. When all sites were compared, the susceptible group had more bleeding, less plaque, greater pocket depths and a much higher bleeding/plaque ratio (1.5 vs 0.26). When all sites of 3 mm or less were compared, the susceptible group had less redness and swelling as well, and an even greater bleeding/plaque ratio (1.64 vs 0.26).

Comment: One of several studies by this group showing a difference in the response to plaque between subjects with proven susceptibility or insusceptibility to attachment loss. There are problems of interpretation because of the age difference.

BLEEDING ON PROBING

The absence of BOP is very useful to us. Can we squeeze anything else from a bleeding measurement? Some have tried using two levels of bleeding to indicate mild or severe inflammation, but even with a constant probing force this has not proved very useful. However, there are two other ways in which BOP may help in our clinical practice.

First, a simple test may help us to examine our patients' adherence to (compliance in) oral hygiene procedures. Usually BOP is elicited by probing the gingival crevice. If the margins of the gingiva frequently bleed with gentle probe pressure in the absence of plaque, then this may indicate a lack of constancy in oral hygiene and we may ask the patient politely whether it is rather difficult to brush or floss every day.

Secondly, BOP in the absence of significant plaque has been investigated as a possible indicator of prognosis (Abstract 5,2).

There is a difficulty of interpretation. The groups differ not only in susceptibility but also in age and perhaps various other characteristics. For instance, it was only just becoming known that tobacco smoking reduces gingival bleeding, and this factor was not reported for the subjects. However, because smoking also causes some periodontitis, it is possible that the resistant older group was not affected by it.

Although the evidence is not clear, many clinicians interpret an increased BOP response to minimal plaque as a warning sign that the patient may have high susceptibility to periodontitis and be difficult to treat. As the authors of the studies pointed out, the question can be answered only by a study comparing the two types of person over a period of many years.

LINEAR PROBING MEASUREMENTS

Not only do we use probes to elicit BOP, but we also make assessments of PD, recession,

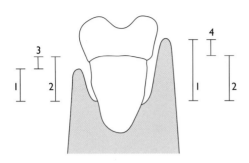

Fig. 5,1

Probing attachment loss = PD + recession. The cemento-enamel junction is the fixed landmark for both recession and attachment loss measurements. The gingival margin and the depth of the pocket are the two movable points that probing aims to measure. 1 = probing depth; 2 = probing attachment level; 3 = recession; 4 = 'negative' recession.

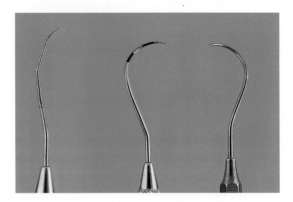

Fig. 5,2

Three assorted furcation probes. It is best to have a selection because furcations vary considerably in shape and accessibility.

probing attachment loss or level, and furcation involvement. Fig. 5,1 illustrates the first three measurements. Recession may be 'positive' or 'negative'.

The prefix 'probing' needs explanation. In literature before the 1970s the usual terms were simply 'pocket depth' and 'attachment loss'. During that decade, studies on probing began to show that the probe often fell short of, or penetrated, the pocket base. Reflecting this uncertainty, common use changed the terms.

Probing attachment loss or level is the clinical estimate of past destruction of the periodontal ligament by disease. Because teeth vary in their length, it is not always a clear guide to remaining support, for which a radiographic assessment is also needed. For long-term certainty that disease is not progressing, attachment level should be monitored, with the CEJ as its fixed landmark.

In contrast, PD does not have a fixed landmark, but is the distance between two alterable points. Gingival recession or enlargement may alter the position of the margin, and progression or healing of the disease alters the base of the pocket. It is an important parameter in making treatment decisions and assessing treatment response.

Recession measurements are used for their own sake, but they are also used in treatment

and research. It is often simpler to record PD and recession, from which attachment level may be calculated, than to attempt to measure the latter directly.

Furcation probing is often performed with a specially shaped instrument such as a 'cow horn' explorer (Fig. 5,2). The measurement is divided into three grades relating partly to prognosis and treatment, which are explained in Chapter 22.

CONFOUNDING OF ATTACHMENT LOSS WITH INFLAMMATION

Abstract 5,3 describes a study of what happens when a periodontal probe is placed into a pocket. It is known as a validity study and tries to answer the question: 'Where does the probe tip end up?'. In other words, is the probe valid in showing us what we think it should, namely the base of the pocket?

The study showed that often the probe ended up at the attachment level, but sometimes, especially in inflamed tissue, it was elsewhere. Either an obstruction prevented full probing or it passed into soft inflamed tissue beyond. The latter therefore represented a simultaneous measurement of two things, with no way of deciding where the dividing line occurred. This is one source of

Abstract 5,3 *Location of probe tip in bleeding and non-bleeding pockets with minimal gingival inflammation*

van der Velden U, *Journal of Clinical Periodontology* 1982; **9**: 421–427

In 13 patients with 21 molar teeth scheduled for extraction, thorough treatment was given to remove plaque and calculus so that marginal inflammation was controlled. From reference grooves made on the teeth, measurements were made in 58 sites, using a 0.75 N constant force probe of tip diameter 0.63 mm. After extraction, teeth were stained to show the attachment level, and the distance to the grooves was measured. Laboratory and clinical measurements agreed on 27 occasions in 32 pockets that did not bleed on probing. In 26 pockets that bled, only 9 pairs of measurements agreed. Bleeding pockets were deeper than non-bleeding pockets (mean 5.65 mm vs 3.38 mm). On average, probe and laboratory measurements of all pockets agreed closely, but the probe was less likely to indicate the attachment level in bleeding pockets.

Comment: This agreed with a previous study by the same investigator. The probes used by most periodontists are thinner and the force is less.

Table 5,1: *The five generations of periodontal probe*

Type	Characteristics
First generation	The usual clinical instrument: a thin tapering tine marked to be read in mm
Second generation: constant force probes (Fig. 5,3)	As above, but with a spring or electronic cut-out when the appropriate force is reached
Third generation: automated probes (Fig. 5,4)	When probe is in place with specified force, a device is activated that reads the measurement accurately
Fourth generation: three-dimensional probes	Currently under development, these are aimed at recording sequential probe positions along a gingival sulcus
Fifth generation: non-invasive three-dimensional probes	These will add ultrasound or another device to a fourth-generation probe

many current problems in periodontal research and development, and has been confirmed by a large number of validity studies with a variety of probing methods.

For the present, we may note that this study suggests that probing is less likely to vary in healthy tissues, and other studies have confirmed this. Where our aim is to treat disease and make the tissues healthy, probing is of great benefit in showing this outcome. However, in the study of disease, there are currently enormous problems. We shall consider these matters further in Chapter 10.

GENERATIONS OF PERIODONTAL PROBE

There are currently three generations of periodontal probe in use. Two further genera-tions are envisaged by the present author, and will be needed to resolve the problems of studying disease. These five generations are all listed in Table 5,1. However, it is worth noting that most researchers who use constant force and automated probes consider them unnecessary for routine treatment of patients. The first-generation probe has clinical advantages, particularly in respect of tactile sensation.

The first three probes are linear devices, customarily used at six points on each tooth to assess PD and probing attachment level (Figs 5,3 and 5,4). On buccal and lingual/palatal surfaces, measurements are made at mesial, middle and distal points selected by the clinician.

The fourth-generation device under development is an attempt to extend linear probing in a serial manner to take account of the continuous and three-dimensional pocket that is being examined. Initial measurements have shown that this may have promise. If the fifth-generation device can be made, it will aim in addition to identify the attachment level

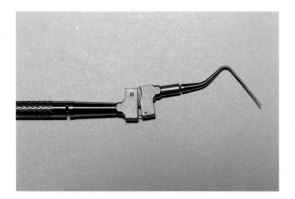

Fig. 5,3

A commonly used constant-force probe opened at its hinge with a force of 0.25 N.

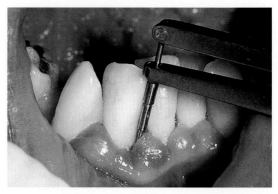

Fig. 5,4

The 'Florida' probe measuring a pocket. When the sleeve reaches the gingival margin the operator will operate a foot pedal, which will record the measurement. (Photograph courtesy of Professor Richard Palmer.)

without penetrating it. Fortunately, we may understand much about treatment without such complicated techniques.

If we are to understand the problems and pitfalls of new diagnostic and treatment procedures, it is essential to have a true concept of the diseases we treat.

OTHER ELEMENTS OF PERIODONTAL EXAMINATION

So far, we have discussed observation, plaque and probing measurements, but three other components of the examination may provide useful information.

First, testing for individual tooth hypermobility may draw attention to either advanced attachment loss or persistent occlusal trauma (Chapter 25). However, there are several other less common reasons for this phenomenon, of which we should be aware (Table 5,2). Adjacent pathology may include cysts, benign or (very rarely) malignant primary tumours or metastases. Apical resorption may be produced by strong orthodontic forces. Other forms of trauma and tumours may produce apical or lateral resorption.

Vitality tests are of use wherever clinical examination suggests pulpal contributions to

Table 5,2: *Reasons for dental hypermobility*

Causes	Related evidence
Common causes	
Attachment loss	Probe measurements, radiographs
Occlusal trauma	Identification of occlusal interference
Rarer causes	
Adjacent pathology	Alveolar/gingival swelling, radiographs
Tooth resorption	Radiographs

an apparently periodontal condition. Isolated severe probing attachment loss on a single tooth is a typically suspect situation, particularly if it is not on a proximal surface.

Radiographs should be neither overestimated nor underestimated. They are no substitute for clinical probing (see Abstract 3,4), but give a useful estimate of remaining support and show some aspects of root morphology and hidden pathology. Both panoramic and paralleling technique periapical views are of help. It is normal to allow for some distortion in these views (Abstract 5,4).

Abstract 5,4 *Selection of the most accurate method of conventional radiography for the assessment of periodontal osseous destruction*

Pepelassi EA, Diamanti-Kipioti A, *Journal of Clinical Periodontology* 1997; **24**: 557–567

In 100 patients receiving flap surgery for periodontitis, 5072 proximal surfaces were assessed for bone loss (BL) by orthopantomographs (OPG), long-cone parallel technique periapical radiographs (PA) and direct measurements (DM) from the cementoenamel junction or restorative margin to the alveolar crest. Mean variation of PA from DM was zero overall, but with a tendency to overestimate maxillary BL and to underestimate mandibular BL by a mean 0.3 mm. The OPGs underestimated BL in both jaws by a mean of 0.4 mm. In relation to DM of 1–4 mm (39% of sites measured), PA underestimated by a mean of 0.4 mm and OPG by a mean of 0.8 mm. For DM of 5–9 mm (54%), PA underestimated by 0.1 mm and OPG by 0.3 mm. Where DM was 10 mm or more (7%), both techniques overestimated by 1.2 mm.

Comment: Long-cone periapicals were more accurate than panoramic views, but both techniques tended to underestimate early disease and overestimate advanced disease. These are mean figures, and in some cases discrepancies were substantially greater.

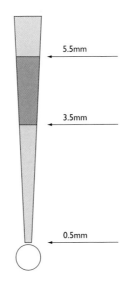

Fig. 5,5

The CPITN probe is used with a recommended force of about 0.2 N (20 g), and each sextant of the mouth is given the highest score identified within it. Table 5,3 shows scores.

PD is 3 mm; when it is partly visible, the reading is 4–5 mm; and when it is out of sight in the pocket, the score is 6 mm or over.

This index is for treatment need (Table 5,3). It has proved useful in surveys to decide on the way in which a population's periodontal needs may best be met, and it is used in the UK National Health Service as a screening test for patients. It does not estimate the level of disease present, for which a measurement of attachment loss is required. People with gingival enlargement may have pockets well over 6 mm deep, for instance, without any

INDICES FOR TREATMENT PURPOSES

An index is a measurement that, as its name suggests, indicates a stage of health or disease. In periodontology, indices are often used both in clinical practice and in research. An example of a widely used treatment need index is the Community Periodontal Index of Treatment Need (CPITN).

The special probe is shown in Fig. 5,5. The ball at the tine end is to help detect subgingival calculus and is 0.5 mm in diameter. The dark band extends from 3.5 mm to 5.5 mm. This means that when it is completely visible, to the nearest whole millimetre the maximum

Table 5,3: *The Community Periodontal Index of Treatment Need (CPITN)*

Score	Finding	Implication
0	≤3 mm PD and no BOP	No treatment needed
1	BOP	Hygiene instruction
2	BOP and calculus	Hygiene and scaling
3	BOP and 4–5 mm PD	Hygiene, supra- and subgingival scaling
4	≥6 mm PD	Full periodontal assessment

Table 5,4: *Essential features of the GI*

Score	Main attributes
0	Health
1	Colour intensifies
2	BOP or hyperplasia
3	'Spontaneous' bleeding

After Löe H & Silness J (1963) Periodontal disease in pregnancy. I. Prevalence and severity. *Acta Odontologica Scandinavica*; **21**: 533–551.

accompanying attachment loss. This is called false pocketing, but the CPITN does not distinguish it from true pocketing.

INDICES FOR RESEARCH PURPOSES

Many research indices have also been used in clinical practice, for instance the Periodontal Index (PI) and the Gingival Index (GI). In the next chapter, we shall see how periodontal epidemiology was initially developed, with two very useful indices. However, we shall explore the shortcomings of indices with a look at the nature and early history of the GI (Table 5,4), developed by Löe and Silness.

The first problem of any index used to describe a biological phenomenon is that of equivalence. Is a score of 2 twice as bad as a score of 1? Perhaps sometimes but not always: this is an answer that tells us nothing. Statisticians deal with this sort of problem by ranking, i.e. they simply say that 2 is worse than 1, without implying how much worse.

Unfortunately, this very point was disputed by an eminent Swiss periodontologist, Hans Mühlemann, who produced his own Sulcus Bleeding Index to emphasize his view that bleeding preceded colour change in the sequence of developing gingivitis. There were some interesting conference discussions when he encountered Harald Löe, who came from Denmark.

After much thought, the international research community came to a consensus that maybe sometimes (perhaps usually in Denmark?) colour change preceded bleeding, and maybe some other times (perhaps usually in Switzerland?) bleeding preceded colour change. The statisticians knew what to do about that, too. The two criteria were analysed separately. In many studies, there was also a trend towards using the presence of BOP as an index of definite inflammation.

A third matter that has not received much attention is that of dissimilar criteria. The GI score of 2 may be given for either BOP or hyperplasia. These are two different processes and perhaps it would be better to deal with them separately. As we shall see in Chapter 6, this affects the PI in a worse way because it combines two diseases – gingivitis and periodontitis – on one scale.

All indices have their shortcomings, but the GI in both original and modified forms has survived trials and tribulation to become one of the most widely used measures of disease in the world.

CONCLUSIONS

Assessment poses many problems, but awareness of the history and shortcomings of clinical measurements is an asset when we evaluate the condition of our patients and seek to understand and apply scientific research in their treatment.

6 FOUNDATIONS OF PERIODONTAL EPIDEMIOLOGY

- What epidemiological findings help perio-dontal practice?
- Is nutrition a significant factor in periodontics?
- Is everyone equally susceptible to perio-dontal diseases?
- Why do tooth surfaces vary in susceptibility to attachment loss?
- What are the main findings from CPITN surveys?

Epidemiology is one of the great detective stories of science. It is the study of diseases within groups of people. Because individuals vary biologically to a greater or lesser extent, studying a defined group enables us to find out more about the diseases from which they suffer, and what factors may influence them.

Broadly speaking, epidemiology covers a wide range of studies, from observations to tests of hypotheses, and from identification of aetiological factors to practical methods of treating them and delivering health care to large populations.

The reader may be aware of the way in which millions of people's lives have been improved following Dean's discovery that a trace of fluoride was essential for optimal resistance of dental enamel to caries (Dean et al, 1942). This early finding led to improvement of many public water supplies, production of toothpastes and other methods of application and the ensuing prevention of huge amounts of caries and all its painful consequences.

Because of fluoride, not only have countless lives been improved, but some young lives may have been saved. Fluoride has averted many of the rare life-threatening sequelae of caries and has avoided large numbers of general anaesthetics, which have always carried a slight risk of death.

In periodontal epidemiology, despite the absence of something as useful and easily applicable as fluoride, studies have increased our understanding of disease processes and enabled large numbers of people to enjoy a happier life. In this chapter, we shall examine a few of the many studies that have helped to establish this science. In later chapters, some other studies will be mentioned, where treatment interventions have controlled disease and thus demonstrated the validity of hypotheses.

THE WORLD HOMOGENEITY OF PERIODONTAL DISEASES

In 1956, Russell, an American dental epidemiologist, published details of an epidemiological index specially designed for recording prevalence of periodontal diseases (Table 6,1).

Table 6,1: *Russell's Periodontal Index (key features)*

Score	Finding
1	Gingival inflammation partly round tooth
2	Gingival inflammation wholly round tooth
4	Radiographic evidence of bone loss
6	Periodontitis with pocket formation
8	Advanced periodontitis; mobility or drifting

Within 10 years, the PI had been used in more than 20 countries in many thousands of people. With the Oral Hygiene Index of Greene and Vermillion ('those colourful gentlemen', according to another eminent researcher), it proved a potent tool in establishing the strong link between oral cleanliness and periodontal diseases.

Since diet had been implicated in caries by earlier classic work such as the Vipeholm study (Lundqvist, 1952), epidemiologists naturally wanted to see whether it was involved in periodontal diseases. Abstract 6,1 summarizes studies of caries and periodontal diseases in eight countries. It shows not only

Abstract 6,1 *International nutrition surveys: a summary of preliminary dental findings*

Russell AL, *Journal of Dental Research* 1963; **42**: 233–244

This review summarizes studies of dental health in 21 559 persons aged 5 to 50+ years in Alaska, Ethiopia, Ecuador, South Vietnam, Chile, Colombia, Thailand and Lebanon over a 3-year period. Blood and urine were tested biochemically in a subsample of 3065 people. The main caries findings were: low disease levels in some nutritionally deprived groups; fluoride inhibited caries. Coefficients of multiple correlation showed that age and oral cleanliness accounted for 90% of the variation in Periodontal Index (PI) scores in all populations. Thus 10% or less of the variation required further explanatory factors. For instance, vitamin A deficiency was correlated significantly with PI ($r = +0.6$; $P < 0.02$) when considered alone, but when included in multiple correlation with age and oral cleanliness, the coefficient was -0.01 and therefore virtually of zero effect. Other nutritional factors were of similar significance. Although the results showed essentially that plaque and time would account for most periodontal diseases, the author was careful not to rule out other possible contributing factors.

Comment: This was the result of a considerable research effort by many people, and all examiners were trained to a high level of consistency.

that age and oral hygiene are the principal factors *associated with* periodontal diseases, but also how much of the latter may be accounted for by the former, in the event that they are also *causative* factors.

Of course, age is not a cause of periodontal diseases, but reflects the irreversible nature of attachment loss. We cannot manipulate time to test this hypothesis, but we can intervene to show that improved oral hygiene reduces disease (Chapters 16 and 17).

When these two factors are accounted for, Russell showed that very little remained to be explained. This did not rule out other factors, and much later it was demonstrated that tobacco smoking was also a significant adverse influence on periodontal health.

The PI is of interest in other ways. As mentioned in the last chapter, it combines two diseases or more on one scale (gingivitis and the various types of periodontitis). It is also quite clear that the scores have no relationship other than by rank. Russell noted later that the two main factors – age and oral hygiene – had been identified by a variety of different studies, performed with different measures of disease, by many different investigators. This is a well-established finding.

HETEROGENEITY OF PERIODONTAL DISEASES WITHIN THE MOUTH

One of the most striking aspects of periodontitis is its site specificity. Less than 2 mm horizontally from intact attachment, there may be 10 mm or more of probing attachment loss. No-one can currently account for such variation within one patient. If we could, we would also be well on the way to predicting sites at risk of attachment loss.

One of the first studies to indicate that risks of periodontal disease varied for different tooth surfaces was the 'Norwegian factory study' (Abstract 6,2). The surfaces least accessible to plaque control were most affected with calculus and periodontal diseases. This explains something of the site specificity question, but it is not by any means the whole answer.

Abstract 6,2 *Incidence of clinical manifestations of periodontal disease in light of oral hygiene and calculus formation*

Lovdal A, Arno A, Wærhaug J, *Journal of the American Dental Association* 1958; **56**: 21–33

This study reports the periodontal condition of 1202 male employees of a Norwegian communications company. Of these, 416 were managerial and engineering staff and the rest were manual workers. Conditions were worse in the latter group. Tooth loss varied from 10% in the 20–25 year-old age group to 70% in those aged 55 and over. Four surfaces were examined on each of 23 584 teeth. Oral hygiene tended to keep only buccal surfaces clean, and this was often restricted to the anterior teeth. The efficiency of hygiene was correlated with disease features. Gingivitis, subgingival calculus and pockets due to attachment loss occurred most commonly on proximal surfaces, next on lingual surfaces and least on buccal surfaces. The authors recommended giving treatment priority to proximal and lingual surfaces.

Comment: The distribution of problems is related to the ease with which particular tooth surfaces may be cleaned by a patient.

Abstract 6,3 *The natural history of periodontal disease in man. The rate of periodontal destruction before 40 years of age*

Löe H, Ånerud A, Boysen H, et al., *Journal of Periodontology* 1978; **49**: 607–620

Periodontal disease progression was compared in cohorts of Norwegians and Sri Lankans over a period of 6–7 years. In the Norwegian group, good health care and personal oral hygiene was usual; in the Sri Lankans, toothbrushing was unknown, but all were healthy and well-built with satisfactory nutrition. Mesial and buccal surfaces of all teeth except third molars were examined for plaque, gingivitis, calculus, caries, fillings and attachment loss. In Norwegians, mean annual attachment loss rates were 0.08 mm per year mesially and 0.1 mm on buccal surfaces; in Sri Lankans, the rates were 0.3 mm and 0.2 mm respectively. The authors considered that this attachment loss was a continuous process, and it appeared to increase in speed in the Sri Lankan group at 25–30 years of age.

Comment: The Norwegians' buccal recession was greater than proximal attachment loss because they used regular oral hygiene; the Sri Lankans had no oral hygiene and the reverse occurred, but with greater destruction.

THE SRI LANKAN STUDY

This ingeniously designed study was started in 1969 with a group of 565 male students and teachers aged 17–31 years in Norway. The next year, the same investigators started work with the 480 male tea labourers aged 14–31 years in Sri Lanka who gave the study its customary name. As is usual in such studies, both groups declined in number, respectively to 245 and 161 at their last examinations.

What made the design so special was the inclusion of subjects over an age range of 15 or more years. This meant that in 6 years, 21 years of disease progression could be covered in the Norwegian group. In the Sri Lankan group, with the prolonged 15-year period, 32 years' progression could be covered.

One of the first papers to be published is outlined in Abstract 6,3. Other papers indicated that the Norwegian group had low plaque and gingivitis scores, whereas in the Sri Lankan group all teeth were covered with plaque from age 14 years onwards and gingivitis was virtually universal. The latter group had a tooth mortality rate 10–30 times higher, and in some people teeth were starting to exfoliate around age 40 years. Because the Sri Lankan group was healthy and well-nourished, the effects are largely the result of undisturbed plaque.

In 1985, the examination of the Sri Lankans showed a further interesting development (Abstract 6,4). Löe and his co-workers were able to identify three levels of susceptibility to attachment loss.

As a result of this and the earlier studies that we have considered, it can be seen that periodontal diseases are complex in the extreme. Over the world, plaque and time

Abstract 6,4 *Natural history of periodontal disease in man. Rapid, moderate and no loss of attachment in Sri Lankan labourers 14 to 46 years of age*

Löe H, Ånerud A, Boysen H, et al., *Journal of Clinical Periodontology* 1986; **13**: 431–445

In 1985, 161 remaining participants of a group of 480 Sri Lankan tea labourers aged 14–31 years in 1970 were periodontally examined. Plaque and gingivitis were ubiquitous and calculus was frequent in all subjects. Three subgroups were distinguished according to attachment loss: rapid progression (RP: 8%), moderate progression (MP: 81%), and no progression (NP: 11%). In the RP subjects, almost all teeth were lost by 45 years; in MP, seven teeth were lost; in NP, virtually no teeth were lost. There were apparent changes in the rates of attachment loss in RP and MP groups; by age 45 years, the mean total loss was, respectively, 13 mm and 7 mm.

Comment: A clear demonstration of differing patient susceptibility to periodontal attachment loss.

Abstract 6,5 *Profiles of periodontal conditions in adults measured by CPITN*

Miyazaki H, Pilot T, Leclercq M-H, et al., *International Dental Journal* 1991; **41**: 74–80

The CPITN data on 35–44 year-olds were scrutinized from nearly 100 surveys in over 50 countries. Very few subjects were healthy, and few showed bleeding only. In most countries, about two-thirds of subjects had calculus or pockets to 5 mm. About 5–50% had pockets over 5 mm, but for most countries this figure was around 10–15%. The main difference between industrialized and non-industrialized countries was that the former had more tooth loss. The authors consider that a severe, irreversible condition that affects 5–20% of people is of high prevalence when compared with other human diseases.

Comment: This shows a picture of widespread developing disease, with potential for significant effects in older populations.

account for most disease. However, within the mouth, sites respond differently. Patients also respond differently.

SURVEYS WITH CPITN

As indicated in the last chapter, the CPITN is not an absolute measure of disease like attachment loss. Its main use is to indicate the level of periodontal resource required to treat a population. It is a reversible index, because treatment can reduce PD, calculus and bleeding. However, increasing periodontal destruction leading to loss of teeth is reflected in the number of excluded sextants (0 or 1 tooth).

Findings with CPITN are illustrated by Abstracts 6,5 and 6,6. This index requires caution when making comparisons between one survey and another. An increase in treatment need may indicate disease progression, but it may also reflect treatment failure at an earlier age.

Abstract 6,6 *Profiles of periodontal conditions in older age cohorts, measured by CPITN*

Pilot T, Miyazaki H, Leclercq M-H, et al., *International Dental Journal* 1992; **42**:23–30

In over 80 surveys from almost 30 countries, CPITN results were described for subjects mainly aged 45–74 years. In many surveys there were substantial numbers (20–90%) of patients with pockets over 5 mm. In younger subjects (45–54 years) 1–2 sextants were missing, and in older people (65–74 years) 2–3 were missing, reflecting continuing tooth loss. This reduced the proportion of CPITN scores of 3 and 4. Of those aged over 45 years, hardly any subjects had a completely healthy periodontium. There were no clear differences between industrialized and non-industrialized countries.

Comment: These are figures indicating treatment need, but they also reveal the progression of periodontitis.

Nevertheless, CPITN studies show that periodontal diseases constitute a significant public health problem and require careful resource allocation. Other treatment need studies have quantified the actual local cost of required care for specific populations, and have assumed specific decisions on the nature of planned treatment.

OTHER ASPECTS OF EPIDEMIOLOGY

As we saw in Chapter 4, there are three main determinants of periodontal diseases: host structures, host response and bacteria. Of these, host response is probably the most susceptible to changes induced by disease or by environmental pollutants. One of the commonest non-dental diseases is diabetes, and by far the commonest environmental pollutant is tobacco smoke ('The number 1 environmental hazard' according to the US Surgeon-General in 1989).

It is well known that diabetics have significantly increased risks of infection, and require careful maintenance of metabolic control. Smokers, too, have increased risks of many diseases because of suppression of parts of the host response, circulatory disturbances and genetic mutations. We shall examine systemic conditions further in Chapter 14, but for an insight into a different type of epidemiological study let us consider Abstract 6,7, which brings together smoking and diabetes.

In this study, the investigators were at pains to gather two random groups that were matched for a longer investigation comparing insulin-dependent diabetics with non-diabetics. At that time, many studies had shown smoking to be damaging to the periodontium. This study showed more clear evidence of the effect, but there was an additional consequence in the diabetic group.

Suppuration is not very common in periodontitis, but in the diabetic smokers it was commoner than in non-smokers. The accumulation of pus is a result of weakening of the neutrophils, the first stage of the host response to bacteria. Diabetic neutrophils tend to have a weaker response, even without smoking. It is unwise to smoke, but more so if you are a diabetic.

Abstract 6,7 *Evidence for cigarette smoking as a major risk factor for periodontitis*

Haber J, Wattles J, Crowley M, et al., *Journal of Periodontology* 1993; **64**: 16–23

Stratified random samples of subjects living in the Boston, Massachusetts area were selected from a diabetic treatment centre and the non-diabetic members of a university-related health maintenance organization. Stratification was for age (19–30 years and 31–40 years) and gender. Consent to participate was given by 132 insulin-dependent diabetics and 95 non-diabetics (response rates 45% and 72%). Separate assessments were made for non-diabetic and insulin-dependent diabetes mellitus (IDDM) groups. No direct comparisons were made between diabetics and non-diabetics, which was the subject of a continuing study. Current smokers, compared to those who never smoked, were more likely to have periodontitis, more BOP, more suppuration in IDDM group only, more PD $\geqslant$4 mm and more PAL >2 mm. Former smokers tended to fall in between. 3/4 heavy smokers were likely to have periodontitis, compared with 1/4 who never smoked.

Comment: Smoking may be the most important single environmental risk factor associated with periodontal diseases. Some effects may compound the already impaired IDDM host response.

CONCLUSION

Epidemiology is a huge subject, and some studies to be discussed later in the book also come under this heading. Some of the snags and difficulties will be examined in Chapter 15, because clinical trials also depend on the principles of epidemiological investigation.

7 ESSENTIALS AND PROBLEMS OF PERIODONTAL MICROBIOLOGY

- Why is bacterial plaque different from mere bacteria?
- How do changes in developing plaque threaten the patient?
- How many types of bacteria live in plaque?
- Why are some bacteria more interesting than others?
- How may bacteria cause periodontal damage?

From birth onwards the mouth is colonized by bacteria. Relatively little is known about the way in which this occurs and how organisms are transferred from relatives and friends of the child. Overall, certain principles of microbiology are likely to determine the oral flora (Table 7,1).

Natural selection operates powerfully and quickly on bacteria. If the surroundings are unsuitable, the organism does not survive. Phagocytic cells and antibodies from a host are a strong discouragement to many oral organisms, and should the occasional bacterium pass into the tissues of the periodontium, it is unlikely to live long.

The environment of a microbe, particularly in the mouth, often contains other organisms that can make their presence felt. This effect may vary from sharing the weapons of defence (e.g. antibiotic resistance) to the opposite extreme of outright hostility. An illustration of how particular periodontal organisms can help each other is given in Abstract 7,1.

One potent defence mechanism employed by groups of microorganisms is the formation

Table 7,1 *Important microbiological principles*

Selection
The environment determines which microorganisms survive and prosper.

Interaction
Some organisms are encouraged by other microbial products
Some organisms inhibit other microbes (specific bacteriocins, non-specific toxic metabolites)
Some microbes assist each other reciprocally (synergy)
Some bacteria transfer resistance to others (conjugation: plasmids; transduction: phages; transformation: important in streptococci)
Some organisms may displace others

Biofilm
A coherent structure more complex than the organisms that live in it
It adheres to a surface in the presence of water
It develops its own rules and properties, which may be different from those of the individual component organisms

of a biofilm. Dental plaque is a biofilm that is firmly attached to teeth like a plaque on a wall. In addition to this adhesion, the film itself is strongly coherent. Because it is not easily penetrated by other substances, there are important clinical implications.

Abstract 7,1   *Nutritional relationships between oral bacteria*

Grenier D, Mayrand D, *Infection and Immunity* 1986; **53**: 616–620

Periodontal bacteria were cultured together: *Bacteroides gingivalis* with *Wolinella recta*, and *B. melaninogenicus* also with *W. recta*. A substance produced by *W. recta* – protohaem – was found to stimulate the growth of the two other organisms. In return, *B. melaninogenicus* produced large amounts of formate, which stimulated growth of *W. recta*.

Comment: A good example of mutual support. Later, *Wolinella recta* was renamed *Campylobacter rectus*, and *Bacteroides gingivalis* became *Porphyromonas gingivalis*.

Abstract 7,2   *Experimental gingivitis in man. II. A longitudinal clinical and bacteriological investigation*

Theilade E, Wright WH, Jensen SB, et al., *Journal of Periodontal Research* 1966; **1**: 1–13

Three phases in plaque development were observed in 11 subjects with excellent initial gingival health, who ceased oral hygiene with the production of generalized gingivitis in 9–21 days. In Phase 1 (days 1–2) an initial sparse Gram-positive flora of cocci and rods proliferated, with the addition of 30% Gram-negative cocci and rods. In Phase 2 (1–4 days), fusobacteria and filaments each occurred up to about 7% each. By Phase 3 (4–9 days) spirilla and spirochaetes were found. There were no further changes up to 21 days. Resumption of oral hygiene removed the gingivitis in 1–2 days. Many polymorphs appeared by about day 4, disappearing rapidly with hygiene resumption.

Comment: Gingivitis appears in response to a mature, complex, predominantly Gram-negative plaque flora.

MICROBIOLOGY OF EXPERIMENTAL GINGIVITIS

Within a few minutes of thorough cleaning, a tooth surface begins to acquire a bacterial dental plaque. The process for smooth surface plaque has been studied in detail, and there are several changes as the biofilm develops and matures.

The first stage is the selective adsorption of salivary proteins to form an acquired pellicle on the tooth surface. This starts rapidly and is complete within 1–2 h. The pellicle is soon colonized by bacterial cells.

The development of microbial plaque from its initial colonization of pellicle may be seen as four related concurrent changes. The first of these is an establishment of differently shaped organisms. This was well described by Löe's group of researchers in 1966 (Abstract 7,2). The significance is that the first organisms to attach to pellicle are less able to provide cohesion to the mass of plaque than some that come later, notably organisms such as *Fusobacterium* species.

Because they used Gram staining, the same researchers were also able to show a shift in the microbial population from mainly Gram-positive organisms to about half positive and half negative after about 7 days. Although many oral microbes have mechanisms whereby they might cause host damage, Gram-negative organisms contain particularly significant substances called endotoxins in their cell walls. These are capable of eliciting a strong host response.

The third change in developing plaque is that as it becomes thicker, good conditions are produced for anaerobic organisms. The spirochaetes are an especially good example of this, because exposure to air briefly will kill them. Indeed, most are still uncultivable. Anaerobes are noted for living in any thick biofilm and for producing many substances likely to damage the host.

A fourth change, highlighted by later workers (Abstract 7,3), is that more motile organisms are present in deeper pockets. Spirochaetes, some rods and vibrios are typical motile morphotypes. Motility is a feature that may help organisms to invade host tissues, although this appears to be a rare event in the periodontium.

Abstract 7,3 *Relative distribution of bacteria at clinically healthy and periodontally diseased sites in humans*

Listgarten MA, Helldén L, *Journal of Clinical Periodontology* 1978; **5**: 115–132

In 12 patients with advanced periodontitis, subgingival bacterial samples from two sites probing ≤3mm and two deep sites (mean 7.3 mm) were examined within 1 h by darkfield microscopy. Following disaggregation of each sample, 100–200 bacteria were classified. At shallow sites, of nine forms, 75% present were cocci. At deep sites, motile rods and spirochaetes (also known to be motile, but killed by the procedure) were 50% of the bacteria present (respectively 13% and 38%).

Comment: This technique has been used widely to show motile organisms, and also shows that many spirochaetes are present in deep plaque.

INTERACTION OF PLAQUE BACTERIA WITH THEIR ENVIRONMENT

What we find in a habitat is whatever is capable of surviving there. Mature plaque contains more organisms capable of causing damage to the host simply because the host has created suitable conditions for their survival. The host has a strong influence on the habitat, and hence on the plaque.

Naturally occurring periodontitis in animals is slow and may be rare. The beagle dog, described well by Lindhe and co-workers in 1973, shows signs of early attachment loss only after 6–8 months of undisturbed plaque. In some captive primates, like *Macaca fascicularis*, it may take up to 20 years before occasional sites develop intrabony pockets such as are commonplace in human beings. If an experimental periodontitis is produced in a beagle or a squirrel monkey, it is usually accelerated by tying ligatures round teeth to help plaque accumulate. This seems to produce a lesion with features of early-onset disease in human beings, including rapid loss of attachment.

Human periodontitis, although relatively common, is usually a slow disease. If the burst theory is applicable (Chapter 10), then much of the time pathogenic organisms are present but are fully controlled by the host; by contrast, the continuous theory implies an almost imperceptible effect whereby attachment is lost. Again, a deep pocket is likely to contain a flora different to a shallow pocket simply because it is a different environment.

None of the above observations is intended to deny the obvious fact that plaque is essential to periodontitis. Remove the plaque and the periodontitis is controlled. But this is very different from saying that the plaque determines periodontitis. As we saw in the Sri Lankan study (Chapter 6), there are some people who do not develop the disease with prolonged exposure to the worst plaque conditions possible.

MATURE SMOOTH SURFACE PLAQUE

It is worth considering the structure of mature plaque, because it has implications for treatment of periodontal diseases. Certain

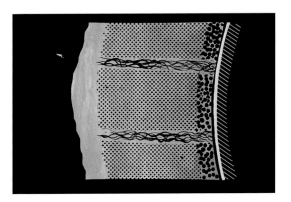

Fig. 7,1

Diagram of mature plaque (green) on a smooth tooth surface (yellow). The condensed microbial layer is next to the tooth and bundles of filaments extend out from the surface, with many other organisms closely associated in a matrix (mainly composed of extracellular polysaccharides) that also covers the plaque.

characteristics among those outlined by Schroeder and de Boever in 1970 may be taken as basic (Fig. 7,1).

At the tooth surface there is a condensed microbial layer of cells that were probably the first to attach to pellicle. There seems to be considerable reproductive activity in these cells.

From the tooth surface, bundles of filamentous organisms extend perpendicularly outwards. These are a significant means of plaque cohesion, and are attached to many coccoid and other bacteria. In early electron microscope studies of plaque, these structures were described as being like corn on the cob.

In between the bacteria and on the surface of the plaque is a large quantity of plaque matrix. Much of this is composed of extracellular polysaccharides produced by the bacteria. These molecules help in cohesion. Salivary components such as proteins are also to be found, and the whole matrix is insoluble and relatively impervious to water.

The main implications are that plaque cannot be washed off a tooth surface with water, and well-established plaque cannot be penetrated with an antimicrobial mouthrinse by more than a fraction of a millimetre. Mechanical means of plaque control, therefore, are currently viewed as essential in most situations.

Abstract 7,4 *Bacteriology of severe periodontitis in young adult humans*

Moore WEC, Holdeman LV, Smibert RM, et al., *Infection and Immunity* 1982; **38**: 1137–1148

Plaque samples were removed from 34 sites in 21 subjects aged 12–30 years (mean 24 years), with at least 5 mm loss of attachment and 6 mm probing depth on eight or more teeth, of which three or more were not first molars or incisors. Altogether, 190 types of microbe were identified. The 11 most frequent organisms accounted for 45% of all bacteria isolated, and included species of *Eubacterium*, *Fusobacterium*, *Lactobacillus*, *Peptostreptococcus* and *Bacteroides*. Spirochaetes were isolated from almost all sites. The flora at sites with severe periodontitis differed from that on the adjacent tooth surface, and in health and gingivitis in other people. The subjects differed significantly from each other in their associated microfloras. *Actinobacillus actinomycetemcomitans* was detected in small quantities in about one-third of subjects, in one case at 15%. Subjects who were antibody-positive for it appeared to have a simpler supragingival flora.

Comment: A complex picture in which many organisms are involved with much individual variation between subjects, and probably more than one kind of periodontal disease. A dominant presence of *Actinobacillus actinomycetemcomitans* and *Pg* (then called *Bacteroides gingivalis*) was not demonstrated.

CULTURING AND THE VIRGINIA POLYTECHNIC INSTITUTE

Early plaque studies produced useful information, but the complexity of the microflora impeded progress. One way of identifying the components of a mixed microflora and their relative proportions is by growing (culturing) the organisms on a suitable medium, and spreading them out (plating) so that different cells are separated. Eventually separate colonies of individual bacteria are produced, and these may be tested to show their identity. This is labour intensive and costly, especially when there are many types of microbe to identify.

There are many problems in such studies. For instance, different organisms grow best on different nutrient media, and although some are aerobic or facultative, others are strict anaerobes. The most detailed studies of periodontal microflora were published by workers at the Virginia Polytechnic Institute (VPI) in the early 1980s. This establishment was noted for its excellent facilities for studying anaerobic organisms. Abstract 7,4 shows a typical study.

The sheer complexity of the plaque is at once apparent. Nearly 200 types of organism were identified. However, no organism dominated the flora, and only 11 were present in quantities exceeding 1%. There were some differences between health and disease, but there were also considerable differences between the 21 individual people examined.

In such multifarious circumstances, the significance of individual organisms is open to question.

Other studies at these laboratories established that: periodontal microflora varied from week to week at clinically unchanged sites; children have a different gingivitis flora to adults; severe periodontitis in mature and young adults had similar microfloras; and the subgingival flora in juvenile periodontitis sites did not differ significantly from that in other types of periodontitis.

Thus, the available data indicate that there is probably a greater effect of the periodontal environment on its microorganisms than viceversa. Because of the many bacterial interactions, notably different microbes may be unable to gain a foothold.

The achievements of the VPI workers should not be underestimated. Nearly 20 years later there is nothing to surpass their thoroughness. At the present time there are new approaches to identifying bacteria, such as genetic probes, which are proving useful.

TAXONOMY PROBLEMS

We should take note that over the past 30 years there has been recurrent confusion over classifying many bacteria. This is based on the behaviour of cultured organisms under specified conditions. Thus, for instance, some *Bacteroides melaninogenicus* gave rise to *B. asaccharolyticus*, of which some were reclassified as *Bacteroides gingivalis* and eventually became the *Porphyromonas gingivalis* (Pg) that we know today. *Bacteroides intermedius* became *Prevotella intermedia*, and *Wolinella recta* became *Campylobacter rectus*. *Actinobacillus actinomycetemcomitans* (often abbreviated to Aa) briefly became *Haemophilus actinomycetemcomitans*, but then reverted.

With so many organisms to choose from, there are naturally some favourites for researchers. Aa and Pg are perhaps the most popular. There is a danger that popularity may be misconstrued to mean significance. The most studied organisms in a mixed flora are not necessarily more important than others.

BACTERIAL DISEASE FACTORS

Periodontal bacteria produce a large range of substances that have potential to cause damage to the host. This may be direct damage by enzymes or indirect damage by triggering host mechanisms with destructive potential. Thus, Pg may produce collagenase, although this may be swamped by collagenase from defending host cells. Aa may also cause neutrophil polymorphs to release collagenase. Endotoxins released from the cell walls of lysed Gram-negative organisms, for instance, can trigger the complement cascade and promote macrophage secretion of cytokines and prostaglandins.

Attention should be drawn to at least two significant matters concerning bacteria and periodontal destruction. One is that some disease mechanisms may not be exhibited by all strains of a species. Thus, some strains of Aa are leucotoxic and others are not. The leucotoxin in question damages neutrophils and can even kill them, consequently undermining the host response and also releasing destructive neutrophil enzymes.

The other important matter is that periodontal destruction may occur in two separate circumstances, and *their distinction is of critical importance*. In all inflammatory lesions there are ongoing destructive processes, and gingivitis is no exception. The destruction that distinguishes periodontitis from gingivitis is loss of connective tissue attachment. However, in a periodontal pocket, there may be considerable inflammation-associated tissue destruction (which may be reversed by treatment) without any progression of attachment loss. This fact has significant clinical implications, but is often overlooked. We shall return to it in Chapters 9 and 10.

CONCLUSION

There are many species of bacteria in the periodontal environment, and most of them probably have the potential for some damaging effect on the host. Bacteriologists estimate that 90% of the cells in a human body are bacterial, and that microorganisms and host cells 'talk' to each other in highly specific ways. The host plays a part in selecting which bacteria are present, and so do the other microbes. With this in mind, we shall turn to a consideration of the highly influential specific plaque hypothesis.

8 THE SPECIFIC PLAQUE HYPOTHESIS

- What is the significance of the SPH?
- How near are we to proving it?
- Why should we be wary of claims that it has been proved?

The specific plaque hypothesis (SPH) was first defined by Loesche in 1976, but a number of experimental findings had directed attention towards such a concept in the previous 10 years. The hypothesis is that some plaque compositions are more likely than others to produce designated periodontal disease conditions. It is not the same as saying that certain individual microbes are the cause of particular diseases.

Before the development of modern periodontal science from the 1950s onwards, it was a consensus view that gingivitis sooner or later would become periodontitis in most untreated individuals. We may compare some of the older views with those that began to

replace them and currently are widely held (Table 8,1).

Although this is a simplification, and some of the 'new' views were long held by pioneers in the scientific revolution, the old concepts really did dominate the thinking of many leaders in periodontology. It took courage for some researchers to stand up at conferences in the early 1970s and insist that periodontitis was primarily inflammation plus attachment loss, when others had been brought up in a long tradition of bone ideas.

The first three 'new' views listed in Table 8,1 underlie the SPH that Loesche first defined in 1976. Although all three observations might be explained by variation in host defence or structure, they might also be explained by variation in bacterial plaque.

Loesche was careful to use the word 'plaque' and not 'bacteria'. His contention was that specific plaques might cause caries or

Table 8,1: *Periodontitis – some older and newer views*

'Old' view	Evidence problems	'New' view
Universal progressive gradual attachment loss	Some have early-onset periodontitis	Variation in disease severity
Gingivitis necessarily leads to periodontitis	Some with gingivitis never develop periodontitis	Only some are susceptible to attachment loss
Disease is generalized	Localized forms in both juveniles and adults	Site specificity
It is essentially a disease of bone	Healthy support without bone (see Chapter 3)	It is essentially a disease of the ligament
Bone loss and mobility are central effects	These may occur in healthy periodontium	Bone loss and mobility are contingent effects
Removal of diseased support tissue is important	Hygiene, scaling and root planing remove disease	Root surface state is of central importance

Table 8,2: *Factors confounding the demonstration of specific plaque effects*

Effect	Example
Influence of habitat on microflora	Deep pockets select more anaerobes
Influence of organisms on each other	Promotion or inhibition of an organism may hide the real culprit
Influence of host defence on microflora	Another opportunity for selection
	Response may hide the real culprit
Variation in host response	Some individuals may cope without attachment loss
Influence of organisms on host defence	Real culprit is allowed carte blanche by another organism inhibiting host
Perhaps 50% of periodontal microflora is uncultivable	Many spirochaetes have never been cultured

periodontal diseases. As we have seen, plaques are complex biofilms with many different components. The hypothesis was received enthusiastically by researchers who have since tried hard to show that specific organisms cause attachment loss.

There are two nightmares hidden in the background for any who might be so bold as to follow the SPH trail. One is the plaque ecology and the other is the demonstration of attachment loss. Table 8,2 lists some confounding factors for the microbiologist, and we shall discuss the horrors of studying disease activity in Chapter 10.

It will help both our patients and us if we can reduce their need for treatment. Unfortunately, the main result of pursuing the SPH so far has been a batch of expensive clinical tests of dubious significance, thereby adding to the patients' costs with but little measurable benefit. Effectively, almost all current treatment is according to the NSPH. Which of these hypotheses is true? Before this question can be approached, we need to ask another, a query of awesome proportions. How can the SPH be proved? This question was approached in 1979 by Socransky, one of periodontology's great thinkers.

BENEFITS AND DRAWBACKS OF THE SPH

If we can prove the SPH, what are the advantages? As Loesche described it, the SPH excludes the normal from treatment. We should only treat where the condition requires it. A birthmark on the face might require plastic surgery, but one on the bottom might not. Similarly, many pockets stay the same for years; the argument is that we should only treat them if they are likely to progress.

The opposite, the non-specific plaque hypothesis (NSPH), means that anyone, anywhere is eligible for treatment. We should realize that our income is paid by our patients. As the cost of personal attention slowly rises, the number of patients who are willing to pay us slowly reduces.

KOCH'S POSTULATES AND SOCRANSKY'S CRITERIA

First, Socransky pointed out that Koch's postulates (Table 8,3) were inadequate to prove causality in dental diseases. In effect, he objected that many periodontal organisms

Table 8,3: *Koch's postulates for identifying causal organisms in infectious diseases*

1. Organism can always be found in the lesions.
2. Organism can be grown in pure culture.
3. Cultured organisms produce similar lesions in susceptible host.
4. Organisms can be found in these new lesions.

Table 8,4: *Socransky's criteria for specificity in dental diseases*

Criterion	Weighting factor
1. Association with lesion	0.3
2. Elimination leading to resolution	0.3
3. Host response to organism	0.2
4. Animal pathogenicity	0.1
5. Specific pathogenic mechanisms	0.1

might fulfil the criteria, that some organisms could not be implanted in the mouths of experimental animals (competition from existing microflora), that the animal disease might differ from the human disease and that the organisms often co-existed with periodontal health.

Next, Socransky derived from the postulates five criteria that were more applicable to dental diseases and to which he assigned relative levels of significance (Table 8,4).

ASSOCIATION WITH THE LESION

Association is the first requirement for a microbe to cause a periodontal lesion. In the absence of plaque, there is no inflammation and no attachment loss. Yet the presence of an organism is proof of very little. In detective story terms, it is circumstantial evidence that amounts to coincidence at the most. But if we really want to be detectives, it would be wise to pay attention to that little word 'lesion'. Just what is the lesion in question? Is it the presence of inflammation, the presence of attachment loss or the process of attachment loss? All three may be involved in periodontitis, but the crucial one is the last of them.

In the change from gingivitis to periodontitis, conditions are made most attractive for a wide range of organisms that could not easily survive before. Which of the many inhabitants of subgingival plaque caused the loss of attachment? Or was it an organism present in gingivitis that has now changed its habitat so that it cannot survive? Thus we see that the organism must be shown to be present before the lesion occurs. It is likely (but not to be taken for granted) that it will also be there afterwards.

However, many studies of microbial association are probably in relatively inactive periodontitis. In this situation we may just as well consider the pocket to be the cause of the microflora in it, by providing a suitable habitat. This is an excellent demonstration of the dictum 'association is not causation'. But the situation is really far worse, as we shall see when we consider disease activity (Chapter 10). We are taking too simple a view if we think that there are only three clinical conditions to be distinguished.

ELIMINATION OF THE SUSPECT ORGANISM

If a lesion is resolved by removal of an organism, causality may be argued. Abstract 8,1 describes the first attempt to remove a single suspect pathogen from periodontal pockets, and marks an interesting new trend in SPH studies. Previously, crude methods used antimicrobial drugs like metronidazole, which is effective against all strict anaerobes and not just Pg, or antibiotics like tetracycline because of its effect against Aa, despite its broad-spectrum activity and acquired resistance problems.

The 1-year follow-up in this passive immunization study is probably not long enough to show a clinical effect in a small number of patients. However, it is clear that individual organisms may be suppressed; but does this constitute evidence of causality if periodontitis is thereby contained?

Referring back to Table 7,1 reminds us that microorganisms are quite interdependent. Removing Pg from plaque should not be assumed to be without effect on the other microbes. We are faced with the need for a detailed study of the plaque in question to show its constituents and their proportions, and how it is changed after the removal of Pg.

HOST RESPONSE TO ORGANISM

Of the main branches of the host response in periodontal diseases, the most studied has

Abstract 8,1 *Passive immunization with monoclonal antibodies against Pg in patients with periodontitis*

Booth V, Ashley FP, Lehner T, *Infection and Immunity* 1996; **64**: 422–427

A monoclonal antibody (MAb) to Pg was selected for its ability to recognize a wide range of strains and serotypes of this organism. Next, a comparison with culture and immunofluorescence methods demonstrated close agreement with MAb recognition of Pg. Fourteen patients were identified who had Pg in their subgingival plaque, and were given thorough treatment with root planing and metronidazole to suppress Pg. Patients were randomly allocated to MAb or saline application 1, 3, 7 and 10 days after Pg suppression. The MAb group showed significantly less Pg recolonization of the sites with worst disease 6 and 9 months later. By 1 year, two MAb patients had recolonization. Numbers of spirochaetes did not differ between groups, indicating a specific effect against Pg. However, there were no differences in periodontal indices between groups during follow-up.

Comment: This very thorough study shows how extremely difficult it is to eliminate one organism from the subgingival microflora, and was the first experiment of its kind. There is also a possibility that eliminating all plaque may lead to a different microflora on recolonization, or even healing of the lesion.

Abstract 8,2 *Longitudinal monitoring of humoral antibody in subjects with destructive periodontal diseases*

Taubman MA, Haffajee AD, Socransky SS, et al., *Journal of Periodontal Research* 1992; **27**: 511–521

Every 2 months for up to 5 years, 51 patients aged 16–61 years with prior periodontal destruction were monitored clinically and immunologically. New attachment loss was found in 33 subjects. Antibody levels were above those for healthy subjects most frequently in diseased subjects with antibodies to Aa, Pg, *Eikenella corrodens*, *Campylobacter concisus*, *Fusobacterium nucleatum* and *Prevotella intermedia*. Major antibody changes were usually limited to one or two species in individual subjects. Some subjects showed prolonged, steady increases or decreases in specific antibodies. The authors suggested that major changes in serum antibody were related to fluctuations in periodontal disease.

Comment: Non-periodontal factors might affect some systemic antibody levels. For instance, *E. corrodens*, *C. concisus* and *F. nucleatum* are found in the intestine.

been humoral antibody production. Polymorphs and macrophages also have been investigated mainly with respect to early-onset periodontitis, of which we will say more in Chapter 11. But several hundred periodontal studies have examined antibodies.

The only indisputable fact about a specific antibody is that it is a response to the antigen; therefore at some time the host has experienced that antigen, or some other antigen with which the antibody cross-reacts. Presence of antibody to Aa means that Aa or a related organism was present in the host (not necessarily in the periodontium) and probably still is.

However, there appear to be some further deductions that researchers make from time to time. A high antibody response is sometimes interpreted as meaning that the organism in question has caused and maybe is causing significant damage, which, being further interpreted by the investigators, somehow seems to imply attachment loss rather than inflammation.

If we examine the literature, a high antibody response may be related to age, at least in child patients, recent exposure to the antigen in question, or exposure to a large amount of the antigen. Nowhere is there any evidence that relates antibody titre to what the organism may be doing to the host periodontal ligament, or even to the surrounding inflamed tissues.

One very intriguing periodontal effect is that crevicular fluid sometimes contains more antibody to local periodontal organisms than serum in the same person. However, even this is no basis for implying some effect of the organisms on the tissues.

Abstract 8,3 *Local and systemic antibody response to putative periodontopathogens in patients with chronic periodontitis. Correlation with clinical indices*

Kinane DF, Mooney J, MacFarlane TW, et al., *Oral Microbiology and Immunology* 1993; **8**: 65–68

Specific IgG, IgA and IgM antibodies to Pg and Aa were measured in crevicular fluid at 5 periodontitis sites in each of 20 patients on a maintenance programme, and also in serum. Local and systemic IgG titres were correlated. Sites with a probing depth of 4 mm and above had significantly lower IgG titres to Pg than shallower sites. A Gingival Index (GI) of 3 also identified sites with a lower IgG response than those with a GI below this. The authors interpreted these findings as an indication of less protection from the humoral response in sites with worse disease.

Comment: It is possible that previous treatment had reduced the host response, but unlikely that this occurred preferentially in the deeper sites.

Exposure to an organism may also occur in other places besides the periodontium, such as the intestine. It is even possible that antigenic components of predominantly oral organisms may elicit a response when transferred to the skin, eye, lung or elsewhere.

Let us consider two very interesting studies from the hundreds available. Abstracts 8,2 and 8,3 are of quite different approaches to periodontal humoral response. The first is a large, longitudinal study from some of the foremost American researchers in this field; the second is a cross-sectional study from some experienced Scottish investigators.

Admittedly, these are very different studies, and yet there is something quite intriguing about them at a simple and understandable level. The first study found higher systemic antibody levels with greater disease; the second found lower local levels in areas of greater disease. In the first study, systemic antibodies were apparently related directly to the amount of destruction; in the second study, local antibodies appeared inversely related to the amount of destruction.

The American group went on to further studies attempting to classify patients with periodontitis according to higher systemic antibody levels to various organisms in subgingival plaque.

The Scottish researchers produced a further study in 1997, which confirmed their results, leading them to suggest that failure to make enough specific antibody might contribute to the process of attachment loss.

Here is a mystery that is not easily solved. For many years, the host response to periodontitis has been viewed as protective and yet destructive. Does a high antibody level really mean that the host is protected, or might it mean that there is a desperately unsuccessful battle against the damage caused by the organism that it is fighting?

It is quite possible that both high and low antibody titres might relate to destruction. For instance, on some occasions, a vigorous humoral response to antigens might be accompanied by a strong neutrophil response with subsequent release of destructive enzymes. On other occasions, a weak humoral response might permit such ingress of bacteria that the same destructive neutrophil response could be evoked in compensation.

Antibody levels presently cannot be interpreted as though they link an organism to a specific disease process in the periodontium.

ANIMAL PATHOGENICITY

There are both advantages and difficulties in using animal models of periodontal disease to investigate the SPH. A major advantage is that known organisms may be introduced into the mouth of a germ-free animal; these two conditions (germ-free and monoinfected) are termed gnotobiotic (Greek: known life). Disadvantages are: the disease may be different in an animal; or the response to bacterial immune challenge may be exceptional because it was previously absent and now involves only one organism.

There may be little point in studying the SPH in an animal that is not gnotobiotic, and yet almost any organism that can survive in the periodontal environment may evoke a response in a germ-free animal. Indeed, there are reports of periodontal disease in apparently

Abstract 8,4 *Histological changes in experimental periodontal disease in gnotobiotic rats and conventional hamsters*

Irving JT, Socransky SS, Heeley JD, *Journal of Periodontal Research* 1974; **9**: 73–80

Germ-free rats were infected with *Actinomyces naeslundii*, *Actinomyces viscosus* or *Streptococcus mutans*. Initial periodontitis began around 28 days, and was advanced by 84 days. There was minimal inflammation but much bone loss. Controls showed no periodontal destruction. A group of hamsters without controls and with their usual microflora were superinfected with *Actinomyces naeslundii* and showed a severe periodontitis that took 160 days to develop.

Comment: Germ-free animals appeared more susceptible to periodontal destruction by organisms not considered prime pathogens.

Abstract 8,5 *Antibody reactive with Actinobacillus actinomycetemcomitans leukotoxin in early-onset periodontitis patients*

Califano JV, Pace BE, Gunsolley JC, et al., *Oral Microbiology and Immunology* 1997; **12**: 20–26.

Serum levels of IgG antibody to Aa leucotoxin, and antibody to a sonicate of Aa, were measured in 119 early-onset periodontitis patients and 59 subjects without periodontitis. Mean levels of antibody to leucotoxin were 3.13 µg/ml for generalized early-onset periodontitis, 2.17 µg/ml for localized early-onset periodontitis and 0.32 ng/ml for controls. Generalized early-onset periodontitis patients with antibody to leucotoxin had less attachment loss than those without. A statistically stronger relationship was found between presence of the sonicate antibody and less attachment loss in these patients.

Comment: If the leucotoxin was neutralized by antibody, there was possibly some protection against attachment loss; but there was apparently greater protection if antibodies to Aa (not just to the leucotoxin) were present.

germ-free animals. In these cases, it seems likely that antigens that are not part of living bacteria evoke an inflammatory response, because other parts of the alimentary tract may also be lined with lymphocytes and plasma cells.

Abstract 8,4 shows that human plaque organisms traditionally more associated with caries than periodontal diseases may cause periodontitis if introduced into germ-free or perhaps even conventional animals.

Such results suggest that this line of study will not contribute much useful evidence for the SPH enquiry. Even if an organism were found to be without damaging effect, and excluded on these grounds, that still would not exclude possible effects of bacterial interaction.

SPECIFIC PATHOGENIC MECHANISMS

Numerous oral organisms are known to have important virulence factors and one of the most interesting is the leucotoxin produced by many Aa strains. A 1997 study of this factor in early-onset periodontitis patients gives some intriguing data (Abstract 8,5).

In the patients with periodontitis, some of those who produced antibodies to the leucotoxin had less attachment loss than those who produced none. However, there was a greater effect in those who had antibodies to Aa sonicate, showing that other protective factors may exist in these patients.

The presence of a specific virulence factor does not necessarily mean that it will always be used, and a study of one organism's activity does not say anything about the other components of plaque and their relationship to the patient. However, the Aa leucotoxin is of special interest in early-onset periodontitis, because many patients show defective phagocyte function.

WHAT IS THE SUM OF THE EVIDENCE?

It is easy to see why Socransky did not consider the five lines of evidence to be of equal weight. All of them have significant problems, and perhaps the least useful are the three to which he attached the least weight.

It is remarkable how much has been discovered about these complex matters, but we still do not have any clear answers. Even the association of Aa and its special virulence factors with early-onset periodontitis does not prove causality. The presence of a defective host response may be the ecological factor encouraging this organism to take up residence. Studies suggest that Aa may be found in 15% or more of the teenage population, and early-onset periodontitis only affects 0.1% according to the best UK data.

VERTICAL AND HORIZONTAL TRANSMISSION OF ORAL MICROBES

Before we leave the subject of plaque and the SPH, there is one further matter to explore. Good evidence shows that spouses may transmit certain organisms to each other and that parents may also pass some organisms to children. The interesting fact is that this does not always occur. Different host-determined factors and resident microflora in different individuals may limit such colonization.

Abstract 8,6 is the longest study in the literature of whether the *periodontal condition* of a spouse may affect that of the other partner. This study asked whether living together for a long time led to actual periodontal deterioration in the healthier partner. If so, the probable cause would be transmissible microbes. Actually, the healthier partners more than resisted any influence towards periodontal decline. Host factors, therefore, were of greater importance in their condition, even though some bacteria were transmitted.

Abstract 8,6 *Longitudinal evaluation of the development of periodontal destruction in spouses*

Van der Velden U, Van Winkelhoff AJ, Abbas F et al., *Journal of Clinical Periodontology* 1996; **23**: 1014–1019

In a remote village in Indonesia where periodontitis had familial occurrence and no regular dental care was available, 23 married couples were examined periodontally in 1987 and 1994. There was a microbiological examination on the second occasion, when they had been married for an average of 10 years. In 1994, the partner with worse attachment loss (PAL) was identified; this group also had a worse condition than their spouses in 1987. Both groups had increasing PAL over the 7 years, but the difference between groups increased. There were no significant differences between the two groups in the bacteria studied in 1994: Aa, Pg and *Prevotella intermedia* were most frequent and were present in both partners in few couples only. These findings suggest that host factors are more important than environmental factors in determining periodontal status.

Comment: This is evidence that living together, with a strong risk of transmission of bacteria between spouses, does not affect periodontal status.

CONCLUSION

There are some indications that particular organisms may be of greater importance than others, but there is no way of deciding that a specific organism is responsible for particular periodontal damage, and no scientific basis for treating any periodontitis as a specific infection. Consequently, all plaque should be controlled.

9

SIMPLIFIED VIEW OF PERIODONTAL PATHOLOGY

- What are the essential actors in periodontal inflammation?
- How does periodontal inflammation develop?
- Why may attachment loss be site-specific?

An American researcher once likened the events of inflammatory periodontal diseases to the sort of scene in a Western movie when the good guys and the bad guys meet in a saloon. Not only do some of the good guys and bad guys get hurt, but there is an effect on the saloon. Every window is broken, every chair is broken, every table is broken, every bottle is broken, every glass is broken, the staircase is damaged, the mirror behind the bar is smashed – you name it and it is broken into little pieces.

This is an excellent picture to start with but, like every good simile, it has limits. For instance, in periodontitis, the good guys (host defences) continue to arrive on the scene in large numbers, and the bad guys (bacteria) multiply. A large army of repair craftsmen also tries to remove the irreparable and restore the structure of the tissues.

In many cases, an uneasy *status quo* is reached, with a grumbling plaque army held at bay by a wall of defence cells; meanwhile the tissues return to a state of relative tranquillity, although with a constant stream of reinforcements to the battle front through enlarged and engorged blood vessels.

Earlier (Chapter 4) we examined the four common manifestations of periodontal disease. Enlargement and recession were explained primarily as inflammatory phenomena. It is now time to consider inflammation and attachment loss in greater detail. This will be a simplified view. In the complex world of immunology and histopathology, it is easy to lose sight of the main questions.

INFLAMMATION IN THE PERIODONTIUM

Many mechanisms are at work in inflammation. However, at least two factors are unique to the periodontal locality. First, the bacteria are substantially on the teeth and hence outside the tissues, and cannot be contained and destroyed as might happen within the body. Secondly, as we have seen, tissue destruction may be limited to the gingiva or may also affect the periodontal ligament: pocket formation creates a haven for a greater mass of plaque and also reduces tooth support.

It is certain that some bacteria enter the tissues and pass into the bloodstream. This is deduced from finding bacteraemia. However, entry to the periodontal tissues is quite different from invasion, where organisms resist host defences to the point of colonizing the tissues and multiplying within them. Invasion probably occurs only with immunosuppression. It has not been demonstrated unequivocally in any other circumstances.

Fig. 3,3 should be compared with Fig. 9,1 to see the main differences between health and moderate periodontitis. In periodontitis, attachment has been lost, leaving the cementum bare; the epithelium has proliferated apically to cover the denuded soft connective tissue, and the pocket wall is the scene of an inflammatory response: cells continually emerge to keep the bacterial threat from invading the tissues.

The bone has receded in front of the inflammation, and usually appears static in histological sections: a thick wall of fibres separates bone from inflammatory tissue. The diagram shows an intrabony pocket, which is of significance in treatment; the pocket ends apically to the coronal aspect of the bone.

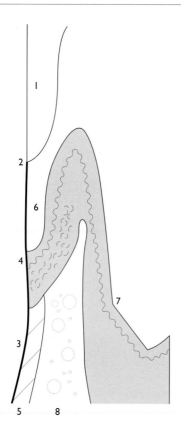

Fig. 9,1

Structure of periodontium that has experienced attachment loss. 1 = enamel; 2 = cementoenamel junction; 3 = cementum; 4 = junctional epithelium; 5 = periodontal ligament; 6 = pocket epithelium, with underlying inflammatory infiltrate; 7 = mucogingival junction; 8 = alveolar bone.

Pocket epithelium is different from sulcular epithelium. Because of the underlying inflammation, it can proliferate into the tissues, and there may be quite large areas of ulceration where cellular movement is intensified.

Comparison of early periodontitis with periodontal health raises a number of questions. How does bacterial plaque initiate periodontal inflammation? What leads some lesions to progress to attachment loss? And when moderate attachment loss has occurred, why does it progress further in certain cases, but remain static in others? The first question has answers. The others remain unsolved but there are many interesting ideas about them.

The framework for our basic understanding of periodontal inflammatory pathology was developed by Page and Schroeder and published in 1976. They described three stages in the evolution of gingivitis, and a fourth lesion with attachment loss (Table 9,1). For convenience, some effects of the main actors on the host response stage are also listed in Table 9,2.

INITIAL LESION

The beginning of gingivitis is dominated by neutrophil activity. Substances from plaque elicit a response indistinguishable from classical acute inflammation. Junctional and sulcular epithelia become less regular with increased intercellular spaces, allowing easy

Table 9,1: *Pathogenesis of chronic inflammatory periodontal disease*

Lesion	Significant cells	Events
Initial (2–4 days)	Polymorphs (neutrophils)	Epithelial disruption, vascular and perivascular activity, beginning of inflammatory cell infiltrate
Early (4–10 days)	Lymphocytes Other mononuclear cells	Further disruption, local collagen breakdown, significant inflammatory cell infiltrate
Established (2–3 weeks)	Plasma cells	Pocket epithelium lines sulcus, marked collagen breakdown with efforts at repair, dense infiltrate
Advanced	Plasma cells	As above plus attachment loss

Based on Page RC & Schroeder HE (1976) *Laboratory Investigation* **34**: 235–249.

Table 9,2: *Significant participants in periodontal inflammation*

Participant	Some activities
Neutrophil	Detection, phagocytosis and killing of bacteria
Monocyte/ macrophage	Control mechanisms; phagocytosis
T-cell	Control mechanisms; cytotoxicity
B-cell/plasma cell	Humoral immunity
Fibroblast	Collagen production and destruction
Osteoclast	Bone resorption
Complement	Chemotaxis; opsonization; anaphylotoxins; histamine release; cytolysis; effects on smooth muscle

passage of large molecules and cells. Breakdown of collagen (starting close to blood vessels) with consequent loss of tissue structure also contributes to freedom of movement.

Although plaque initiates a strong neutrophil response, this effect is compounded by the neutrophils themselves as they release chemical attractants for yet more to follow them. These cells are short-lived, typically with a life of 12–24 h, and a human being produces about a million of them every second. They adhere to and pass through vascular endothelium, migrate through the tissues, phagocytose microbes and kill them. We will consider them further in Chapter 11.

EARLY LESION

As the initial lesion begins, other cells start to detect substances that they recognize as foreign. A process of antigen recognition is started, involving T-cells and macrophages. The latter are much longer-lived cells than neutrophils, with a life in the tissues of about 3–4 months. They are derived from blood monocytes.

As antigens are recognized and processed, the mechanisms of cellular and humoral immunity come into play. The early lesion is considered to be an example of the phenomenon of delayed hypersensitivity.

ESTABLISHED AND ADVANCED LESIONS

The established lesion is the final phase in developing gingivitis, and is therefore what is most often seen in a microscopic section from inflamed tissue. The plasma cells, characteristic of all chronic inflammation, dominate the lesion, and produce large amounts of Ig antibodies. In the gingiva, these are primarily IgG, with lesser outputs of IgA and IgM.

In chronic inflammation, processes of repair coexist with destruction. Because of the altered environment, repair processes may differ from those of normal tissue turnover. For instance, it has been shown that a different form of collagen occurs in inflamed gingiva. This shows that fibroblasts can be affected by the presence of inflammation.

The histological features of the established lesion persist in the advanced lesion, but with the addition of attachment loss.

CYTOKINES AND COMPLEMENT

Leucocytes and some other cells produce proteins that convey messages to their neighbours. These cytokines include lymphokines (produced by lymphocytes), growth substances (affecting cell growth and differentiation), chemokines and interferons.

Cytokines add considerable complexity to the picture of periodontal inflammation. For instance, at least 16 interleukins (ILs) are known. They are produced mainly by lymphocytes, macrophages and monocytes, but some also by epithelial cells and fibroblasts. Several are intimately involved in periodontal inflammation. Their many effects include: T-cell activation (IL-1), B-cell differentiation (IL-4 and IL-5), activation and attraction of neutrophils (IL-8) and initiation of cell-mediated immunity (IL-12).

Table 9,3: *Possible reasons for site specificity of attachment loss*

Main factor	Some evidence
Plaque quantity	Epidemiological studies (Chapter 6): Russell and co-workers, Norwegian factory study
Plaque specificity	See Chapter 8
Local anatomical predisposition Local host defence	Localized juvenile periodontitis (see Chapters 11 and 14); Sri Lankan epidemiological study (Chapter 6)

Complement involves at least 20 serum proteins and has a wide range of activities that contribute to the effectiveness of inflammation as a defence (Table 9,2).

The intricacy of immune mechanisms has two human effects: it often puts off the clinician who seeks to understand periodontal disease; but it may also hypnotize the researcher into a state of hypersuggestibility about one small corner of the big picture.

SITE SPECIFICITY

As was noted in Chapter 4, there are plenty of mechanisms for collagen destruction. Collagen is destroyed as part of the turnover of healthy tissue, in gingival inflammation and in periodontal ligament attachment loss. Why should some sites be more susceptible than others to this latter phenomenon? Table 9,3 lists some possible reasons.

Although plaque quantity varies greatly in people who practise some oral hygiene procedures, it is clear that it is a definite factor in attachment loss. The studies of Russell and other workers in many countries showed a clear association of this factor with the prevalence of periodontitis (Chapter 6). The

Norwegian factory study also showed that this related to specific tooth surfaces. It should be noted that an increase in plaque quantity will necessarily alter the environment for its organisms, for instance favouring more anaerobes. An effect on plaque specificity, therefore, cannot be ruled out.

The question of specific plaques was discussed at length in Chapter 8. Although the hypothesis is not provable at present, it cannot be dismissed for precisely the same reason.

Finally, there may be rare anatomical factors that could weaken the resistance of a site to attachment loss, or the local host defence may vary either to cause damage directly or to allow bacterial invasion.

CONCLUSION

This chapter has briefly examined the main aspects of inflammatory periodontal pathology. It has suggested that we know very little about why periodontal attachment is lost in any specific site. However, many studies have centred on the matter of periodontal disease activity. This is a huge subject and requires a chapter of its own.

10

PERIODONTAL DISEASE ACTIVITY

- What is disease activity?
- How many clinical conditions can be distinguished with respect to inflammation and attachment loss?
- How likely is apparent disease activity to be mere probing error?
- Is there any possibility of predicting sites at risk of disease?

The term 'periodontal disease activity' has not been defined clearly throughout its period of currency. In 1981, Hancock reviewed the literature and made a distinction between gingival inflammation and 'progressive, destructive periodontitis'.

The definition implied in Hancock's review, although marking a forward step in thinking at that time, had certain difficulties. First, he identified activity and inactivity with the traditional pathological distinction between acute and chronic inflammation. Secondly, there was an implication that progression of disease occurred as a 'burst' of activity. Neither idea is certain.

Periodontal disease activity may be defined simply as the progression of connective tissue attachment loss. As far as current knowledge goes, this may be in any direction where there is such tissue, at any speed and by either burst or gradual progression, or both.

DISTINGUISHABLE CLINICAL SITUATIONS

Given that the diagnosis of individual forms of periodontitis may be problematic, there is a need at least for identifying the currently distinguishable situations that may be the subject of clinical measurement. The nature of a clinical site may not be clear at examination, but there are at least 12 possibilities, each of which carries certain implications for the study of disease activity.

Unfortunately, as Table 10,1 makes clear, we can clinically distinguish only three things: health, inflammation and attachment loss. Let us consider the 12 periodontal clinical conditions and their significance. Table 10,2 lists some of their features.

Table 10,1: *Possible periodontal states according to basic clinical findings*

Clinical status	Without probing attachment loss	With probing attachment loss
Healthy	Health	Reduced support health: receded attachment, repaired periodontitis, regenerated periodontium
Inflamed	Gingivitis	(True) periodontitis, arrested periodontitis, false periodontitis, retrograde periodontitis, disease activity, recurrent periodontitis, recurrent disease activity

Table 10,2: *Main features of 12 clinical states of periodontal sites*

Condition of site	BOP	PAL	Other features
Health	–	–	
Receded attachment	–	+	No long junctional epithelium
Repaired periodontitis	–	+	Long junctional epithelium
Regenerated periodontium	–	+	Significant new attachment
Gingivitis	+	–	Inflammation
(True) periodontitis	+	+	Pocket; progression of attachment loss possible
Arrested periodontitis	+	+	Pocket; progression unlikely
False periodontitis	+	+	Inflammation; no true AL or pocket
Retrograde periodontitis	+	+	Endodontic origin of lesion
Disease activity	+	+	Progressing AL lesion
Recurrent periodontitis	+	+	Breakdown of healed lesion
Recurrent disease activity	+	+	AL lesion progressing further

HEALTH

This may be defined by the absence of detectable inflammation or attachment loss, and is probably the condition about which the greatest certainty exists. Traditional probing measurements are more reliable in this situation. However, the condition of health does not preclude the presence of active host defence mechanisms, such as macrophages in the tissues and neutrophils passing in random movement from the blood vessels to the crevice.

REDUCED SUPPORT HEALTH

Health may be present in sites with reduced support after treatment for previous attachment loss. The significance of this is that the site has proven susceptibility to disease activity, although its freedom from inflammation suggests that microbial initiating factors are under control. There are three subdivisions of this category: receded attachment, repaired periodontitis and regenerated periodontium.

Receded attachment refers to the apical movement of the attachment level, but without long junctional epithelial attachment. It may occur most frequently with gingival recession and is less likely when pockets heal. If it results from recession, it may not represent the same type of susceptibility as when a pocket forms.

In cases of repaired periodontitis, the control of plaque following treatment may lead to the eradication of inflammation, and the formation of a long epithelial attachment. In some situations, there may be little difference between repaired periodontitis and receded attachment.

There is currently no clear evidence that repaired periodontitis is any more susceptible to further disease than a site where disease has healed without a long epithelial attachment. Nevertheless, these situations must be distinguished from each other because the recurrence of disease may involve different mechanisms. Where the coronal attachment lacks cementum and periodontal ligament, persistent inflammation may re-establish periodontitis without true periodontal disease activity.

Regenerated periodontium refers to sites where the attachment has been partly reconstructed, for instance by techniques of guided tissue regeneration (GTR), or with enamel matrix derivatives (EMDs). Although these techniques have been shown to achieve this result, there may sometimes be doubt about the individual result.

Currently, there is little evidence as to whether regenerated periodontium sites are more protected than repaired sites against further disease activity (Chapter 20). This is partly because of the difficulty of distinguishing between recurrent disease activity and recurrent periodontitis as defined below.

GINGIVITIS

The presence of inflammation without true attachment loss sometimes may be quite difficult to determine. Because a probe may penetrate inflammation, its passage past the cementoenamel junction may give rise to a false diagnosis of early periodontitis. Abstract 10,1 shows another validity study (see

Abstract 5,3), this time in gingivitis and early periodontitis. Only in two out of 82 sites did the probe penetrate intact gingiva. In this study, measurements were rounded to the nearest mm, which effectively means a threshold of 0.5 mm for accepting the presence of attachment loss.

(TRUE) PERIODONTITIS

To determine the presence of the earliest stages of attachment loss with inflammation is likewise difficult. Attachment loss is usually obvious in the more advanced lesion, although its degree is subject to a high level of uncertainty. However, there is one occasional confounding factor which may be called 'false periodontitis'.

Abstract 10,1 *The attachment level as a measure of early periodontitis*

Clerehugh V, Lennon MA, *Community Dental Health* 1984; **1**: 33–40

Seventy-nine teeth were extracted, mainly because of caries, in 57 subjects aged 14–61 years. Before extraction, a probe was used to measure the position of the CEJ and clinical attachment level (CAL) on buccal (75 sites) and mesiobuccal (71 sites) surfaces. A reference mark located these sites. The exclusions were because of extraction trauma or CAL > 3 mm. After extraction, laboratory measurements (LM) were made and compared with CAL. There was 99% and 96% agreement of CAL and LM on buccal and mesiobuccal surfaces, respectively, regarding whether attachment loss was present or absent. About one-third of surfaces showed attachment loss, and in 30% of these the CAL differed from LM by 1–2 mm. In two cases, CAL showed attachment loss where LM did not.

Comment: This study shows that clinical probing is more than 95% likely to show whether attachment loss is present or not when measurements are to the nearest millimetre. The level of error for where attachment loss is present is similar to other studies (30–40%).

ARRESTED PERIODONTITIS

This is a condition that many clinicians have suspected, for instance, when so-called 'burnout' occurs in some patients after rapid loss of attachment in localized juvenile periodontitis. It also appears to be the case that some lesions may progress and others stay the same for long periods of time in chronic adult periodontitis. However, arrested disease needs to be distinguished from a reduction in the speed of attachment loss. Arrest may be a satisfactory outcome for treatment, for instance, in some patients with refractory disease.

FALSE PERIODONTITIS

This term may be applied to the situation when a probe passes down the root surface of a tooth that has not lost attachment, on account of the presence of inflammation associated with true periodontitis on the next tooth. Such conditions cannot be diagnosed at present, but are presumed when extraction of the adjacent tooth leads to apparent healing of the attachment apparatus.

RETROGRADE PERIODONTITIS

This describes periodontitis arising from the spread of a lesion of endodontic origin, either at an apex or from lateral or accessory canals. There are distinct differences described between periodontal and endodontic microflora, and cases of false retrograde periodontitis are known where the lesion has apparently healed completely with resolution of inflammation.

DISEASE ACTIVITY

To date, this condition has not been described convincingly, although there have been some tantalizing glimpses where it cannot be ruled out. Its identification is inextricably linked to that of the lesion that is not progressing, and because progression may be very slow and continuous, or a short and sudden burst, this condition is likely to prove elusive for some time to come.

RECURRENT PERIODONTITIS

This may be described as the breakdown of repaired periodontitis by inflammation only. It may be apparent by comparison of previous periodontal charts for the patient in question. As mentioned above, it is a condition of great significance because it may confuse attempts to identify true disease activity in patients who have been treated and are on a maintenance programme.

RECURRENT DISEASE ACTIVITY

This may be said to have occurred where a lesion has reappeared at a repaired or arrested periodontitis site but has progressed significantly beyond any previously charted disease. It is possible that different mechanisms may account for the previous and recurrent disease activity.

IMPLICATIONS OF THIS CLINICAL COMPLEXITY

The above conditions probably constitute a minimum consideration for the study of periodontal disease activity. Greater complexity may occur with combination of some conditions: for instance, both true and false periodontitis may be present at a site, and so may true and retrograde periodontitis in a periodontal-endodontic lesion. The greatest difficulties may relate to distinguishing between conditions in the mouths of patients who have had previous limited periodontal treatment.

At this point, the reader may begin to suspect that all is not clear and straightforward when enthusiastic researchers advocate monitoring various microbial, immunological or biochemical factors in the routine treatment of periodontal diseases. Such suspicions are more than justified. Not only is there turmoil over the SPH and great uncertainty about why collagen should be destroyed in the ligament instead of just in the gingiva, but there is absolutely no assurance that we can detect disease activity in the periodontium.

ATTEMPTS TO IMPROVE CLINICAL DETECTION OF DISEASE ACTIVITY

Researchers certainly have not been idle with regard to clinical measurement. As described in Chapter 5, three generations of probe now exist. However, with the benefit of hindsight we may ask why the research workshop that led to the development of automated probes (Parakkal, 1979) did not question the existing approach to measurement, instead of merely stating rigorously exact and precise requirements for that approach.

Probing at six points on the tooth has established, without doubt, that a number of periodontal treatments are very effective, but has helped little in the study of disease. Table 10,3 shows some of the ways in which researchers have tried to overcome the manifold defects of unidimensional probing.

Table 10,3: *Attempts to improve probing as a method of assessing periodontitis*

Method	Aim	Defects
Operator practice and calibration with others	Improve consistency	30–40% inconsistency at best in advanced disease
Constant force and automated probes	Reduce error levels	Unfortunately, high levels of error still occur
Use of stents and onlays with guides for probing	Increase the likelihood of probing the same site	Similar inaccuracy, and by missing active site may increase Type II error
Duplicate probing	Accept average as better indication of 'true' status	May be average of two different sites, and reduces precision
Threshold for accepting disease activity	Only accept definite cases (reduce Type I error)	Failure to recognize sub-threshold cases (increased Type II error)
Statistically guided decisions	Use probabilities to reduce Type I and Type II error	Statistics depends on assumptions, some of which may not be testable

MEASUREMENT ERROR GREATLY REDUCES THE CHANCE OF DETECTING DISEASE ACTIVITY

Suppose that we probe six sites at each of 28 teeth in a patient, wait half an hour and then repeat it. If there is an advanced level of periodontitis, perhaps two out of five sites will give a different reading the second time. Studies show that 10% of sites will differ by 2 mm or more, and 2% by 3 mm.

With these error levels, what chance have we of correctly identifying a real change over a period of, say, two months? If such changes were very frequent, affecting all sites within that time, and we set a threshold of 2 mm for accepting real change, then we would have a 90% chance of the change being real. In reality, these changes appear much rarer, perhaps affecting 5% of sites in 2 years or longer, giving a comparable probability of 0.42% between two examinations. An altered measurement over 2 months is therefore 24 times as likely (10% divided by 0.42%) to indicate an error as it is to indicate a real change.

TWO TYPES OF ERROR

This is a good point at which to consider the two main errors that we may encounter when seeking to identify an event such as disease activity. Type I error means that we wrongly identify a supposed change, and Type II error means that we wrongly conclude there has been no change. It is easy to see the very significant problem of Type I error from the last example, but what about Type II error? Alas, there are even more difficulties here.

The risk of Type II error is increased by every increase that is set in the threshold to avoid Type I error. Consequently, it has long been appreciated that periodontal measurements need to be accurate to as small an interval as possible: the 1979 workshop leading to the development of third generation probes recommended the interval of 0.1 mm (Parakkal, 1979). However, the measurements that we use are so error-prone that large thresholds for change are advocated, e.g. 2 mm.

THE EXACT POSITION OF THE PROBE IS A MAJOR PROBLEM

Consider Figs 10,1–10,6. If the attachment level can be measured exactly (which it cannot in reality), then we can only identify disease if we happen to probe vertically at the same place. If the disease occurs horizontally, we may miss it entirely. If a threshold is involved,

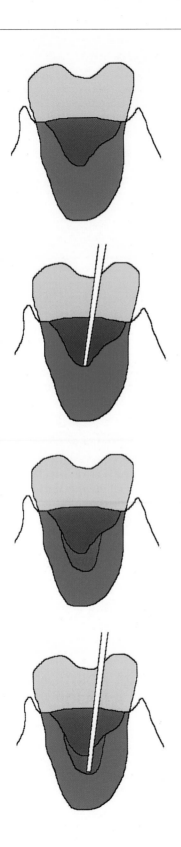

Fig. 10,1

Diagram of a pocket (green) on a proximal surface of a lower molar.

Fig. 10,2

We make the assumption that the probe validly identifies the attachment level on all occasions. (In reality, there is confusion between the attachment level and accompanying inflammation.)

Fig. 10,3

The red area marks an increase in attachment loss through disease activity.

Fig. 10,4

The probe identifies increased attachment loss, thereby showing that disease activity has occurred.

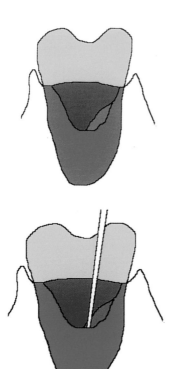

Fig. 10,5

We suppose that disease activity has occurred in the position shown.

Fig. 10,6

The probe does not identify this disease activity. The problem is that we are using unidimensional measurements in an attempt to identify changes in three dimensions.

then the position is even worse. Every increase in the threshold rules out detection of an increased subthreshold level of disease activity.

If we probe at one point on one occasion and at a slightly removed point on the next, we may either miss a change or wrongly conclude that there has been one, simply because of the error of positioning the probe. If we actually do probe the same point twice, and miss a change that occurs 1–2 mm away from it in a horizontal direction, then this is yet another sort of Type II error. For instance, the contents of such a pocket will be associated with disease activity but the researchers may wrongly consider it to have a stationary attachment level. If they identify some change in bacteria or crevicular fluid, they will assume that it has nothing to do with disease activity.

Having seen some of the problems, let us move on to a consideration of some of the interesting ideas that have been suggested regarding disease activity.

CONTINUOUS OR BURST?

For many years, dentists considered that slow, gradual loss of attachment was the rule in periodontitis. This was perhaps unconsciously fostered by epidemiological surveys in which data for many sites were averaged. The experienced investigators in the Sri Lankan study (see Abstracts 6,3 and 6,4) considered attachment loss to be a continuous process in most of their subjects who suffered from it.

However, another view was gaining support at that time, and Abstract 10,2 shows a relevant early study. It is interesting that over 1 year more sites became shallower than deeper in this study. We might account for shallower sites by saying that the probe penetrated areas of inflammation early in the study and subsequent resolution made them less easy to enter, or perhaps the examiner reduced probing pressure as time went on.

If we make allowances for the many possibilities of probing error and assume that they

Abstract 10,2 *Patterns of progression and regression of advanced destructive periodontal disease*

Goodson JM, Tanner ACR, Haffajee AD, et al., *Journal of Clinical Periodontology* 1982; **9**: 472–481

Attachment levels were monitored at two sites per tooth in 22 subjects (total 1155 sites) every month for an average of 13 months, using a first-generation periodontal probe. For each site, a regression line was calculated and a statistical significance of $P<0.01$ for this line was used as a threshold to determine whether the site had changed over the period of study. According to this criterion, 83% of sites were unchanged, 6% became deeper and 12% became shallower. Where depth increased, about half the sites showed spontaneous recovery to their original level. The authors interpreted their results as showing frequent stability of lesions, with some exacerbation and remission.

Comment: There is a problem in the method of this study: measurements repeated over a period may vary in force, so today a second- or third-generation probe would be used.

Abstract 10,3 *The microflora of periodontal sites showing active periodontal destruction*

Moore WEC, Moore LH, Ranney RR, et al., *Journal of Clinical Periodontology* 1991; **18**: 729–739

Every 2 months, 25 patients aged 26–55 years (mean 42 years) with evidence of previous periodontitis were monitored for PAL changes. A duplicate measurement system with thresholds was used to reduce the likelihood of false-positive results (but by implication increasing the risk of false-negative results). Twelve patients were found who experienced at least 2 mm of attachment loss at 42 sites during several years of monitoring. Within 7 days of the finding, microbial samples were taken from these sites and from 36 matched control sites within the same patients. Analysis showed 137 taxa at active sites and 134 taxa at control sites, with no detectable difference in the microbial flora present.

Comment: Despite the large high-quality research effort, it is difficult to interpret studies such as this. Do we say that the presence of similar microflora at 'active' and 'inactive' sites rules out a specific plaque effect? Or should we say that setting a probing threshold for 'activity' means that many less-active sites are included among the 'inactive' group? Some might also say that the previous microflora is more relevant than that present after attachment loss. Indeed, the researchers started with an attempt to identify prior organisms, but the rarity of attachment loss events led them to abandon the approach.

balance each other and do not affect the overall result, then there are two statements of the authors that command acceptance: 'existence of periodontal pockets alone cannot substantiate the existence of active disease',

and the detailed results 'suggest that disease activity may be a transient phenomenon', i.e. a 'burst'.

The main problem with accepting bursts of disease activity is related to measurement, just like the continuous theory. As the latter may be an artefact of averaging many epidemiological measurements, so the former is entwined with individual measurement error. At present we must assume that both exist (Fig. 10,7).

If we add the problems of measurement error to all the possible variations in disease activity, there is obviously great difficulty in

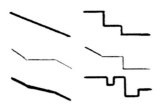

Fig. 10,7

Possible variations in disease activity with time. (Left) Top downwards: continuous constant progression, continuous intermittent, continuous variable progression. (Right) Top downwards: repeated burst, continuous with burst, burst and remission.

store for anyone who tries to identify factors that relate to the progression of attachment loss. A good example of this is given in the very thorough study in Abstract 10,3. No microbiological difference could be found between sites that apparently lost attachment and clinically matched sites, in the same patients, that did not. The enormous amount of research effort needed to identify and examine 12 subjects means that comparable studies are unlikely to be attempted on a larger scale.

THE SLY TRICKS OF INFLAMMATION

We interpreted the remissions in Abstract 10,2 as perhaps showing resolution of inflammation rather than attachment loss. In Abstract 10,4 there is another example of the crafty

tricks that inflammation may play. When a patient has been treated, in many cases a site shows what we have defined as repaired periodontitis (Table 10,2). In studies such as this, involving maintenance patients, there is therefore an unresolved question: does subsequent probing attachment loss result from disease activity or from recurrent periodontitis, which does not involve real attachment loss? This fact has been overlooked in some studies of disease activity in more recent times.

Another problem of inflammation concerns the pocket wall. The larger the pocket, the greater the quantity of inflammation. Large pockets do not just mean more anaerobic organisms but they also mean more of most inflammatory substances. Nor is there any way of knowing just how inflamed a pocket wall is. Consequently, there is no way in

Abstract 10,4 *Positive correlation between the proportions of subgingival spirochetes and motile bacteria and susceptibility of human subjects to periodontal deterioration*

Listgarten MA, Levin S, *Journal of Clinical Periodontology* 1981; **8**: 122–138

Nineteen subjects who had received full treatment for periodontitis, including surgery, took part in a 1-year study during maintenance follow-up. Every 2 months they received a full periodontal clinical examination, and plaque was sampled from the deepest pocket in each sextant. The six samples were pooled for each patient, and the percentages of motile organisms and spirochaetes identified by darkfield microscopy were recorded. If a tooth showed an increase of 3 mm in probing depth, then it was taken out of the study and treated. There was a strong correlation between the percentage of motile organisms and spirochaetes and the clinical deterioration of subjects.

Comment: This investigation aimed to identify patients who were at risk of further periodontal breakdown, and led to numerous studies with darkfield microscopy of plaque. However, the research did not clearly identify disease activity.

Abstract 10,5 *Clinical parameters as predictors of destructive periodontal disease activity*

Haffajee AD, Socransky SS, Goodson JM, *Journal of Clinical Periodontology* 1983; **10**: 257–265

Every 2 months for a year, periodontal measurements were made at 3414 sites in 22 subjects. The attachment level measurements were repeated within 7 days of each examination. If a threshold based on any pair of measurements was exceeded at a subsequent examination (which happened 242 times), then this event was interpreted as disease activity. Various clinical parameters (including plaque, gingival redness, bleeding or suppuration on probing, assorted probing depths and attachment levels) immediately before these events were compared with parameters at sites where no event was found, to see whether any were related to the event, either alone or in combination with each other. In all cases, these parameters had low sensitivity (ability to predict an event) or specificity (ability to exclude a non-event) or both.

Comment: The main problem in this study was the measurement of disease activity. Using a pair of measurements allowed different sites to be probed, and thresholds also raise the probability of Type II error.

which the quantity of an inflammatory substance can be related to possible disease activity.

There is also a relationship between the inflammatory response and the pocket microflora. Variations in the microflora, therefore, may be unrelatable to possible disease activity.

Finally, if inflammation-related clinical measurements are used to attempt to predict clinically estimated disease activity, none are found to be useful (Abstract 10,5).

Where does all this leave us?

THE CURRENT STATUS OF TESTS SUPPOSEDLY IDENTIFYING DISEASE ACTIVITY

It has been a difficult journey, but let us attempt to summarize the arguments of this chapter. At the root of all the problems is the 'gold standard' for disease activity. We depend on inadequate clinical measurements even when we think disease has obviously increased. Studies have shown that when we measure healthy periodontium the errors are less, but they may still be there.

In the light of this, we should cultivate a degree of humility when we assess a patient. If there are 12 possible clinical conditions of a site and we can only distinguish 4 (Tables 10,1 and 10,2), and if there are many ways in which probing may err, then our knowledge is only approximate. The patient should be told this during any case presentation.

Are there any tests that might help to identify those sites that require special attention in a patient? The answer again must be negative, because no-one knows how to recognize disease activity. Whether the test is based in microbiology, immunology or periodontal biochemistry, it is presently impossible to validate.

How should we interpret a test, say, that accurately identifies the amount of Aa or Pg in a crevicular sample? Unfortunately, we do not know how it relates to periodontitis, and all the patient can be told is that we think the organism may be of importance but no-one has yet demonstrated this clearly.

11

EARLY-ONSET PERIODONTITIS

- How do early-onset diseases differ from other forms of periodontitis?
- What are the differences in the underlying pathology?
- How are these diseases best treated?

The early-onset group of diseases constitutes a fascinating enigma for dentists (Table 11,1). The first of these diseases to receive separate attention was the localized form of juvenile periodontitis (LJP). Why are teeth so selectively involved (Figs 11,1–11,4)? Not only teeth, but also their surfaces are selected – perhaps only one or two surfaces of a tooth may be affected.

In LJP we have a radical example of site specificity. Is it the result of preferential colonization by organisms with significant virulent factors? Does some host factor lead to that colonization? Is there a variation in the host response at the affected sites only, and if so, why? Is there a developmental weakness in the tissues that renders them more susceptible to breakdown of the periodontal ligament? Is a combination of some of these factors responsible? At present, none of these questions has been answered.

Table 11,1: *Characteristics of early-onset periodontal diseases: prepubertal periodontitis (PPP), localized juvenile periodontitis (LJP), generalized juvenile periodontitis (GJP) and rapidly progressive periodontitis (RPP)*

Characteristic	Disease PPP	LJP	GJP	RPP
Aggressive attachment loss				
before 10 years	+			
10–25 years		+	+	
10–35 years				+
Characteristically minimal plaque, frequent minor phagocyte defects (chemotaxis or phagocytosis), familial but transmission mode uncertain.		+	+	+
Occasional major phagocyte defects, but also minor ones.	+			
Duration				
usually several years	+	+	+	
usually less than 1 year				+
Few teeth affected		+		
Most teeth usually affected	+		+	+
Often significant systemic disease	+			
Prognosis more likely to be good		+		?
Prognosis more likely to be poor	+		+	

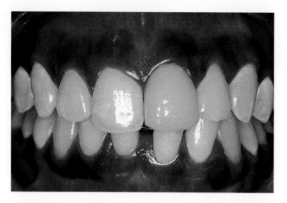

Fig. 11,1

Anterior view of 13-year-old female with localized juvenile periodontitis. Gingival tissues appear healthy externally but tooth 31 has drifted.

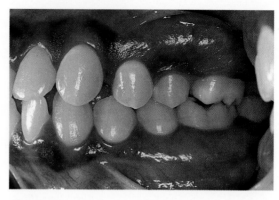

Fig. 11,3

A mirror view of the left side shows a healthy appearance in the patient of Fig. 11,1. Only periodontal probing would indicate that all is not as it seems.

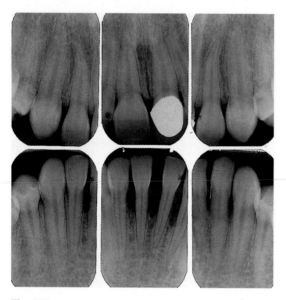

Fig. 11,2

Radiographs of the same patient, showing marked bone loss on teeth 31, 32 and 41. This approximately matches the probing attachment loss.

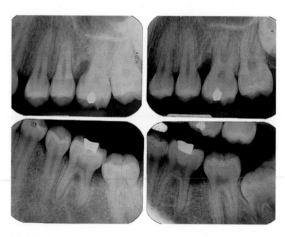

Fig. 11,4

Radiograph of the same patient indicating bone loss on the mesial surface of tooth 26, but this is related to probing attachment loss of 8 mm. Tooth 36 had a significant distal pocket and lingual grade II furcation involvement. The right posterior teeth were unaffected by juvenile periodontitis.

FAMILIAL OCCURRENCE

Early-onset diseases are grouped together because they are early and aggressive in comparison with chronic adult periodontitis. Studies have shown that the different varieties of disease may occur within the same family, and there is a well-recognized transmission of these diseases between generations.

What is not known is how and why the transmission occurs. It could be through an inherited weakness in the tissues or an inherited variation in the host response, or through transmission of specific virulent micro-

Abstract 11,1 *The prevalence and sex ratio of juvenile periodontitis in a young racially mixed population*

Melvin WL, Sandifer JB, Gray JL, *Journal of Periodontology* 1991; **62**: 330–334

In 5013 young military recruits, 31 juvenile periodontitis cases were diagnosed in 1052 black subjects, three in 3459 white Caucasians and four in 502 members of other ethnic groups. Of 3158 males, 23 were affected; of 1855 females, 15 were affected. The prevalence was 3.8% in black males, 2.0% in black females, 0.04% in white males and 0.2% in white females. Because of the small numbers of Caucasians affected, the authors warned of possible bias in the results for this group.

Comment: As the authors stressed, this was not a random sample but consisted of military volunteers. The data on gender variation may not be fully representative, but the ethnic differences are in agreement with other research studies.

Abstract 11,2 *No female preponderance in juvenile periodontitis after correction for ascertainment bias*

Hart TC, Marazita ML, Schenkein HA, et al., *Journal of Periodontology* 1991; **62**: 745–749

In a group of 211 subjects with juvenile periodontitis, 24 were identified who were known to have at least one sibling aged more than 13 years with the disease. Of these, 18 were female and 6 were male, which gave the often-quoted 3:1 ratio for gender prevalence. A further 143 siblings and other close relatives were identified, of whom 110 were examined. Of these, 31/54 males and 33/56 females had the disease, giving similarly affected proportions in each gender.

Comment: In this study, not only did the male and female proportions appear similar for all families examined, but this was also true for white and black subjects considered separately.

organisms, or a combination of any of these. Different genetic studies have indicated possible autosomal recessive, autosomal dominant and X-linked dominant modes of transmission in different groups of people. Perhaps this reflects the fact that there may be a number of possible causes for the same clinical disease presentation.

There is good evidence that these diseases have differing prevalences in different ethnic groups. However, the long-standing belief that females are three times as likely as males to have juvenile periodontitis has recently undergone some revision. Abstracts 11,1 and 11,2 relate to both of these matters.

HOW MANY DISEASES?

In Figs 11,5–11,7 the progress of periodontitis can be viewed in three panoramic radiographs of the same patient taken at ages 18, 26 and 30 years. She attended a dental hospital for examination on each occasion, but did not return for treatment, although she plainly received some restorative treatment and extractions elsewhere. A question is raised as to the likely periodontal diagnosis for this patient.

At age 18 years there is little radiographic indication of any problem, but by age 26 years there has certainly been some juvenile periodontitis. By age 30 years, further marked attachment loss raised a question of RPP, since juvenile periodontitis is not considered likely after 25 years. However, the progression is not characteristic of rapidly progressive disease either, because this usually affects many teeth for a short time only.

It is clinically apparent that early-onset periodontitis may be divided as shown in Table 11,1. Some clinicians have occasionally assumed that GJP and RPP are the same disease, but there is no clear evidence to support this. The diagnosis of RPP depends on the speed with which it has occurred. Patients similar to the example in Figs 11,5–11,7 imply that more than one type of disease may affect the same person.

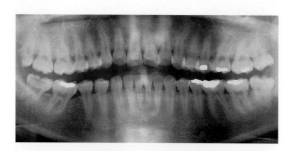

Fig. 11,5

There are no obvious periodontal problems visible in this dental panoramic tomogram of an 18-year-old female. Tooth 46 has been lost, probably much earlier. Teeth 18 and 48 appear to have severe caries.

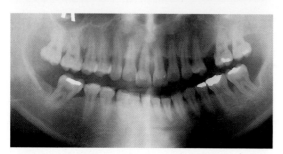

Fig. 11,6

By the age of 26 years, the patient has lost teeth 18, 25 and 48, perhaps from caries, and also teeth 28 and 38 (pericoronitis?). There appears to be significant bone loss on teeth 11, 12, 13, 15, 16, 21, 22, 23, 26, 36 and 37. By some definitions, this would be GJP, and by others, the localized form.

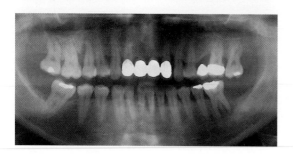

Fig. 11,7

By age 30 years, the patient has clearly seen someone who does bridgework but does not use a periodontal probe. Teeth 11, 21 and 37 have been lost and bone loss has progressed on teeth 15, 27 (which is also overerupted), 36 and possibly 46. It is totally amazing that the bone loss on the abutment teeth 12, 22 and 26 does not appear to have progressed, and testifies to the highly site-specific nature of the disease.

THE PHAGOCYTE LINK

In the developing science of immunology during the 1970s, after some disappointing forays into lymphocytic phenomena, researchers into juvenile periodontitis found some interesting results when they examined neutrophils.

The typical neutrophil has a short (12–24 h), very active life, as outlined in Chapter 9. It is the first cell on the scene in inflammation and randomly changes direction as it moves and searches for bacteria, which it devours. When its granules have gone, it dies and releases substances such as collagenase, which may cause tissue damage. Its primary role is to protect the host's body, rather than the periodontal tissues. Absence of neutrophils (agranulocytosis) is a serious, life-threatening disease.

The first indication that these cells might be involved in early-onset disease was the discovery of reduced neutrophil chemotaxis in some, but not all, patients. This meant that the wandering cells were less strongly attracted towards bacteria on their travels.

Unfortunately, the usual method of measuring chemotaxis *in vitro* (Boyden chamber) is not very exact; it is indirect and prone to error. A study *in vitro* using a direct method was unable to identify this defect in a group of patients with early-onset periodontitis (Kinane et al, 1989). Neutrophil chemotaxis cannot be studied in the patient *in vivo*, but the overall movement of the cells can, as they migrate through a membrane over a mild abrasion on the skin (Figs 11,8–11,11); in the very few studies of this phenomenon in such patients, there appears to be less activity and fewer migrating cells.

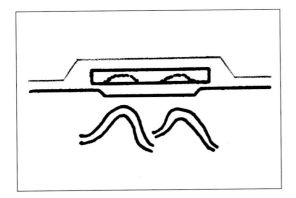

Fig. 11,8

A skin window for assessing neutrophil migration from cells that actually do migrate, without the possible confounding factor of periodontal bacteria. A mild abrasion is made in the skin without causing bleeding, a filter is placed over it for neutrophils to enter and the whole area is covered. Capillaries are shown under the skin, and two leading fronts are shown in the filter.

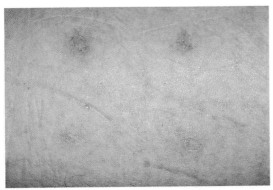

Fig. 11,9

Typical skin abrasions. There is no bleeding but small vessels can be seen. The mild trauma excites a speedy neutrophil response.

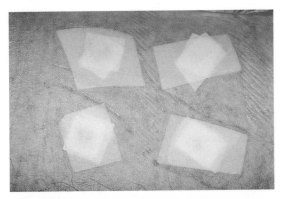

Fig. 11,10

Millipore filters are placed over the abrasions and filter papers are placed on top. All are soaked in physiological saline. The whole is covered, and left in place for 90 minutes, by which time a regular flow of neutrophils is established. Then the filters are replaced, usually for a test period of 20 min, when they are removed for study. For macrophages, a similar technique takes 12–24 hours.

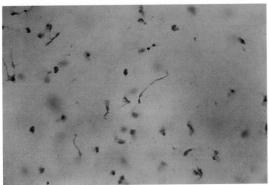

Fig. 11,11

The filters are fixed and stained after a specified time for migration, and a special microscope is used to measure the leading front – the greatest distance the neutrophils have travelled.

Abstract 11,3 *Immunologic profile of juvenile periodontitis. II. Neutrophil chemotaxis, phagocytosis and spore germination*

Suzuki JB, Collison BC, Falkler WA Jr, et al., *Journal of Periodontology* 1984; **55**: 461–467

This study compared 29 subjects with LJP (incisors and first molars only), 24 with GJP (more than 14 teeth affected) and 24 healthy controls. Using neutrophils recovered from peripheral blood, a chemotactic defect was identified in all LJP and 14 GJP patients, a phagocytic defect in 18 LJP and 7 GJP patients, and induction of bacterial spore germination (hence protection of the bacteria) in 13 LJP and 3 GJP patients.

Comment: The definition of defects in these patients was reasonable, but at the same time, arbitrary. It excluded all the healthy subjects, but there is clearly a difference in the JP patients. The other point worth noting is that not all peripheral neutrophils are the same, and ideally the migrating gingival cells need to be studied.

Abstract 11,4 *Phagocytic cells in periodontal defence. Periodontal status of patients with chronic granulomatous disease of childhood*

Cohen MS, Leong PA, Simpson DM, *Journal of Periodontology* 1985; **56**: 611–617

Periodontal examination was performed for five patients with this exceptionally rare neutrophil and monocyte defect. Patients had a variety of severe infections and plaque was profuse in all of them. In three patients aged 17, 21 and 25 years, there was no evidence of attachment loss; the other patients, aged 27 and 32 years, had early attachment loss consistent with a diagnosis of chronic adult periodontitis. There were no signs of early-onset forms of periodontitis. All patients were receiving antibiotics but none were taking tetracycline or metronidazole.

Comment: If any major neutrophil defect could cause early onset aggressive periodontitis, it should have shown up in these subjects. The authors mention another paper in which nine patients with the disease similarly showed no sign of early-onset disease. It is unlikely that the antibiotics taken by these patients had any effect on the periodontal microflora.

However, the neutrophil link has extended to include reduced phagocytosis, reduced cellular adherence and some defects in the other phagocyte – the macrophage – which is far more difficult to study. All the early-onset diseases may have these problems, which suggests that phagocyte effects may be important in attachment loss and not just in the associated inflammation. Abstract 11,3 gives details of one of the larger studies on neutrophils, showing that all patients do not appear the same.

One interesting fact is that patients with chronic granulomatous disease – a serious and rare defect in which the neutrophil phagocytoses but fails to kill bacteria – apparently have no significant susceptibility to early-onset periodontitis (Abstract 11,4). Why should the other neutrophil defects be linked to these diseases? Several possibilities have been suggested.

For instance, if the neutrophils fail to reach bacteria in the crevice, but stop and die in the appropriate part of the tissues, that may be responsible for the damage. Alternatively, perhaps the combination of virulent microorganisms and weakened host defence may lead to the lesions. The same could apply where macrophages are involved. However, where bacteria are phagocytosed, perhaps they are inactivated without killing. Other reasons could be more complex, involving signalling molecules such as ILs, effects on fibroblasts and other phenomena.

Before we conclude this discussion of pathological factors involved in early-onset periodontitis, brief mention should be given to another rare condition – leucocyte adhesion deficiency syndrome. In patients who are severely affected, a generalized prepubertal periodontitis occurs, followed by aggressive disease in the permanent dentition. In this disorder, neutrophils appear unable to leave blood vessels, despite being present in large numbers. They need to adhere to vessel walls before passing through and migrating into the tissues.

From the brief insights gained from rare diseases and studies of phagocyte defects, it is apparent that there may be several ways in which they predispose to early-onset disease, and that some very severe defects, such as chronic granulomatous disease, may not carry this additional burden.

FAVOURITE MICROBES

Early on in the study of juvenile periodontitis microbiology, Aa aroused considerable interest, and still does. Some strains may damage neutrophils, and if this is added to the host defence defect a credible explanation of the disease begins to emerge. However, initial studies overstated the presence of Aa in these patients (see Abstract 7,4 for a clearer picture).

It is now quite clear that many people harbour Aa without any associated periodontitis of early-onset or other varieties. So far, it has not been clearly associated with diseased sites, as opposed to healthy sites, in the mouths of susceptible patients. Nevertheless, it still remains possible that strains with special virulence factors may be found only in close association with the disease, which is the first requirement for incrimination of this organism.

Other organisms do not seem to fare any better. *Capnocytophaga*, which was also discovered in the 1970s, does not seem to be associated with disease so much as with health; yet this organism also carries virulence factors that may inhibit neutrophils.

However, the interest in Aa provided a spur towards the investigation of tetracycline in periodontal treatment. The organism is a facultative anaerobe, and in early studies proved immensely susceptible to tetracycline, with very little evidence of resistance developing. But tetracycline affects a broad spectrum of organisms, any of which also might be involved in early-onset periodontitis, and success in treatment therefore does not imply that Aa is causally implicated.

THE TETRACYCLINE FACTOR

Since the interest in neutrophils, Aa and tetracycline all began in the mid-1970s, it is curious that 20 years later almost nothing was known about the clinical effects of adding tetracycline to the treatment of early-onset disease. Several studies had shown that treatment with tetracycline could produce satisfactory results, but it was not known whether the drug added anything at all to the outcome of normal therapy.

At this point, we shall leap ahead of the rest of this book and consider what we may learn from the results of adding tetracycline to the treatment of early-onset periodontitis. Abstract 11,5 describes the largest and, at the time, almost the only randomized controlled trial to be published.

From this trial, it is apparent that the addition of a 2-week course of systemic tetracycline to non-surgical treatment nearly

Abstract 11,5 *A double-blind trial of tetracycline in the management of early onset periodontitis*

Palmer RM, Watts TLP, Wilson RF, *Journal of Clinical Periodontology* 1996; **23**: 670–674

Full periodontal treatment was performed for 38 patients (30 with LJP, 8 with GJP), with randomization to 2 weeks of adjunctive tetracycline or placebo in conjunction with non-surgical treatment, and the same adjunct again with surgical treatment, which 26 required. In the test group, 3 months after non-surgical treatment, mean probing depths for proximal surfaces reduced from 5.3 mm to 3.8 mm and attachment levels improved from 3.7 mm to 2.7 mm. This differed significantly from the control group (PD: 5.3 mm to 4.3 mm; PAL: 3.2 mm to 2.7 mm). In the test group 58% of teeth required surgery, but in the control group 75% required surgery. There were no significant differences between groups after surgical treatment, however.

Comment: Tetracycline added 50% to PD reductions and 100% to PAL improvements on proximal surfaces after non-surgical treatment. The need for surgery was also reduced.

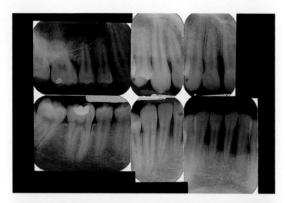

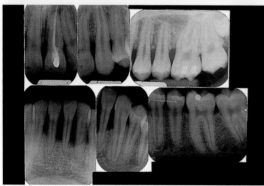

Fig. 11,12

Right-side radiographs of a 13-year-old male with GJP. It is probable that the disease is very recent, and the bone has not yet caught up with the lesions which can be probed already.

Fig. 11,13

Left-side radiographs for the same patient. Again, with the exception of the lower anteriors, little bone loss can be seen.

Fig. 11,14

PD charts reveal the real state of the right side of the patient. The charts closest to the tooth numbers across the centre (in black) are pretreatment. The charts at top and bottom are 1 year after oral hygiene education and surgery with adjunctive tetracycline. (For note on how to read PD Charts, please see Conventions and Abbreviations, p. xi.)

Fig. 11,15

Left-side PD charts reveal a similar picture.

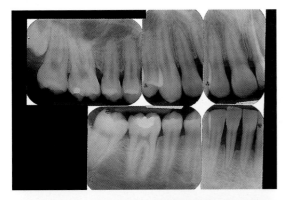

Fig. 11,16

The patient of Fig. 11,12, 1 year post-treatment: radiographs suggest very stable periodontal support, with crestal lamina dura on interdental septa; before treatment the indistinct bone outline suggested the presence of inflamed tissue.

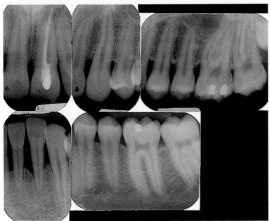

Fig. 11,17

The left-side radiographs show a similar picture. Five years after treatment, the periodontal tissues were clinically healthy with virtually no bleeding.

doubled its effect on patients who have experienced this form of periodontitis. Even so, the overall result was not enormous and there was no further effect on those patients who went on to a surgical phase of treatment.

In Figs 11,12–11,17 we see the results after 1 year in a patient treated before the results of this trial were known. There are periodontists who would argue that the elimination of organisms such as Aa contributed to this result.

Do the results of the trial in Abstract 11,5 mean that the drug acted primarily as an antibiotic and enhanced results by removing some bacteria? Or is the explanation perhaps that the interesting effect of tetracycline against collagenolysis (see Abstract 2,2) encouraged tissues to reform?

The plaque biofilm is not easily penetrated by any substances, and the effect was ultimately in the tissues. Either we postulate that there was bacterial invasion and the invading microbes were removed, or we are forced towards the belief that tetracycline acted on the tissues.

Bacterial invasion is extremely difficult to prove. Apart from the problem of contamination when periodontal tissue is removed for examination, there is the well-established fact that many oral microrganisms cause bacteraemia, but that is not invasion. Invasion means that cells take up residence in the tissues at least for a while, and some investigators have defined it as colonization and multiplication within the periodontium.

Consequently, the mere presence of bacteria in these tissues does not mean that they have invaded. We can see a little of what invasion means if we consider acute necrotizing ulcerative gingivitis (ANUG), where it clearly does occur. This process seems completely different from other forms of periodontal disease, and therefore it may be that tetracycline's main periodontal effect is on the tissues. Certainly it can be shown to reduce bacteria, but this may be a marker of its presence rather than a cause of the change in the tissues.

Tetracycline will be discussed as a drug in Chapter 24.

SUMMARY

The early-onset diseases are relatively easy to identify and they provide an interesting subject for researchers. It is clear that they involve defective phagocyte behaviour but it is not so clear whether specific microbes are causally involved, although they seem to be associated with many cases. For the present, the very attractive idea that a weakened anatomical site determines disease seems to have fallen into abeyance and, although tetracycline enhances some aspects of treatment, the reasons for this are not certain.

12   ACUTE PERIODONTAL DISEASES

- What are the main acute periodontal diseases?
- What is the underlying significance of some acute problems?
- How are acute diseases best managed?

The term 'acute' is applied clinically to diseases that are of short duration and often uncomfortable. In the practice of periodontics, these diseases signify comparatively rare occasions when patients know that something is wrong and seek help. There are four main sorts of acute periodontal lesion.

Just as the early-onset periodontal diseases seem associated with certain types of phagocyte defect, so does ANUG with immunosuppression. In this disease there is definite invasion, and in some patients it may continue into a very unpleasant form of periodontitis, and even further (cancrum oris or noma).

Other acute periodontal diseases are not strongly linked to immunosuppression, although the two may coincide on occasions. Apart from the necrotizing diseases, either bacterial or viral diseases may cause acute problems, and trauma may also occur.

The bacterial group is represented by various forms of acute periodontal abscess, which is usually a mechanically induced phenomenon. A deep pocket becomes blocked by inflammation or repair, or both, in its coronal aspect and the enclosed microorganisms induce a swift phagocyte response. Even without such blockage, small abscesses form frequently in deep pockets, and probing elicits pus instead of, or in addition to bleeding. Pus is largely a collection of neutrophil debris, including collagenase; therefore such events may be important in the development of sporadic attachment loss.

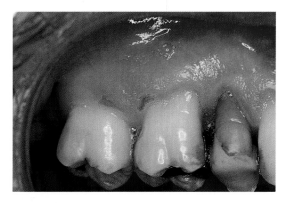

Fig. 12,1

Marginal gingival ulceration caused by vigorous toothbrushing adjacent to teeth 16 and 17.

Viral diseases may cause short-lived upset in the periodontal tissues, whilst usually spilling over into the other parts of the oral mucosa. Acute herpetic gingivostomatitis is a typical example of this, but other diseases (e.g. hand, foot and mouth) may have a similar oral appearance.

Finally, the effects of trauma are manifest both directly, such as ulceration from toothbrushing (Fig. 12,1), and indirectly, such as when occlusal interference from a recent restoration causes severe discomfort.

ANUG

In a classic study, Listgarten showed clearly the invasive nature of this disease (Abstract 12,1). Spirochaetes are motile organisms and they appear in large groups in the deepest zone of the lesion. This appearance is not

Abstract 12,1 *Electron microscopic observations on the bacterial flora of acute necrotizing ulcerative gingivitis*

Listgarten MA, *Journal of Periodontology* 1965; **36**: 328–339

Biopsies were obtained from proximal papillae with typical clinical lesions of ANUG. From the surface of lesions inwards, four zones were apparent, although adjacent zones occasionally merged. Most superficial was the bacterial zone: a layer of numerous organisms in which a few spirochaetes could be distinguished. Next was the neutrophil zone, with a few phagocytosed organisms and some other leucocytes. A necrotic zone was below this, with many spirochaetes and a few other organisms, predominantly fusiform in shape. Mononuclear and polymorphonuclear leucocytes were also present. The deepest zone, of spirochaetal infiltration, showed these organisms well beyond all other bacteria, up to 250 µm below the ulcerated tissue surface. These spirochaetes were usually of the larger sizes and often surrounded by an area of lysis.

Comment: In this study, spirochaetes showed clear leadership in the process of invasion. Because they are present in all plaque, they might be expected to act similarly in any other lesion where invasion is really present. However, papers that purport to describe invasion in non-ANUG types of periodontitis centre on other morphotypes, which suggests that true invasion is not present.

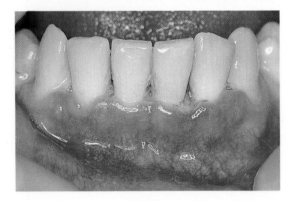

Fig. 12,2

Typical clinical appearance of ANUG, in a 17-year-old female with poor oral hygiene.

12,2), and may spread if host resistance is sufficiently impaired.

The lowering of host resistance may be accomplished in many ways. The commonest is probably by tobacco smoke but this factor is linked to psychological stress, which may also play a part. Patients on immunosuppressive drugs also may develop ANUG. Severe protein deficiency in famine areas may so reduce the plasma immunoglobulins and other defence factors that ANUG spreads to involve alveolar bone and other adjacent areas, including the cheeks. This is known as cancrum oris.

Because ANUG is not primarily a simple plaque-induced disease, it is pointless as well as unkind to start treatment with thorough oral hygiene instruction (OHI). The state of lowered resistance permits invasion by strict anaerobes, so the eradication of these organisms from the tissue will stop the necrosis and remove the pain. The drug of choice is metronidazole, and a 3-day course (200 mg t.i.d.) will suffice in most cases. Penicillin also may be used (250 mg q.i.d. for 5 days is usual).

At the end of the antimicrobial drug treatment, the patient should be reviewed to ensure that tissues are healing and comfortable, and at this point OHI and scaling may be given. If possible, any immunosuppressive trigger factor should be identified and dealt with (e.g. smoking cessation).

characteristic of any other group of periodontal diseases, although spirochaetes frequently are closest to host tissues in the depth of adult periodontitis pockets.

This disease is characterized by pain and halitosis. The pain is due to release of inflammatory mediators, and the halitosis is from necrotic and putrefying tissue. In more severe cases, the cervical lymph nodes are enlarged and tender and there is moderate pyrexia. Commonly, patients are in the second and third decades of life.

The trigger for ANUG is lowered host resistance, permitting invasion primarily by spirochaetes but with a contribution from fusiform (cigar-shaped) bacilli. Invasion begins in the tips of interdental papillae (Fig.

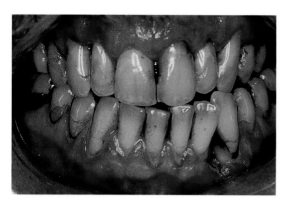

Fig. 12,3

NUP in a patient who was HIV positive but did not know it. A portion of alveolar bone very recently sequestrated from the labial and proximal aspects of the septum and buccal plate between teeth 32 and 33. The very white appearance of the root of tooth 33, with coronal stain present from tobacco, wine and coffee, is a pointer to what has happened. (Photograph courtesy of Mr Guy Palmer.)

Abstract 12,2 *Necrotizing ulcerative periodontitis: a marker for immune deterioration and a predictor for the diagnosis of AIDS*

Glick M, Muzyka BC, Salkin LM, et al., *Journal of Periodontology* 1994; **65**: 393–397

Over a 4-year period, 700 HIV-positive patients were enrolled in a dental care study and were followed regularly. Of these, 44 presented with NUP. These patients were more than 20 times as likely to have a CD4+ cell count below 200 cells/mm^3 (laboratory definition of AIDS) than above this figure. There was a 73% probability of death within 24 months of an NUP diagnosis. Patients with a clinical AIDS diagnosis tended to die earlier.

Comment: HIV-positive patients with NUP are likely to deteriorate rapidly, and need particularly compassionate management.

In the longer term, after the acute phase has been fully dealt with, there is occasionally a need for surgical recontouring of tissue either to facilitate plaque control or for aesthetic reasons.

NECROTIZING ULCERATIVE PERIODONTITIS (NUP)

Sequestration of portions of alveolar bone is characteristic of NUP, which sometimes occurs in marked states of immunosuppression such as AIDS (Fig. 12,3). These patients also report considerable discomfort, and NUP onset is an indicator of progression from HIV-positive status to frank AIDS (Abstract 12,2).

NUP requires treatment with metronidazole and appropriate oral hygiene and debridement measures (Figs 12,4–12,7). A chlorhexidine mouthrinse may increase comfort and can be used to maintain plaque control if mechanical hygiene is painful, provided that plaque is removed first (Chapter 24).

ACUTE PERIODONTAL ABSCESS

This commonly occurs as a lateral abscess (Figs 12,8 and 12,9) but alternatively may be located in a furcation. It is usually precipitated by a strong host response to the initiating pathogens, often when these are enclosed temporarily within a pocket.

Because of the possibility of an abscess originating in the pulp (especially in the furcation area), vitality tests are a mandatory diagnostic test. Radiographs contribute little to diagnosis.

Traditional treatment (drainage through the pocket, followed by thorough root planing) may save more than half of all teeth with abscesses (Abstract 12,3), and there is a distinct variation in the response of patients to therapy.

Small abscesses may constitute one form of disease activity in periodontitis, and there is considerable interest in their nature. One recent study (Abstract 12,4) suggests that if abscesses are *not* given root planing immediately after drainage is established, then they have substantial healing potential.

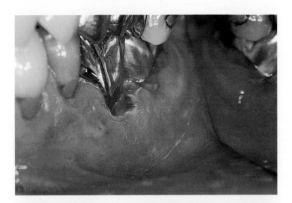

Fig. 12,4

NUP in a male aged 55 years. Ulcerative lesions with marginal bone loss adjacent to teeth 36 and 37 at presentation.

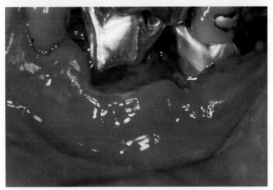

Fig. 12,5

The same lesions from the buccal aspect.

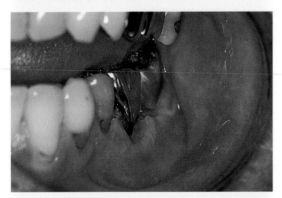

Fig. 12,6

Four days after one week of metronidazole treatment, the lesions have healed.

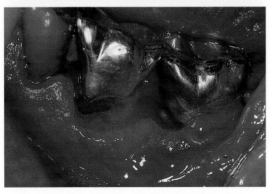

Fig. 12,7

From the buccal aspect, the healed, shrunken periodontium reveals the white appearance of the roots that have recently lost the attached marginal bone, adjacent to areas stained by tobacco, wine and coffee.

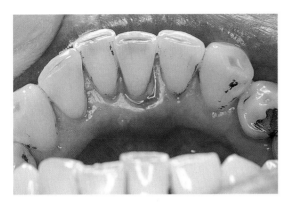

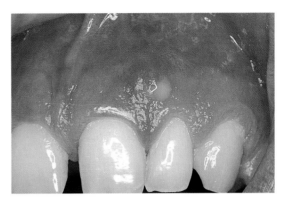

Fig. 12,8

Periodontal abscess on tooth 31. Because this is pointing through the pocket, drainage is established and the tooth requires thorough planing to remove plaque and calculus, with appropriate oral hygiene.

Fig. 12,9

An enclosed periodontal abscess, originating on tooth 21, that has pointed on the buccal gingiva. If the pocket can be probed down to the abscess source, it may be instrumented to remove causal factors.

Abstract 12,3 *Tooth loss due to periodontal abscess: a retrospective study*

McLeod DE, Lainson PA, Spivey JD, *Journal of Periodontology* 1997; **68**: 963–966

Patients treated by one periodontist at a US dental school and on regular recall for 5–29 years were identified retrospectively during a 6-month period. Of 114 patients, 42 had presented with periodontal abscess during maintenance after a full programme of active periodontal treatment. This amounted to 109 out of 2899 teeth. Of these, 60 teeth were maintained indefinitely (average 12.5 years, range 5–29) and 49 were extracted. Risk factors for loss were furcation involvement and hopeless prognosis given by clinician. Patients were divided into groups according to the number of teeth lost after active treatment: in the well-maintained group (0–3 lost), 19 of 63 teeth were lost because of periodontal abscess; in the downhill group (4–9), 20 of 35; and in the extreme downhill group (10–23), 10 out of 11.

Comment: This is rare evidence that many teeth with periodontal abscesses may be maintained for many years. These results may be compared directly with the 1978 study of Hirschfeld and Wasserman, who defined the three categories of patient (see Abstract 4,1 and Table 22,1). As in that study, most tooth loss occurred in a few patients.

From Abstract 12,4 it appears that a suitable alternative sequence of treatment is: establish drainage (usually with a sharp instrument through the pocket); scale only the entrance to the pocket; prescribe a 2-week course of tetracycline; wait at least 6 weeks (6 months was possible in the study); and then institute normal non-surgical treatment for the residual pocket along with any other lesions.

For many years, it has been said that diabetics are more susceptible to periodontal abscesses, but there is no clear evidence on this matter. It is clear that diabetics as a group are more susceptible to infections if they are not in a state of good metabolic control, but this does not necessarily translate into the specific condition of a periodontal abscess.

ACUTE HERPETIC GINGIVOSTOMATITIS

A primary attack of this unpleasant disease is commonest in the first few years of life, although primary cases have been reported in old age. In many cases, parents are very concerned about the condition of a child, and need reassurance that it is a simple viral disease.

Abstract 12,4   *Effect of treatment on some periodontopathogens and their antibody levels in periodontal abscesses*

Hafström CA, Wikström MB, Renvert SN, et al., *Journal of Periodontology* 1994; **54**: 1022–1028

This is a rare longitudinal study of the treatment of 20 patients with abscesses of well-defined periodontal origin. In addition, one shallow and one deep pocket was chosen for comparison in each patient. Abscesses were treated with drainage, scaling only to the pocket orifice (i.e. not subgingivally), saline irrigation and a 2-week course of tetracycline. All patients were followed for a minimum of 6 weeks. In two cases where drainage was not established, recurrence occurred within 4 months, and five other patients dropped out before 6 months had elapsed. Clinical results showed mean PD reduction from 8 mm to 4 mm in abscess pockets, with a PAL gain of 4 mm, compared with minimal improvement in deep pockets. Eradication of Pg and marked reduction in *Prevotella intermedia* accompanied the improvement, but serum antibody levels remained similar throughout the study. The authors note that tetracycline may have assisted healing as well as combating microbes, and that where drainage was not achieved, there was recurrence. The remarkable clinical gains are ascribed to the survival of ligament cells despite the adjacent abscess inflammation (a form of false periodontitis, described in Chapter 10) and subsequent resolution of inflammation.

Comment: The title and published abstract for this paper actually conceal some of the most fascinating clinical findings in the literature. Most periodontists would have thoroughly planed the tooth roots at the earliest opportunity (in addition to establishing drainage) and, if an antibacterial was needed, would have used a penicillin or metronidazole rather than tetracycline.

Abstract 12,5   *Treatment of herpes simplex gingivostomatitis with aciclovir in children: a randomised double-blind placebo-controlled study*

Amir J, Harel L, Smetana Z, et al., *British Medical Journal* 1997; **314**: 1800–1803

In a paediatric hospital in Israel, 72 children with this disease were randomized to aciclovir or placebo within 72 h of onset. The active dose was 15 mg/kg of the suspension five times daily for 7 days. In children receiving aciclovir, the median duration of oral lesions was 4 days (placebo, 10 days), with earlier improvements in pyrexia, extraoral lesions and eating and drinking difficulties. Viral shedding (linked to infectivity) was also shortened.

Comment: This is an expensive treatment that may be of benefit in some cases diagnosed early.

Management of the primary attack requires strong support for the patient. Dehydration is an avoidable complication, and frequent fluid intake should be encouraged. If the mouth is too painful for normal foods to be taken, a

Abstract 12,6   *Herpes simplex and mood: a prospective study*

Dalkvist J, Wahlin TB, Bartsch E, et al., *Psychosomatic Medicine* 1995; **57**: 127–137

Self-reports from 38 patients with genital herpes and 28 patients with oral herpes were studied with respect to recurrent disease over a 3-month period. Decreased emotional well-being occurred for 10 days before genital recurrence, with apparent short-lived improvement in the middle of this period. Females showed a more marked trend that was not related to the menstrual cycle. In males, a sleeplessness trend was reported, with least sleep on the 8th and 3rd preceding days. In oral herpes, however, the common cold was the major preceding event, with a possible associated mood factor.

Comment: The two types of infection appeared to have different factors that might play a part in precipitating recurrence.

Pyrexia, loss of appetite and lassitude are common presenting signs and examination of the mouth will usually reveal the typical vesicles and erythema associated with a viral infection. These may affect all parts of the mucosa, and not just the gingiva (Figs 12,10–12,13). In an adult, oral hygiene will usually cease.

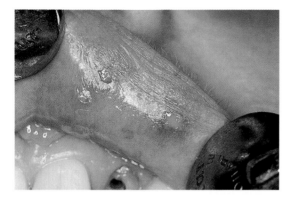

Fig. 12,10

Acute herpetic gingivostomatitis in a 52-year-old female. Typical vesicles with erythema on upper lip.

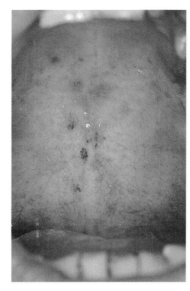

Fig. 12,12

Some vesicles have burst in the palate with slight bleeding.

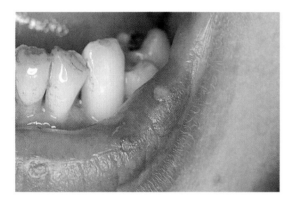

Fig. 12,11

Vesicles on lower lip of the same patient.

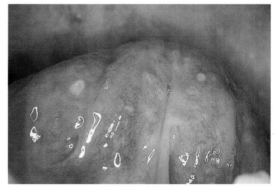

Fig. 12,13

Vesicles on inferior surface of tongue.

suitable processed soft diet should be prescribed. A mild hypnotic, such as promethazine, also may be prescribed for children.

Until recently, it was generally believed that specific antiviral therapy achieved little once vesicles had appeared, but this is not the view of the authors of a recent large study (Abstract 12,5), in which the disease duration was more than halved provided that treatment was started early enough. Aciclovir prevents *Herpesvirus* replication, which is why it may have this effect. Given that the disease is suffi-

ciently unpleasant, such treatment may be appropriate in the absence of specific contraindications if diagnosed early.

As with some other viral diseases, the organism persists in a latent state in the tissues and can be reactivated by a stimulus. In a recent study, the common cold was the most frequent factor involved (Abstract 12,6). Avoidance of known contagious viral diseases, therefore, may be of benefit to patients who have frequent and severe recurrences.

OTHER ACUTE PERIODONTAL DISEASES

Other forms of acute infection or trauma may be a rare event in the periodontal tissues. It is advisable to take a broad history when faced with some lesion with no specific diagnosis, and to use appropriate supplementary tests.

It is worth remembering that local oral pain rarely crosses the midline, and that generalized bilateral pains may relate to systemic factors such as hormonal imbalance after the menopause or anaemia, or to drug effects such as gingival enlargement produced by cyclosporin. Menopause-related oral discomfort can be relieved often, but not always, by hormone replacement therapy, but this should be prescribed only by a physician with due regard to all relevant factors.

Where no periodontal or oral cause can be found for an acute complaint, referral to an oral physician is desirable. The physician is the appropriate person to decide whether the pain is organic or functional in origin, and to arrange suitable attention.

13 LOCAL PLAQUE RETENTIVE FACTORS AND PERIODONTAL DISEASES

- How is calculus involved in periodontal diseases?
- What is the effect of overhanging restorations on the periodontium?
- Can unsatisfactory appliances damage the periodontium?
- How can we manage less than satisfactory previous restorative work?

A number of factors may play a part in plaque retention. This is not the same as causing periodontal diseases. There are two plaque factors that may relate to disease: amount and composition.

More plaque is associated with more disease at the population level (Chapter 6), but we have seen that plaque may vary in its effects at different sites. Although the SPH (Chapter 8) cannot be proven at present, neither can it be ruled out. Different periodontal sites also may vary in disease susceptibility. For these reasons, it is not always possible to identify the specific effect of a retentive factor.

We may group plaque-retentive factors under three headings: anatomical, i.e. built into the structure and development of teeth and jaws; of pathophysiological origin, such as calculus in all its variety; and iatrogenic (literally 'physician-produced'), such as restorative margins and dental appliances.

ANATOMICAL FACTORS

These may be tooth-, mucosal- or jaw-related. Anatomical plaque-retentive factors in general relate to the difficulty that may be encountered in removing plaque, rather than to any other effect.

TOOTH-RELATED ANATOMICAL FACTORS

Gemination (Fig. 13,1) may cause an uncleanable groove at the junction between the two parts of the tooth. Sometimes this is associated with a deep local periodontal pocket. If no other attachment loss is present, this may suggest defective attachment formation. Fusion of two teeth may give the same result.

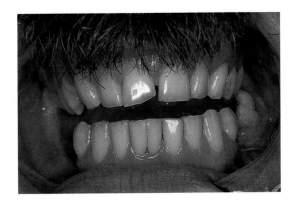

Fig. 13,1

Tooth 41 is geminated – two joined teeth have formed in place of the normal single incisor. There is calculus in the root groove at the join. In this case, the patient was not particularly susceptible to attachment loss, and scaling with oral hygiene was all that was needed to maintain periodontal health.

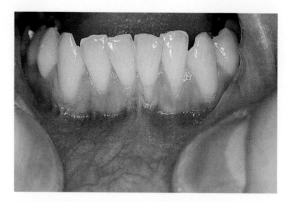

Fig. 13,2

Fraenal 'pull'. Tension on the fraenum leads to blanching of the marginal and papillary mucosa adjacent to tooth 31. There is associated recession on this tooth, but it has now been maintained with good hygiene for 3 years without progression. The fraenum interfered with the patient's original oral hygiene practices; a little help with this was all that was needed. The fraenal 'pull' was no problem.

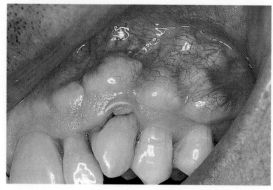

Fig. 13,3

Multiple exostoses present for over 30 years. They were covered with reflected mucosa, but good oral hygiene has been maintained without difficulty and the maximum PD on these teeth was 2 mm. Note that there is no attached gingiva at all on tooth 25 where the exostosis extends right up to the alveolar margin.

Other developmental grooves are to be found in a variety of sites, including the palatal aspect of upper incisors and the proximal aspect of upper premolars.

Additional roots may be present on certain teeth and if attachment loss reaches them, the extra furcation may be involved (Chapter 22). Lower molars may have two distal roots, for instance, and lower incisors and canines may have mesial and buccal roots.

MUCOSAL-RELATED ANATOMICAL FACTORS

The commonest mucosal factor contributing (but indirectly only) to plaque retention is the lower labial fraenum. Where this impedes the use of a toothbrush, there occasionally may be a need for intervention (Chapter 23).

Another alleged problem that has been wrongly attributed to the fraenum is so-called 'fraenal pull' (Fig. 13,2), which is said to be a force that somehow causes gingival recession. Some clinicians used to diagnose 'fraenal pull' by pulling out the lower lip and noting

whether this caused blanching of the marginal gingiva. However, in normal lip movements, the fraenum does not cause tension.

It was thought at one time that a lack of attached gingiva was likely to predispose to problems of gingival inflammation, but there is no evidence to support this view (Chapters 4 and 23). It is difficult to see how it could happen if plaque control is maintained. In a rare case of longstanding multiple exostoses (Fig. 13,3), there was excellent periodontal health despite the presence of no attached gingiva and an obstructive exostosis over one tooth.

JAW-RELATED ANATOMICAL FACTORS

Orthodontic problems may cause difficulties in plaque removal, but if plaque can be controlled then so can the periodontal condition. Crowding is a common condition impeding plaque control in the anterior regions.

It is not always recognized that some teeth may be placed so far posteriorly that hygiene

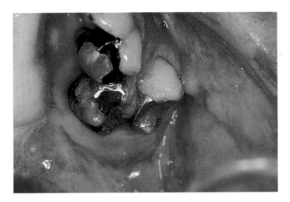

Fig. 13,4

Tooth 28 is malpositioned and the main periodontal difficulty is caused by the coronoid process of the mandible when the mouth is opened for toothbrushing. There has been sufficient access for a dentist to place a restoration in this tooth, but the patient is physically unable to control plaque.

Abstract 13,1 *Tissue response in the guinea pig to sterile and non-sterile calculus*

Allen DL, Kerr DA, *Journal of Periodontology* 1965; **36**: 121–126

Sixty milligrams of calculus was retrieved from each of 30 male inpatients. Each sample was divided in two and half were autoclaved. Thus, 30 sterile and 30 plaque-covered samples were implanted in the peritoneum of 60 animals, with 10 more animals as untreated controls. The animals were sacrificed at intervals over the next 90 days and the tissue reaction was examined. With sterile calculus, the reaction was typical of that to foreign bodies; with non-sterile calculus, it was suppurative with a tendency towards abscess formation.

Comment: This early classic study showed that what matters about calculus is the plaque that it retains. Only the plaque can produce a strong host response.

access is permanently impeded by anatomical factors (Fig. 13,4). The upper third molar may also tilt to the buccal side and, as the mouth opens, movement of the coronoid process may make it impossible to use a toothbrush or even a periodontal probe. In this situation it is wise to remove a tooth with significant periodontitis or caries, because its future is unpredictable and likely to cause problems for the patient.

A severe overbite may cause regular direct trauma to the upper palatal or lower labial anterior gingival tissues (Chapter 25). In some patients orthognathic surgery may be considered, but this is unwise if the teeth have a proven susceptibility to periodontitis, because their loss may complicate the situation.

RETENTIVE FACTORS OF PATHOPHYSIOLOGICAL ORIGIN: CALCULUS

Calculus originates in the calcification of the plaque biofilm. In this elaborate biochemical environment, precipitation of a complex crystalline deposit that adheres to the tooth ensures that there is an irregular surface adjacent to the periodontal tissues. On this surface, plaque organisms maintain their output of biologically active and tissue-damaging substances.

It was shown many years ago that the living microorganisms on the calculus are the crucial factors that cause disease (Abstract 13,1). Calculus does not force its way into the tissues; its formation is rather a passive process in whatever space happens to be available.

However, there are two other considerations about calculus that need to be borne in mind. Particularly when it is supragingival, calculus may impede oral hygiene; and on some occasions toothbrushing may force the gingival tissues against subgingival calculus, with resultant prolonged inflammation and occasional recession. When marginal tissues remain inflamed despite apparently good supragingival plaque control (Chapter 18) a careful search should be made for small subgingival calculus deposits. When they are removed, the tissues heal as the plaque control is continued.

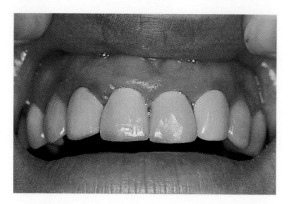

Fig. 13,5

Margins of crowns on teeth 11 and 21 and on bridge abutments 12, 14, 22 and 24 are maintaining gingival inflammation by plaque retention.

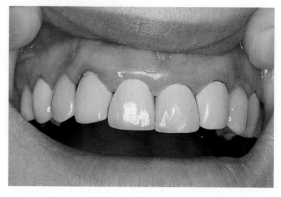

Fig. 13,6

One year later, subgingivally directed plaque control has virtually eliminated gingival inflammation. No other treatment was needed.

IATROGENIC PLAQUE-RETENTIVE FACTORS: RESTORATIONS

Any form of restorative treatment may contribute to plaque retention, particularly if placed below the gingival margin. However, good plaque control may fully resolve such problems, albeit with a degree of gingival shrinkage and recession (Figs 13,5 and 13,6). The material of a restoration is of significance: porcelain has long been considered to have minimal plaque-retentive properties (Abstract 13,2), whereas aging composite resin has a greater potential for damage (Abstract 13,3). However, any restoration with a good margin can enhance the potential for plaque control where a cavity is present (Figs 13,7 and 13,8).

Abstract 13,2 *Plaque retention on teeth restored with full-ceramic crowns: a comparative study*

Chan C, Weber H, *Journal of Prosthetic Dentistry* 1986; **56**: 666–671

Plaque indices were recorded for 150 crowns in 19 patients. These were compared with the average plaque index for the quadrant in which each crown was inserted. As controls, 242 natural teeth were included. The least plaque was found on full-ceramic crowns, followed by ceramometal crowns, natural teeth, cast gold and acrylic resin crowns.

Comment: The smoother the surface, the less the plaque. However, this study did not record any differences in gingivitis.

Abstract 13,3 *The effect of different types of composite resin fillings on marginal gingiva*

van Dijken JWV, Sjöström S, Wing K, *Journal of Clinical Periodontology* 1987; **14**: 185–189

Plaque and gingivitis and crevicular fluid were measured in 18 patients with 108 composite subgingivally-extended restorations placed 1 year before, and in 24 patients with 228 similar restorations placed 3–4 years before. Enamel surfaces were used as controls, and three different composite types – conventional, hybrid and microfilled – were compared with enamel in each patient. There were no significant differences in plaque and gingivitis between enamel and any composites in the 1-year-old restoration group, nor between the three types of 3–4-year-old restorations. However, the latter restorations had substantially more plaque and gingivitis than the enamel controls.

Comment: Surface wear rendered these restorations more vulnerable to plaque accumulation, with consequent increased gingival inflammation.

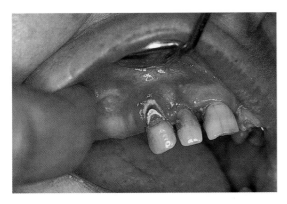

Fig. 13,7

Caries on teeth 11, 12 and 13 make oral hygiene difficult for this 75-year-old patient.

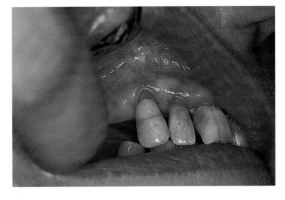

Fig. 13,8

Following restorations in these teeth, good oral hygiene was achieved.

Marginal discrepancy is a common restorative problem. However, it may be possible for plaque to be controlled, for instance, by

Abstract 13,4 *Clinical and microbiological effects of subgingival restorations with overhanging or clinically perfect margins*

Lang NP, Kiel RA, Anderhalden K, *Journal of Clinical Periodontology* 1983; **10**: 563–578

In nine dental students with clinically healthy gingivae, 10 MOD gold onlays were placed, of which five had 1-mm proximal overhangs and the other five had clinically perfect margins. After 19–27 weeks, each inlay was replaced with the other type for a similar period of time. Sulcular microbial samples yielded a microflora characteristic of health or initial gingivitis adjacent to onlays with clinically perfect margins. However, adjacent to overhanging onlays, the microflora was similar to that associated with chronic periodontitis, with increased Gram-negatives, anaerobes and black-pigmented *Bacteroides*, and increasing gingival inflammation.

Comment: Because the provision of a gold onlay with an overhang was followed by alteration of the plaque flora, cause and effect have been reasonably established. However, it is not clear whether the changed microflora has significant potential for attachment loss in these subjects.

slipping floss past an overhang. The problem is greater if subjacent plaque is not accessible. One study has indicated what may happen if this occurs (Abstract 13,4).

However, what is not known for certain is whether long-term presence of an overhang contributes to progressive attachment loss. It is clear that the attachment retreats a suitable 'biological' distance from an overhang, but perhaps that is the only effect of the margin and its associated plaque. Clinically, many overhangs seem to co-exist with this situation for many years.

Nevertheless, it is undesirable to maintain the gingiva in a state of inflammation for a long time: it may be a persistent concern for the patient, and interfere with provision of other aspects of dentistry. Furthermore, because it is not possible to return the gingiva to health, there will always be doubt over whether attachment loss will progress. It is therefore desirable to place restorative margins supragingivally.

RECESSION AND ROOT CARIES

There are two other matters of concern if restorative margins are placed subgingivally. First, in some labial situations this may encourage gingival recession, which is a particular problem if the restoration was placed to improve aesthetics because of previous reces-

Abstract 13,5   *Association between root caries occurrence and periodontal state*

Vehkalahti M, Paunio I, *Caries Research* 1994; **28**: 301–306

A representative sample of 4777 Finnish adults aged over 30 years was examined for root caries and periodontal factors relating to it. Only 4% of subjects with healthy periodontium (163 subjects) had root caries, but 15% of those with gingival inflammation and 17% of those with deepened pockets did so. Men (but not women) showed more root caries with deeper pockets. In all age groups and both genders, root caries was more frequent in dentitions with retention of subgingival plaque by calculus or restorative overhangs. This factor had the strongest association with root caries (odds ratio 3.7) out of those investigated.

Comment: This study provides evidence that root caries may be viewed partly as a complication of subgingival plaque retention by calculus or restorative overhangs.

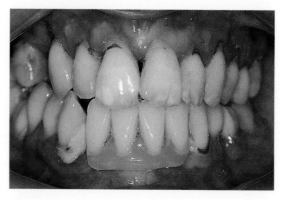

Fig. 13,9

A combination of a nervous patient, a rarely removed mucosal-borne lower prosthesis and poor plaque control has led to extensive calculus formation, especially on tooth 43. There are also extensive, formerly subgingival calculus deposits now revealed through gingival recession.

sion. Patients do not appreciate treatment that makes them longer in the tooth without solving their problem.

Secondly, it appears that subgingival plaque retention may increase root caries – a problem of increasing concern in patients with chronic periodontal diseases (Abstract 13,5). It is not good practice to replace one problem with another. The complication of root caries requires attention that is beyond the scope of this book. Remineralization with nightly applications of a strong fluoride gel for 2–3 weeks is one option in the early stages. Where restorations are needed, glass ionomers seem to provide a useful option, provided that they are replaced when appropriate.

prosthodontic circles. A mucosal-borne partial denture (often in the lower jaw) without rests and with marginal gingival coverage has been seen as periodontally damaging. However, there is no direct evidence of such damage where good oral hygiene has been maintained. If plaque can be controlled, then it is difficult to see how attachment could be lost.

Any orthodontic appliance may impede oral hygiene, and this is to be avoided particularly in those patients who have a proven susceptibility to attachment loss. For reasons that are not clear, many patients with appliance-associated gingivitis have a hyperplastic appearance to the tissues (Chapter 26). The treatment for these lesions is in principle exactly the same as for any other plaque-induced lesion.

IATROGENIC PLAQUE-RETENTIVE FACTORS: REMOVABLE DENTURES AND ORTHODONTIC APPLIANCES

The 'gum-stripper' design of denture (Fig. 13,9) has long been condemned in orthodox

CONCLUSION

The answer to many local plaque-retentive problems may lie in the modification of oral hygiene techniques, but in a few cases there will be a need for further action. Related matters such as root caries may also require attention.

14 INTERACTION BETWEEN SYSTEMIC FACTORS AND PERIODONTAL DISEASES

- How may systemic factors affect the periodontium?
- What factors are known to exacerbate periodontal diseases?
- Can systemic treatment affect periodontal health?
- Can periodontal diseases affect systemic health?

The periodontium is a robust part of the body with a structure that is rarely altered by major systemic diseases. However, it is notably prone to inflammatory phenomena, and in this lies a much greater possibility that systemic factors may alter it. Host response factors have some marked effects on the progress of periodontal diseases. The oral environment, particularly the microorganisms and their regulation by human behaviour, is another source of systemically mediated variation. Finally, there is also a possibility that the periodontium, which often contains a relatively large volume of chronic inflammation, may have an effect on other parts of the body.

In the overview of periodontal diseases in Chapter 4, we saw some of the systemic factors that might affect the periodontium. Gingival recession has no clear link to systemic diseases. Table 14,1 lists the main

Table 14,1: *Examples of some systemic factors that may alter periodontal tissues and diseases*

| Nature of factor | Affected aspect | | |
	Tissue structure	Host response	Oral environment
Genetic	Down syndrome	Down syndrome	
Developmental	Hypophosphatasia		
Endocrine and metabolic	Diabetes mellitus Pregnancy	Pregnancy Diabetes mellitus	
Haematological	Leukaemias	Leukaemias Phagocyte defects	
Respiratory		Mouthbreathing	
Behavioural		Tobacco smoking Personal stress	Depression Anxiety Health beliefs
Nutrition	Scurvy	Protein deficiency	
Infection		HIV and AIDS	Microbial transmission
Medication	Phenytoin Calcium channel blockers Cyclosporin		

types of systemic factor that may modify periodontal diseases. Some of these are quite common: 1 in 700 pregnancies is of a Down syndrome foetus; diabetes affects 1–2% of people; and 25–50% of adults smoke tobacco, depending on their social class, country and how much smoking and its promotion is discouraged. Other factors, such as hypophosphatasia and scurvy, are very rare in the UK.

FACTORS AFFECTING TISSUES

The principal component of tissue structure that is modified by systemic factors is the ubiquitous collagen fibre. In Down syndrome, abnormal patterns of collagen synthesis may be linked to the increased prevalence of periodontitis, but this is not the only possible factor. There is no doubt that patients with Down syndrome have an increased periodontal treatment need (Abstract 14,1).

Abstract 14,1   *Caries levels, Streptococcus mutans counts, salivary pH and periodontal treatment needs of adult patients with Down syndrome*

Shapira J, Stabholz A, Schurr D, et al., *Special Care in Dentistry* 1991; **11**: 248–251

Caries and periodontal problems were examined in a Jerusalem hospital. Twelve patients aged 20–48 years with Down syndrome (D) were compared with two control groups: healthy patients (H) and patients with other forms of mental handicap (MH) living in an institution. There was no difference in pH, but MH had double the microbial count of the other groups. Both D and MH groups had a higher CPITN score than H (respectively: 2.1; 1.9; 0.9). The D group had far less caries than MH and H (respective DMF scores: 16; 30; 34). Caries-free D patients also had lower CPITN scores than patients with caries.

Comment: This is a characteristic study showing that patients with Down syndrome have more periodontal disease and less caries than other patients.

Abstract 14,2   *Scurvy – a mistakenly forgotten disease*

Hurlimann R, Salomon F, *Schweizerische Medizinische Wochenschrift* 1994; **124**: 1373–1380

In a Zurich hospital, four cases of scurvy were diagnosed over 2 years. They were typical of the patients who are seen with this disease in developed countries. Two male patients had heavy nicotine and alcohol abuse, a woman in her 4th decade had malnutrition for dietary phobic reasons and an elderly woman had dementia and was socially isolated. A variety of signs was present, including anaemia, fatigue, other deficiencies and haemorrhagic problems. In two cases, there were periodontal complaints. All problems resolved with restitution of deficient nutrients.

Comment: This disease is rare, but certain types of patient are clearly at risk.

Defective collagen formation and maturation in scurvy is the reason why the tissues are fragile and easily overwhelmed by plaque. However, it takes 4–6 months of vitamin C deprivation for periodontal manifestations to develop. If scurvy is suspected, the patient should be referred to a physician because other abnormalities may be present, such as alcoholism or food fads (Abstract 14,2).

Collagen overproduction in response to plaque may occur with three types of medication. This is probably never a hyperplasia because the number of cells remains constant, as far as experimental studies can show. However, far more collagen is produced than is usual, and perhaps it is also broken down more slowly.

In a proportion of leukaemias, the engorgement of tissues with the culpable form of leucocyte is the reason for a firm enlargement of the gingiva. This effect may occur partly in response to plaque but can be reduced by successful treatment of the leukaemia. There have been amazing developments in treatment of several types of leukaemia since the 1970s, but one of the more informative studies on oral manifestations comes from before that time (Abstract 14,3).

Abstract 14,3 *Oral manifestations of leukemia: a postdiagnostic study*

Lynch MA, Ship II, *Journal of the American Dental Association* 1967; **75**: 1139–1144

In 155 patients with leukaemia admitted to a Philadelphia hospital over a 10 year period, the main oral manifestations were recorded and related to acute and chronic cases. Initially, in acute cases, 36% presented with petechiae or bleeding (rising to 56% postdiagnosis); 27% with ulcers (53%); and 25% with gingival enlargement (36%). Corresponding figures for chronic cases were: 10% (28%); 10% (22%); and 4% (10%).

Comment: Gingival enlargement is relatively infrequent but quite characteristic when it occurs. This study suggests that about one-third of patients with acute leukaemia and one-tenth of patients with chronic leukaemia are affected.

Abstract 14,4 *Mouthbreathing, lip seal and upper lip coverage and their relationship with gingival inflammation in 11–14 year-old schoolchildren*

Wagaiyu EG, Ashley FP, *Journal of Clinical Periodontology* 1991; **18**: 698–702

One examiner assessed gingival health and crowding of incisors and first molars in 201 subjects aged 11–14 years. Plaque, mouthbreathing and lip relations were assessed by another examiner. A careful analysis, allowing for plaque and other factors such as crowding, suggested that lip coverage affected gingivitis on palatal and labial aspects of upper anterior teeth, and that mouthbreathing had an effect limited to palatal gingiva.

Comment: As was pointed out in subsequent correspondence, mouthbreathing is hard to assess. However, this study presents a plausible result. The effect is small.

The rare disorder of hypophosphatasia is linked to cemental dysplasia and the early exfoliation of deciduous teeth, but individuals with this rare disorder may not have any effect in the permanent dentition. A hypothesis has been put forward that defective formation of cementum arising in mild cases of hypophosphatasia may be one reason for the development of early-onset periodontitis (Page and Baab, 1985); this would help to explain site specificity in localized juvenile periodontitis, for instance, but there is no clear evidence on the matter.

FACTORS AFFECTING THE HOST RESPONSE

As we have seen in Chapter 11, phagocyte dysfunction is strongly implicated in early-onset forms of periodontitis. It follows therefore that some disorders that affect cells such as neutrophils will be likely to enhance attachment loss. Examples in Table 14,1 include Down syndrome, diabetes mellitus, and tobacco smoking. However, this is not the sole aspect of immune pathology that could be implicated in such disorders. As we saw above, Down syndrome has collagen abnormalities that also might be implicated.

Likewise, tobacco certainly affects neutrophils, but it has a wide range of adverse effects on the whole of the immune system, some of which may be implicated in more serious matters such as oncogenesis.

Mouthbreathing is a behaviour of complex origin. It was long suspected to contribute to gingival inflammation, but the first study to implicate it whilst considering other factors in gingivitis came up with unexpected results (Abstract 14,4). Only the palatal aspect of the upper anterior gingivae was affected, whereas it was primarily the labial appearance that previously had made people suspect the phenomenon.

Personal stress is difficult to study. However, one interesting approach is seen in Abstract 14,5, where stressful life events appear to be associated with increased periodontal disease.

As referred to in Chapter 12, the transition from HIV seropositivity to AIDS may be marked by the invasive and unpleasant disease of NUP. A variety of other periodontal manifestations have also been associated

Abstract 14,5 *The relationship between life-events and periodontitis. A case-control study*

Croucher R, Marcenes WS, Torres MCMB, et al., *Journal of Clinical Periodontology* 1997; **24**: 39–43

A sample of 100 patients was recruited at a London hospital: 50 had at least one pocket of 6 mm or more, and 50 had none over 3 mm. Both groups had the same number of reported life events over the previous 12 months. The periodontitis group had more negative life events with a greater perceived impact and fewer positive events than the control group, using a version of the Social Readjustment Rating Scale.

Comment: This is an interesting study that points to a possible effect of stressful events, but it would be unlikely for the differences in periodontal status to have occurred as a result of the reported events over the previous year. It may be that the subjects' experience over that year reflected their previous life and their feelings.

Abstract 14,6 *Actinobacillus actinomycetemcomitans, Capnocytophaga and Porphyromonas gingivalis in subgingival plaque of adolescents with Down syndrome*

Barr-Agholme M, Dahllöf G, Linder L, et al., *Oral Microbiology and Immunology* 1992; **7**: 244–248

This study compared 37 patients with Down syndrome against age- and gender-matched healthy controls. The patients with Down syndrome had significantly more gingival bleeding, pocketing and bone loss. In subgingival plaque, Aa and *Capnocytophaga* were significantly more frequent in subjects with Down syndrome. However, patients with Down syndrome with and without these organisms did not differ in gingival inflammation, pocketing or bone loss; nor were there differences according to sites with and without the organisms.

Comment: As the authors state, this study is evidence that certain periodontal organisms are associated with Down syndrome. However, because the patients with Down syndrome differed in periodontal status from the controls, and since Down patients without these organisms had similar periodontal disease, it is also evidence that these organisms are not essential to periodontitis.

with HIV infection, and all have been seen in patients without HIV infection.

FACTORS AFFECTING THE ORAL ENVIRONMENT

As emphasized in earlier chapters, the specificity of the oral microflora is a highly contentious matter in periodontology. However, there is no doubt that organisms may pass between people living in close association, such as families. There are also examples of some members harbouring interesting organisms that have not passed to the others. The study in Abstract 8,6 showed both of these situations, whilst indicating that such transmission was probably not of major aetiological significance.

Attempts to link a specific microflora to particular diseases have not been successful on the whole. For instance, although a different microflora was found in Down syndrome in the study of Abstract 14,6, this could be explained in other ways. For instance, deeper pocketing provides better conditions for colonization by the organisms found more frequently in the patients with Down syndrome.

Behavioural factors may affect plaque control and host response. In regular attenders, a higher score on a depression questionnaire was associated with poorer plaque control (Abstract 14,7); and in new patients, the expressed intention to comply with OHI was associated with subsequent improvement (Abstract 14,8).

PREGNANCY AND GINGIVA

The greatest single alteration in gingival tissues in pregnancy is the increase in epithe-

Abstract 14,7 *Psychological mood of regular dental attenders in relation to oral hygiene behaviour and gingival health*

Kurer JRB, Watts TLP, Weinman J, et al., *Journal of Clinical Periodontology* 1995; **22**: 52–55

A Hospital Anxiety and Depression (HAD) Scale questionnaire was completed by 51 regular dental attenders, who each brought a salivary cortisol sample taken at 1030 on the day of initial examination. Subjects were instructed in Bass technique toothbrushing and asked to use it regularly. At full re-examination 5 weeks later, 47 subjects returned. Plaque was reduced by 20% and gingivitis by 40%, but no other parameters were changed. Mean anxiety scores at both examinations were associated with gingivitis, and mean depression scores with plaque. Neither mood nor salivary cortisol predicted change in plaque or gingival health.

Comment: It is interesting that plaque was correlated significantly with gingivitis, and anxiety with depression, but that the disease parameters were correlated separately with mood scores. In fact, gingivitis nearly reached a significant correlation with depression, and plaque was only a little lower in relation to anxiety. This sort of finding always needs further experimental study.

Abstract 14,8 *The relationship of health beliefs and psychological mood to patient adherence to oral hygiene behaviour*

Borkowska ED, Watts TLP, Weinman J, *Journal of Clinical Periodontology* 1998; **25**: 187–193

Full periodontal examination was performed for 52 subjects, of whom 47 completed the study. All subjects completed a dental beliefs questionnaire (DBQ) and HAD Scale (Abstract 14,7) questionnaire, following which they received instruction in Bass technique brushing and small loop flossing. The main significant result was that a component of the DBQ, Adherence Intent (AI), correlated well with initial and final plaque scores. Thus, subjects who expressed a strong intention to comply with OHI were those who achieved the best plaque scores. There was also a moderate correlation between initial AI scores and final gingivitis scores. Mood did not correlate consistently with plaque and disease scores.

Comment: These were different patients from those in Abstract 14,7 – those were regular attenders, and these were new patients who had received little, if any, OHI. It is clear that the intention and expectation of these patients was related to their plaque control both before and 5 weeks after OHI. A positive outlook may relate to future success.

lial and endothelial permeability. Research many years ago showed that both progesterone and oestrogens were involved. The result is only apparent if plaque is not controlled adequately: the inflammatory effects are magnified (Fig. 4,19). Paradoxically, when the hormonal effect is taken into account, pregnant women may have a higher real level of periodontal health than controls (Abstract 14,9).

In pregnancy, both oedematous and proliferative chronic inflammation may occur, and the latter type is sometimes apparent as an epulis (Fig. 4,7). If an epulis is not too large, it does not have to be removed if the patient prefers this. When left, the epulis usually shrinks or drops off shortly after parturition. If it does not, surgical removal is simpler at this stage because the tissues are more fibrous and do not bleed as easily as in the earlier stages of pregnancy.

There is no doubt that pregnancy may affect the gingiva; whether the periodontal condition may affect the pregnancy, however, is more controversial.

DIABETES AND THE PERIODONTIUM

Diabetes has long been known to exacerbate periodontal diseases. In both principal types of diabetes, inflammation and attachment loss are increased (Abstracts 14,10 and 14,11). Diabetes is a complex disease that may have effects on blood pressure, kidney, heart and eye.

Attempts to show a different microflora in diabetes have not been successful when the

Abstract 14,9 *Periodontal condition of pregnant women assessed by CPITN*

Miyazaki H, Yamashita Y, Shirahama R, et al., *Journal of Clinical Periodontology* 1991; **18**: 751–754

In this Japanese study, the CPITN was assessed for 2424 pregnant women and 1565 non-pregnant female controls. Both groups had a mean age of 28 years. In the pregnant group, codes 0–4 were the highest scores in 5%, 5%, 70%, 19% and 1% of cases, respectively. In the control group, the respective figures were 4%, 4%, 75%, 15% and 2%. The mean number of sextants with scores 0–4 in the pregnant group were 2.4, 0.8, 2.6, 0.4 and 0.0, which was similar to the control group: 1.9, 0.6, 3.2, 0.3 and 0.0. The number of sextants with healthy tissue tended to increase to a peak of 2.5 after the first trimester, from 0.5 in the 2nd month.

Comment: This is a large robust study, and the results suggest no special need for periodontal attention in pregnancy. Whether pregnancy is a time when we should encourage improved oral hygiene because of the mother's increased awareness of health matters, is another question. It is also uncertain whether periodontal ill-health affects the foetus in pregnancy (see Abstract 14,14).

Abstract 14,10 *A site-by-site follow-up study on the effect of controlled versus poorly controlled insulin dependent diabetes*

Seppälä B, Ainamo J, *Journal of Clinical Periodontology* 1994; **21**: 161–165

At 0, 1 and 2 years, a group of insulin-dependent diabetics was examined for periodontal health. At 1 year, 38 subjects were seen, and at 2 years, 22 subjects. The age range at baseline was 35–56 years and mean duration of diabetes was 18 years. After 1 year, 26 subjects were identified as having poor metabolic control, and after 2 years, 16 subjects. All patients received thorough periodontal treatment, including extraction of teeth with poor prognosis. Results suggested that treatment did not improve metabolic control, and that increased bleeding and bone loss occurred in the patients with poor metabolic control.

Comment: Subjects with poor metabolic control benefited less from periodontal therapy. Although not a controlled trial, this study also suggests that poor metabolic control does not benefit from periodontal treatment over a longer period of time than the studies in Abstract 14,13.

extent of disease has been taken into account. Patients with better metabolic control have fewer complications, which may include periodontal diseases. When periodontal diseases are treated in well-controlled diabetics, their response to therapy is similar to non-diabetics. However, poor metabolic control affects periodontal conditions (Abstract 14,10). There is also evidence suggesting that diabetics who develop periodontitis are more liable to acquire other diabetic complications.

TOBACCO SMOKING AND PERIODONTITIS

The earliest studies on smoking and periodontal diseases reached the conclusion that smokers had more disease because they had worse oral hygiene, perhaps because they were a group of people with a poor self-image. However, in the early 1980s a different picture began to develop as researchers took an interest in the effects of this addiction which was known to produce immunosuppression.

It has since become apparent that smoking tobacco reduces BOP in the gingiva, which means that inflammation is underdiagnosed. It also increases attachment loss, PD and bone loss. Overall, the effects on periodontitis of smoking tobacco are worse and far more widespread than those of any other systemic factor, including diabetes (see Abstract 6,7). But the response to treatment of all types is less as well (Abstract 14,12). These are good reasons for dentists to involve themselves in activities against this unfortunate addiction, which has been shown in the USA to be exacerbated by corporate greed and deceit on an unprecedented scale.

Abstract 14,11 *Periodontal disease in non-insulin-dependent diabetes mellitus*

Emrich LJ, Shlossman M, Genco RJ, *Journal of Periodontology* 1991; **62**: 123–130

The Pima Indians of the Gila River Indian Community have the highest incidence and prevalence of type II diabetes (non-insulin-dependent diabetes mellitus (NIDDM)) in the world. Half of those over 35 years are affected. In a sample of 1342 subjects aged 15 to more than 55 years, 254 had NIDDM, 158 had impaired glucose tolerance (IGT: plasma glucose concentration between diabetes and normal) and 930 were normal. The age distribution was skewed, with more of the younger subjects. From age 15 to 55 years, the NIDDM subjects had approximately 1 mm greater mean periodontal attachment loss than IGT or normal subjects, and corresponding bone loss scores. Above 55 years, the three groups had similar periodontal disease prevalence, which the authors attribute to loss of severely affected teeth.

Comment: This is an impressive study that clearly shows how type II diabetes leads to increased periodontal attachment loss. A mean increase of 1 mm means that there will be considerably more attachment loss on some teeth and less on others. The greater attachment loss certainly will lead to some tooth loss.

Abstract 14,12 *The effect of smoking on the response to periodontal therapy*

Ah MK, Johnson GK, Kaldahl WB, et al., *Journal of Clinical Periodontology* 1994; **21**: 91–97

A comparison was made between 46 smokers (mean age 43 years: 10 or more cigarettes/day) and 28 non-smokers (46 years: not smoking at the initial examination) who participated in a trial comparing different treatments in a split-mouth study. Following treatment, patients were followed up for 6 years of a maintenance programme. There were minor but statistically significant differences in plaque between the two groups up to 5 years (10–20% more surfaces with plaque in smokers). However, there was 30–50% less attachment level improvement in smokers, and 30% less probing depth reduction in smokers from 1 year onwards. The differences were similar for all modes of treatment, both surgical and non-surgical, and greatest in deeper pockets.

Comment: These results are a clear example of how smoking reduces the improvement after all forms of periodontal treatment. In fact, the results are even more striking because the authors tell us in the discussion that 16 smokers gave up the habit during the 6-year maintenance period, at least for the rest of the study.

PERIODONTAL DISEASE AFFECTING SYSTEMIC HEALTH

There has been a recent renaissance of the idea that periodontal inflammation may have a 'focal infection' effect on other parts of the body. At present, the evidence is questionable and centres on diabetic metabolic control, preterm low-birthweight babies and cardiovascular disease.

METABOLIC CONTROL AND PERIODONTAL DISEASE

First, let us consider a question of some importance. We know that diabetics with less satisfactory metabolic control are subject to more periodontal diseases. Can it also be true that periodontal diseases adversely affect metabolic control? What is the likely result if two damaging bodily processes reinforce each other? More periodontal disease means worse metabolic control, which produces still more periodontal disease, which produces still worse metabolic control, and so on. If this scenario actually occurred, it would imply that there was a vicious circle tending to make matters worse. Yet there are diabetics who have inflammatory periodontal diseases and whose metabolic control is fully stable. This line of evidence is in conflict with the theory.

What is the actual evidence that periodontitis makes metabolic control worse? In fact, it depends on cohort studies and not on randomized trials. In the cohort studies, there seems to be some improvement in metabolic control after periodontal treatment. Unfortunately, this might be the result of a metabolic 'Hawthorne effect' (Chapter 15): it cannot be ruled out that the participants might have improved their compliance with diabetic therapy as a result of being included in a clinical study.

However, in one significant longitudinal study that separated out the poorly controlled subjects (Abstract 14,10) and in the first randomized controlled trials there was no such change. These were small trials in relatively well-controlled and metabolically stable insulin-dependent diabetics and they

Abstract 14,13 *Single-blind studies of the effects of improved periodontal health on metabolic control in Type 1 diabetes mellitus*

Aldridge JP, Lester V, Watts TLP, et al., *Journal of Clinical Periodontology* 1995; **22**: 271–275

A first trial randomly assigned 41 IDDM subjects with gingivitis and early periodontitis to oral hygiene and scaling (16 completed) or no treatment (15 completed). After 2 months, there appeared to be similar plaque control improvement in both groups. No other change or difference between groups was apparent, and metabolic control was unaltered. In a second trial, full non-surgical treatment was performed for 12 subjects randomized from a group of 23 with advanced periodontitis (one subject was dropped out during the trial). The treated group improved significantly in all periodontal parameters, but not in metabolic control. Indeed, the statistically non-significant trend was for this group to become less metabolically controlled than the untreated group. The power of this trial to detect a real difference of 3% in glycated haemoglobin (a measure of metabolic control over the past 4–6 weeks) was 90% (see Chapter 15).

Comment: The problem of these studies is their short duration, and what appears to be a Hawthorne effect on untreated subjects in the first trial. However, the results give no support to the idea that periodontal improvement will enhance metabolic control in stable patients with reasonable diabetic health.

may have had confounding factors (Abstract 14,13). However, they had absolutely no trend in the direction suggested.

So far, the evidence suggests no clear causal link in the direction suggested, namely that periodontal health influences metabolic control. Rather, metabolic control seems to be the dominant factor in this relationship. If the disease is well-controlled, periodontal complications are less likely. However, there are other matters to be checked before the idea is dismissed. Larger controlled studies are needed in both major types of diabetes, and somehow a safe and accurate way has to be devised of looking at the matter in poorly controlled diabetics. At present, their metabolic control may be so variable that it is not certain why a particular alteration has occurred.

PRETERM LOW-BIRTHWEIGHT BABIES

In diabetes, there is a question mark over the relative influence of metabolic control and inflammatory periodontal disease on each other. No such question arises when we consider whether a mother's periodontal disease may affect her child by premature birth and low weight.

However, there are certainly many important confounding factors (such as smoking and other health-related behaviour) to be considered. The link is tenuous at present, and is related to attachment loss rather than the amount of pocketing or gingival inflammation (Abstract 14,14). Other studies may show whether there really is a relationship. One problem is that with a multivariate statistical analysis we may be misled if our mathematical model does not fully represent the real-life situation.

CARDIOVASCULAR DISEASE

This is another matter of some significance but it has a number of confounding factors. Again, smoking is a common link between periodontal and cardiovascular diseases, and other adverse health behaviour also may be

Abstract 14,14 *Periodontal infection as a possible risk factor for preterm low birth weight*

Offenbacher S, Katz V, Fertig G, et al., *Journal of Periodontology* 1996; **67**: 1103–1113

The periodontal status of 93 mothers giving birth to babies of less than 2.5 kg and with gestational age < 37 weeks, or premature labour or membrane rupture (PLBW group), was compared with that of 31 mothers giving birth to normal weight babies (NBW). Examiner-blind assessment was performed either during a prenatal clinic or within 3 days of delivery. Mean probing depth was similar in both groups: 3.17 mm in PLBW mothers, and 2.99 mm in NBW. Clinical attachment levels just reached a significant difference: 3.1 mm in PLBW and 2.8 mm in NBW. A measurement of the extent of periodontal disease suggested that it was moderate over many sites, rather than affecting a few sites severely. A multivariate logistic regression analysis using this measure gave an odds ratio of 7.5 for greater periodontal disease in the PLBW mothers.

Comment: This study was an enterprising 'first' that caused considerable controversy. The actual difference between the groups was rather small at 10% of attachment loss scores, and there was no difference in probing depth, which might be viewed as an indicator of the amount of inflammation. It is hard to understand why 0.3 mm mean extra attachment loss over and above nearly 3 mm in the normal group should make such a great difference in the health of a baby.

Abstract 14,15 *Periodontal disease and cardiovascular disease*

Beck J, Garcia R, Heiss G, et al., *Journal of Periodontology* 1996; **67**: 1123–1137

From 1968 to 1971, periodontal pocket and bone loss was measured in 1147 men of mean age 43 years. Subjects were followed up every 3 years for 18 years. By then, 207 had coronary heart disease (CHD), 59 of them had died of it and 40 had strokes. Complete data were available for 1094, of whom 203 were in the disease group. The presence of 1 mm or more bone loss gave adjusted odds ratios of 1.5 for CHD over the next 18 years, 1.9 for fatal CHD and 2.8 for stroke.

Comment: This thorough research shows an association borne out by other studies. What especially needs further study is the contribution of adverse health behaviour (including smoking, plaque control, dental treatment and diet) to either disease or both diseases. Causation, if it exists here, will be exceptionally hard to demonstrate.

ASSOCIATION, CAUSATION AND STATISTICAL MODELS

It is very important not to assume that because two diseases are associated, one must

involved. This means that it is very difficult to sift out the causal 'wheat' from the 'chaff' of mere associations. The association (Abstract 14,15) may be explained in several ways. The evidence for causality in this study is quite strong, given that only about 10% of cardiovascular disease is accounted for by currently known risk factors.

However, although theories of causality have been advanced, it is very difficult to produce concrete evidence for them. Perhaps the best approach at present is to advise our patients that both diseases tend to occur in the same people, and encourage them to take appropriate preventive measures.

Table 14,2: *Association and causation in respect of two synchronous health problems*

Possible explanation	Evidence needed
1. Coincidence	More studies showing no association
2. First condition causes second	Longitudinal studies of subjects with first condition at start
3. Second condition causes first	Longitudinal studies of subjects with second condition at start
4. Both caused by common factor(s)	More evidence of aetiology
5. Independent, but both time-based	Preventing one does not affect the other

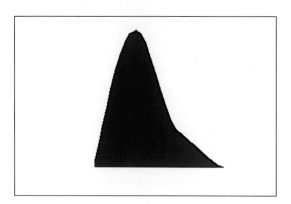

Fig. 14,1

Suppose we find that our data have a positive skew. This is a very common event in periodontal studies, because there are many shallow pockets, and few deep ones.

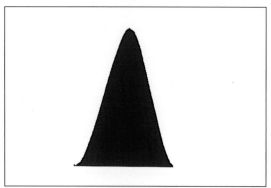

Fig. 14,2

The statistician would like to apply a transformation to make our data conform more to a normal distribution. Then the most powerful statistical tests can be used, and give the best results.

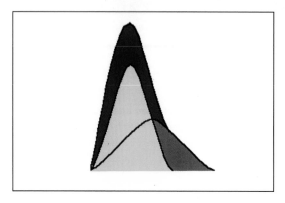

Fig. 14,3

Unknown to both periodontists and statisticians, this skewed data distribution really includes two different distributions which relate to two different phenomena. Transforming the data is going to hide this and give a false sense of security about the results.

cause the other. When a study reveals an association between preterm low-weight birth and periodontal disease, or cardiovascular and periodontal diseases, there are at least five possibilities (Table 14,2).

To say that periodontitis is a causal factor in preterm low-weight births or cardiovascular disease, the other four possibilities of the association must be ruled out. Statistical models alone cannot do this. So far, for

cardiovascular disease the first possibility seems to be excluded because several studies have shown the association. However, the evidence of the study in Abstract 14,15 does not exclude the second possibility, even though it goes some way to countering the third.

There is a tendency among periodontal researchers to assume that because a first-rate statistician participates in a study, the interpretation of the results is straightforward. Unfortunately, the statistical model also matters a great deal. If we know that a 20-cigarette-per-day smoker is likely to double a particular risk, this can be allowed for; but other confounding factors may not be so easy to incorporate in the model. In Figs 14,1 to 14,3 we see a potential problem of some statistical models: what if a skewed distribution is really the sum of two different distributions? What is needed here is evidence, not a statistical transformation. Statisticians are essential and very helpful people, but the periodontists need to be aware of conceptual pitfalls.

Associations are tantalizing things. We may be able to produce a good explanation of how one problem might lead to another, but in the end it is evidence that counts, not theoretical argument. It may take a long time to unravel some very interesting associations that have occurred in relation to periodontal diseases.

15

CLINICAL TRIALS

- What is the relevance of clinical trials to periodontics?
- How can the importance of a trial be judged?
- What are the main weaknesses in published trials?
- How may trials be misinterpreted?

The clinical testing of treatment is arguably the most important research area for any dental clinician to understand and yet this subject is rarely taught adequately. People have only a hazy idea about what they should take home as the message of a trial. There is often confusion over the mathematical aspects, even though these are subservient to the ideas that are under test.

If we dental clinicians do not understand these matters in a simple and relevant way, then we are at the mercy of anyone who wishes to manipulate us. As we saw in Chapter 1, there is a large publicity industry promoting all kinds of treatments to our patients through the popular press and in other ways. The professional's first duty is to give advice, and that is not possible if we do not appreciate how treatments are properly evaluated.

THE PURPOSE OF A TRIAL

A case history may give valuable and informative evidence on a specific disease and its treatment. However, it always lacks certain important information. What would have happened if the treatment had not been administered? Might the patient's condition have improved without treatment? The first stage in answering these questions is the recruitment of a control patient with a similar problem.

There are two types of control in a clinical trial: negative and positive. The negative control is where no actual treatment is administered. For instance, a drug formulated in a vehicle preparation may be given to patients receiving active treatment, and the vehicle only to the controls.

Obviously, the situation may be such that a control patient ethically cannot be left without treatment. It is not ethical to leave periodontitis for several years without treatment simply in order to watch things get worse. In this situation, a positive control patient would receive another treatment that had been regarded hitherto as beneficial for the condition. The question to answer then would be whether the test treatment was as good or better.

Before clinical trials were well-defined entities, opinions decided how patients should be treated. Where there was a drastic difference between outcomes with and without treatment, this was sometimes valid. No-one would question the need to remove or destroy a cancer or to use antibacterial drugs against tuberculosis, for instance. However, opinions do not tell us reliably which of two treatments is better or whether a new treatment actually works.

THE QUESTION OF BIAS

What makes a trial different is that it involves a determined effort to exclude mere opinions from the evaluation of a treatment. A clinical trial was defined accurately by Duncan Vere, a noted professor of pharmacology, as 'a device to prevent bias'.

The first bias that must be avoided in a trial arises from the biological variability of patients. A treatment may be followed by improvement in one patient and by deterioration in another. Yet the decline does not necessarily mean that the treatment had no effect: without it, the deterioration might have been worse. It is important to have a sufficient number of patients in the trial to average out their varying responses to treatment.

Biological variability creates another problem. Given that we have sufficient patients in the trial, how do we know that the test and control groups are similar? One way (in theory) would be to make them both random samples from the population of all patients with the disease. This is not usually possible because: we do not know who constitutes the whole population; some patients will not wish to participate for various reasons; and quite large numbers of patients may be needed. There are three other ways in which a periodontal study may ensure comparable test and control groups.

The first way is by matching the groups in some way. For instance, Abstract 15,1 describes a study in which patients were recruited to the two groups in pairs, each of whom had the same gender, ethnic group, smoking status and similar age and disease experience.

A good way of matching test and control groups is to compare both treatments in the same patient. Secondly, therefore, systemic drugs might be used in a cross-over study, with a period of time between the two treatments. Thirdly, a special dental version of the cross-over study is the split-mouth trial, in which one side receives active treatment and the other side receives the control treatment.

Abstract 15,1 *A randomized controlled trial of a 2% minocycline gel as an adjunct to non-surgical periodontal treatment, using a design with multiple matching criteria*

Graça MA, Watts TLP, Wilson RF, et al., *Journal of Clinical Periodontology* 1997; **24**: 249–253

From about 100 consecutive patients in a periodontal department, 30 subjects were selected by pairing for gender, age, ethnic group, smoking habits and probing depths. A constant force probe was used for measurements. Each group received thorough OHI and root planing with local anaesthesia. Subjects were randomized to receive active or placebo gel subgingivally at sites immediately after planing and 2 and 4 weeks later. Two subjects dropped out during the trial and their pairs were excluded from analysis. At 6 and 12 weeks, the active gel significantly improved bleeding from the depth of pockets and improved PAL but not PD. Mean active PAL at baseline, 6 and 12 weeks was 6.9, 4.9 and 4.9 mm respectively; control PAL was 6.8, 5.3 and 5.3 mm respectively.

Comment: Subjects were specially selected for the trial so that they were closely matched; however, they were then allocated randomly to use active or placebo gel on a double-blind basis. The mean PAL improvement was significant at $P<0.05$ but was less than 0.5 mm in size.

THE ETHICAL BASIS FOR CLINICAL TRIALS

We shall examine some other sources of bias later. It is time to consider why clinical trials are not only desirable but essential for ethical treatment. Table 15,1 lists the present author's approach to this important matter.

In essence, some people have argued that trials are wrong because usually the patient has no choice over the treatment or even (when a placebo is used) whether they are actually given a treatment. This view has been expressed by some jurists who follow the Napoleonic Code – meaning that, according to them, it is wrong for persons to put themselves at risk.

Such an opinion takes no account of the context in which a trial is performed. If we do not know whether a treatment works, then using it is irresponsible in the extreme. If it is wrong to perform a trial, then it is also wrong to use the treatment. If a plausible treatment is suggested, then is it not putting people at

Table 15,1: *The ethics of therapeutics*

	Explanation
1. Principle of theoretical consistency	Treatment for a disease should agree with knowledge about the disease or at least not be in conflict with it
2. Principle of experimental validity	Treatment aimed at a material change in body structure (e.g. anatomy or chemistry) should be supported by evidence for the effects claimed
3. The toxicological assumption	Treatment that has any healing effect on disease may be expected to have effects that are at least occasionally adverse
4. Principle of efficacy testing	Where scientific evidence of efficacy is lacking but the treatment has a reasonable basis (theoretical consistency), reasoned experiments may be performed to test it
5. Principle of toxicological investigation	Any treatment undergoing examination for potential therapeutic use should be investigated also for adverse effects
6. The experimental imperative	Where significant improvement may be reasonably expected from a hitherto untested treatment, there is an *obligation* for those who are qualified to test it to do so, given time and resources
7. The experimental priority	It follows from the principle of theoretical consistency and the experimental imperative that treatment in the absence of known experimental validity should be given only in conditions that are likely to establish or negate it, usually within a properly designed clinical trial

greater risk if we do not test it to see whether it works?

However, if there are grounds for thinking that it might be of use where no treatment exists, or that it might provide a better result than other treatments, then it is irresponsible if we do *not* test it. It is utterly wrong to use a proposed new treatment in clinical practice without subjecting it to a properly designed clinical trial.

If patients do not wish to take part in a trial, that is their right, but they should not be given an untested treatment outside a trial.

Some forms of periodontal treatment have been introduced without this safeguard and have cluttered the literature with biased reports. It is unfortunate, to say the least, if the earliest use of a new treatment in human beings is not designed to test its therapeutic potential. Furthermore, a collection of case histories put together as a cohort study is no substitute for a properly designed trial. Such studies do not show what would have happened without the treatment in question.

DIFFERENT TYPES OF TRIAL OBJECTIVE

Consider the two studies in Abstracts 15,1 and 15,2. In the first, a small study of 26 carefully matched subjects was used to test a treatment adjunctive to root planing. In the second, a study of over 400 patients was used to test another adjunct. What are the differences between these trials? Obviously the first involved far fewer resources and was carried out in one centre, but it also gave a statistically significant result. Why not simply do a small trial and forget about the larger, expensive one?

For a start, no trial is ever simple. The first trial required screening of about four times as many subjects as eventually participated, and the second trial used a form of within-subject matching similar to a split-mouth trial. But why introduce variables such as different centres for treatment by different operators? A large study becomes essential to deal with

Abstract 15,2 *Adjunctive use of a
subgingival controlled-release chlorhexidine
chip reduces probing depth and improves
attachment level compared with scaling and
root planing alone*

Jeffcoat MK, Bray KS, Ciancio SG, et al., *Journal of
Periodontology* 1998; **69**: 989–997

In two trials, each with five participating centres,
447 patients were recruited, each with at least 10
natural teeth and 4 of these with pockets of 5–8 mm.
Conditions of treatment were meant to approximate to those in dental practice. Following 1 h of
scaling and root planing for all periodontal
problems (SRP), two sites in each patient received a
biodegradable chip, either releasing chlorhexidine
over 7–10 days (225 subjects) or a placebo (222). The
other two sites served as SRP controls. All patients
were stratified according to smoking status, and
sites were assigned randomly to treatments. Active
and placebo groups each lost 14 patients. Chips
were replaced at 3 and 6 months if pockets were
still 5 mm or more at those dates. Initial mean
probing depths were: SRP, 5.6 mm; placebo + SRP,
5.6 mm; active + SRP, 5.7 mm. Respective reductions 9 months later were 0.65 mm, 0.69 mm and
0.95 mm. Initial mean clinical attachment levels
were: 5.1 mm, 5.1 mm and 5.3 mm. Reductions after
9 months were 0.58 mm, 0.55 mm and 0.75 mm.

Comment: This was a well-performed large trial
aimed at realistic practice conditions, but some
would say that 1 h was too short for effective whole-
mouth SRP. The extra improvements with the chip
were very small but might be of clinical significance
in some cases. Because the study was so large, small
changes reached statistical significance.

such variability. The answer is that the two
trials had different objectives.

The first was an experimental trial. It aimed
at testing the treatment under conditions that
largely excluded other sources of variation.
The second trial was a community study that
tested a treatment known to have an effect, as
the authors said, under realistic conditions of
practice. This classification of trial objectives
was first proposed in 1976 by O'Mullane in
the context of caries preventive agents (Table
15,2).

The experimental trial is an attempt to let
the treatment show its therapeutic potential in
as few subjects as possible, the subjects being
specifically chosen to provide as little variation as possible. At the same time, careful note
is taken of whether any adverse effects ensue.
Experimental trials are suited to the first test
of any new therapeutic measure, and ensure
minimal risk with close supervision. They are
intended to indicate quickly and relatively
inexpensively whether a treatment is worth
further investigation.

Community trials are for treatments that
are known to have useful effects, to ascertain
whether those effects make any difference in a
realistic population under the normal conditions of practice by a wide range of operators.

Some manufacturers apparently do not
know the difference between these two types
of trial and spend huge sums of money before
they know whether a treatment is worth that
sort of investment.

Table 15,2: *Some differences between experimental and community clinical trials*

Factor	Experimental trial	Community trial
The agent or method	Does it work?	How well does it work?
Trial conditions	Specially selected	Normal practice
Theoretical basis	Null hypothesis	Decision theory
Controls	Negative, e.g. placebo	Positive, or comparative
Operators	Academic researchers	Practitioners
Subjects	Specially selected	Patients in the community

After O'Mullane DM (1976) Efficiency in clinical trials of caries preventive agents and methods. *Community Dentistry and Oral
Epidemiology* 4: 190–194.

STATISTICAL AND CLINICAL SIGNIFICANCE

It was quite apparent in the two trials discussed (Abstracts 15,1 and 15,2) that there were statistically significant differences. This means that there was only a small probability of the difference occurring by chance. The probability is expressed as the 'P' level: for instance, a chance of less than 1 chance in 20 is stated as P<0.05. This is a statement about the reality of the difference. The lower the value of P, the more likely it is that the difference is real and not an experimental error.

The 'P' level tells us absolutely nothing about the *size* of the difference. It may be a real difference but very, very small. The present author found a difference of P<0.0000000001 in one of his studies, meaning that there was less than one chance in ten billion that the difference arose from experimental error. However, the percentage difference between the two effects under comparison was about 20%, which means that it was rather small.

The clinical difference in the two trials (Abstracts 15,1 and 15,2) was real but small. How do we interpret it? Unfortunately for manufacturers, the best interpretation takes into account cost-effectiveness. How much does it cost to produce a 20% improvement in the depth of a pocket? If it doubles the cost of treatment, it is plainly exorbitant. Consider the trial in Abstract 11,5: what is the cost of a 2-week course of tetracycline capsules? It is very low, and the benefit is to increase the effect of non-surgical treatment by 50% of PD and 100% of PAL. In absolute terms, the PD reduction of 1 mm was enhanced by 0.5 mm and the PAL improvement of 0.5 mm was enhanced by a further 0.5 mm. This is minimal cost for maximal benefit, and plainly in the interest of the patient.

In the trial in Abstract 15,2 the benefit was around 45% in PD and 30% in PAL. This benefit is difficult to assess: perhaps, in the more realistic conditions of dental practice, the scaling and root planing does not reach the level of results produced in good research studies; alternatively, it might be said that the reduced effect of instrumentation actually helps the adjunct to show an effect, and that it is of most help in this situation. But the chlorhexidine chip also is expensive. Does an improvement of 0.2–0.3 mm make any clinical difference?

What is the ultimate criterion by which such treatments should be judged? Plainly, the patient's objectives (see Table 1,2) are of importance. Does the treatment make any difference to any of these? If tooth retention is the ultimate aim of periodontics, does spending £40 or more on treating one site with a local application make the difference between keeping and losing a tooth?

There is good evidence that mechanical and surgical treatment of periodontitis will help to keep teeth that otherwise would be lost. However, some adjunctive treatments are very expensive and contribute very little. The decision to use them must be made in the light of all known evidence about the effects of such treatments. There may be some situations where the expected benefit is appropriate for the cost.

TRIALS AND COHORT STUDIES

There are many cohort studies in the literature. These studies are essentially collections of case histories regarding one particular treatment. Their results sometimes seem rather optimistic in comparison to the results of trials, and there may be several reasons for this.

The best cohort studies take a consecutive series of cases and assess them, but there is always a temptation to omit those cases that seem to respond atypically to treatment. Thus, someone who simply deteriorated might be omitted and even written up as an exceptional case in another paper, instead of being included with the others who improved. A trial imposes a discipline on the investigators.

Some excellent cohort studies appear in the literature. One of the best is given in Abstract 15,3: a 14-year follow-up of a group of patients given thorough periodontal treatment. For ethical reasons, of course, no control group was possible. However, it is possible to compare the results with those of epidemiological studies where no treatment was given.

Abstract 15,3 *Long-term maintenance of patients treated for advanced periodontal disease*

Lindhe J, Nyman S, *Journal of Clinical Periodontology* 1984; **11**: 504–514

In 1969, 75 patients were treated thoroughly for very advanced periodontitis and 61 were followed up for a full 14 years (3 died and 11 moved). Mean individual plaque and gingival indices were reduced during treatment from around 1.3 to 0.3 and maintained there. Mean attachment levels improved slightly during treatment (6.1 to 5.4 mm) and remained constant thereafter, along with bone scores. Deeper pockets improved more, but shallow pockets lost clinical attachment. Over the whole period, 43 surfaces in 15 patients had significant recurrent periodontal disease, leading to the loss of 16 teeth in seven patients. Caries and periapical pathology led to the loss of 14 other teeth.

Comment: This cohort study reflects a number of findings in other investigations. Because no control group was ethically permissible, the authors compared their results with those of epidemiological investigations in Sweden and the USA. They suggested that progression of disease affected 20–30 times as many sites in untreated populations.

Trials frequently seem to give smaller improvements for active treatments than some cohort studies. It is possible that bias is the main reason for this. The absence of a control group means that other reasons for improvements go unnoticed.

RANDOM SAMPLES AND BLINDING

A random sample is quite a precise concept. It means that in any population, each member has an equal chance of being selected. This is fine where the population is really large and a random number table, coin-tossing or similar method is used for selection of the sample.

But what does random mean in any trial where matching is involved to make sure that the two or more samples are equivalent?

The randomization appropriate to testing a treatment against placebo in matched pairs is that each member of the pair has an equal chance of being given the treatment. By this important technique, the two samples are equivalent but one possible bias is avoided. This was the method used for the trial in Abstract 15,1, for instance.

Hand-in-hand with randomization, 'blinding' is another technique for avoiding bias. If the patient knows which treatment is used, a biased response may ensue. If the operator knows, bias may affect the treatment or its assessment, or both. In some situations, a single-blind trial is all that is possible, such as when the patient is either undergoing treatment or not, as in Abstract 14,13. The operators making the essential measurements in that trial did not know whether the patient had been treated or not. The patients, however, were aware of whether they had received treatment.

In a double-blind trial, neither the patients nor the operators know who has received the treatment, as in the studies in Abstracts 15,1 and 15,2. There is a joke among researchers about a 'triple-blind' trial, which means that the trial administration is so bad that no-one knows which patient has had which treatment.

NOT-SO-OBVIOUS BIAS: HAWTHORNE EFFECT AND OPERATOR BIAS

In a large workshop in the late 1920s, a fascinating effect was demonstrated for the first time. It was in the Hawthorne workshop of the Western Electric Company in the USA, and so it was called the Hawthorne effect. The company interviewed a large number of workers to ask them how they thought workplace improvements could improve the industrial output. The results showed that many workers had significant ideas on this matter, but before anything was changed, productivity improved. The natural interpretation of this phenomenon was that someone was taking an interest in the workers and they felt better as a result and worked more efficiently.

In the world of dentistry, the Hawthorne effect is most likely to be manifest when patients can do something to alter their clinical condition. The most obvious situation for this is when they may improve plaque control and so affect dental diseases. The example in Abstract 14,13 is not absolutely clear, although the authors interpreted it this way. What they said in effect was 'These control patients have reduced their plaque, because they have simply been enrolled in a clinical trial. Someone has measured their plaque, and directed their attention to this matter, and they have improved as a result.'

However, there are other possible explanations; for instance, the scoring of plaque is an operator activity, and the operator might have felt (subconsciously) that the scores should get less, and so they did. This might easily have happened because there is always a decision to make about which of two adjacent scores should be recorded. If it is between a score of 2 and 3, then operators might round down to a 2 under certain conditions, and round up to a 3 under other conditions. We are all more subjective than we like to think.

Another problem is hidden operator bias. The simplest example of this is when an adjunct is added to surgical periodontal treatment. A very good example of how it may be avoided is given in Abstract 19,11. In this study, paired clinical lesions were subject randomly to flap surgery or to flap surgery with a GTR membrane. Now if the operator thinks that GTR is a good thing, this might result in better debridement of the lesion before the membrane is placed, and vice versa.

To prevent this possibility, these researchers ensured that the operator prepared both sites in a patient before the decision was made as to which site should have the membrane. Many studies have appeared in the literature where some adjunct to surgery has been tested, but without this obvious precaution against operator bias.

TWO TYPES OF ERROR AND THE POWER OF THE TRIAL

In clinical trials, two types of mistake are possible. We have already seen the two types of error in relation to clinical measurement in Chapter 10. The trial is an attempt to find out whether there is a difference between treatments. If there is in reality no difference, and the investigators conclude that the trial shows one, then they have made a Type I error. Most trials are carefully designed to avoid this error, and set a level of risk – usually 1 in 20, or less – above which there is said to be no difference. The actual level of risk can be calculated from the trial results, and is stated in the form 'P<0.05'.

In relation to a trial, Type I error is of considerable significance. In a trial, we test a 'null hypothesis' that two treatments do not differ in their outcome. If we reject the hypothesis, we examine the result to see which treatment is better.

However, acceptance of the null hypothesis (H_0) may also involve an error. If the investigators conclude that there is no difference (accept the null hypothesis) on the basis of the results of their trial, and there actually is a difference in reality, then they have made a Type II error. The result is to discard a useful treatment or to conclude that something has no effect, when in fact it does. The main cause of this error is where there are too few subjects in a trial. Where no difference is found, the best trials contain a calculation of how likely this error was, usually stated as the 'power of the trial', or alternatively as the probability of Type II error.

Statisticians have developed ways of assessing the risk of being wrong when we consider the results of a clinical trial. They give the symbol α to the probability of Type I error, setting a risk, say, of a 1 in 20 chance of making this error. Then they can calculate from the trial results the probability of wrongly saying that there is no effect in the treatment under test, i.e. of Type II error (β). This can all come out of the data from the trial (Table 15,3).

Then they calculate the power of the trial. This is 1-β, and is defined as the probability of

Table 15,3: *Type I and II errors and the power of a clinical trial*

The situation in reality	The result of the clinical trial	
	No difference	Difference
No difference	Correct (accept H_0)	Type I error (wrongly reject H_0) (α)
Difference	Type II error (wrongly accept H_0) (β)	Correct (reject H_0) (1-β)

rightly rejecting the null hypothesis. The study in Abstract 14,13 shows the use of this quantity. The power of the trial (1-β) is dependent on numbers: the larger the trial, the more likely we are to be right when we conclude that the treatment has no effect. But if we want actual probabilities, then 1-β gives them to us. If a study concludes there is no effect in a treatment, always ask what the power of the trial was. In other words, if the trial shows no effect for the treatment, what are the chances that it was a wrong result?

HAVE THEY FUDGED THE STATISTICS?

One of the best examples of statistic fudging comes from a fringe trial. It was a study of a so-called dietary supplement called coenzyme Q10. The present author reviewed the whole question of this substance and its effects on periodontal diseases after patients came back saying that they did not want to go on with their periodontal treatment because they were convinced that this substance was a new miracle cure.

The review was published in the *British Dental Journal* (Watts, 1995) and it pointed out that only one of numerous studies quoted by the manufacturers gave enough detail for an assessment of its evidence. In this study, there was a large baseline difference between the patients who took the supplement and those who took placebo. Four weeks later, the difference had increased by the tiniest of amounts and as a result was now statistically significant.

Of course, it was nonsense to claim that this was a significant result for the treatment,

because the baseline difference was almost as large. No details of the statistics were given in the study and it was obvious that the correct technique had not been used.

LONGITUDINAL CHANGES AND CONTROL GROUPS

When someone claims that a beneficial change has occurred in a control group in a periodontal trial, it is time to take a long hard look. One interesting study many years ago was performed by researchers of the highest calibre (see Abstract 16,2).

In this study, after 3 years of controlled oral hygiene in a test group of children, with a suitable control group, the experiment stopped. One year later, there was a surprise re-examination of both groups. We will discuss the actual result in Chapter 16, but for now there is one particular claim of the researchers that we should examine.

In essence, the difference between the groups, which became substantial over the 3 years of the experiment, had declined to non-significance 1 year afterwards. The researchers noted that the test group had declined in its scores. But they also said that the control group had somehow improved, and went to some lengths to try to explain this.

The study did not show any improvement of the control group nor, for that matter, any deterioration of the test group. The measurements used were not up to that level. What they unambiguously showed was that at 3 years there was a better condition in the test group, and that 1 year later the difference had vanished. This is the whole purpose of having a control group. Our measurements are subjective and we vary in making them. However, we can tell if there is a difference between groups at any stage in the study. Longitudinal differences are much harder to pin down and more elusive when using subjective periodontal measurements.

When probes are used in a trial, any probing measurement – bleeding or PD, etc. – may vary over the time of the study. However, there are occasions when a longitudinal comparison may be made. If the trial investigators used a constant-force or automated probe, and tried to probe the same points by using a stent or onlay, then we may attach some credence to longitudinal change. Otherwise, we should not do so: the trial is simply not up to it.

CONCLUSION

The perfect trial has not been performed. Many very good studies have appeared in the periodontal literature, but all good researchers in this field find fault with their own work. The Cochrane Collaboration is performing a painstaking and difficult long-term task in reviewing systematically the trials literature to analyse the evidence on many forms of treatment. An example of a Cochrane-style review is given in Abstract 2,1.

The difficulty is that researchers, although disciplined in their own trials, do not conform to each other's approaches. In time it may be possible for people to agree on what they measure in clinical trials and how they design their studies. For the present, we may read what is published and apply our own critical and analytical talents to them.

16

BEHAVIOURAL FACTORS IN PERIODONTAL TREATMENT

- How do people learn?
- What factors influence patients' behaviour?
- What are the main barriers to periodontally favourable behaviour?
- How may we encourage patients towards such behaviour?

Much periodontal disease is behaviour mediated. Plaque control, smoking and various other behaviours may affect the onset, presentation and severity of periodontitis. Even where other factors affect the progress of disease, as in early-onset periodontitis, the control of relevant behaviour is central to treatment.

To understand the determinants of a person's behaviour is not always possible. Yet the clinician should be aware of what may help and what may hinder the task of treatment. Case History 3 shows an unusual situation in which a patient's behavioural history was the key to correct treatment.

CASE HISTORY 3: an obsessive patient with oral ulceration

A 23-year-old patient was referred by her general dental practitioner, presenting with ulcers resembling major apthae and varying from 5 to 15 mm diameter on the attached and marginal gingiva in all parts of her mouth. She was accompanied by both parents and had a history of psychiatric treatment, apparently for depressive illness. There was no further significant medical history; the patient had received no medication either then or in the recent past. The ulcers had occurred repeatedly over a period of 3 months, without any relation to menstrual cycle or other factors. Examination revealed no significant

dental problems of any sort. The periodontal findings included a plaque score of virtually zero, minimal labial gingival recession of 1 mm on several anterior teeth, no other attachment loss and gingival bleeding on probing only adjacent to ulcers. In other respects, the patient appeared healthy. Special tests gave results within normal limits for differential blood cell counts, haemoglobin and indices, and there were no abnormal film appearances. Urine tests revealed no abnormality. At the next appointment, on further review of the dental history, it was found that the patient had been instructed in oral hygiene a short time before the onset of the ulcers. She used a version of the scrub technique and proximally, an interdental brush and woodsticks. What was unusual was the excessive vigour and frequency of her brushing, which she performed five or six times daily, for more than 5 min on each occasion.

DIAGNOSIS

Traumatic ulceration resulting from excessive toothbrushing.

MANAGEMENT

She was advised to cease all toothbrushing forthwith, and to use a 0.2% chlorhexidine mouthrinse 12-hourly for 3 weeks. At that time, all ulceration had disappeared. The patient was then instructed to stop using the mouthrinse and to brush firmly only once each day, and to use a gentle technique for the application of fluoride toothpaste on no more than two other occasions each day. When reviewed 3 months later, she had well-maintained healthy periodontal tissues and there had been no recurrence of ulceration.

COMMENT

It was apparent that the patient responded with extreme obedience and deference to her parents and to other authority figures such as dentists, and had a strong obsessional tendency. This apparently caused her ulcers and was also the key to resolving the problem.

Two further case histories (Case Histories 4 and 5) are strong testimony to the effects of stress in many human lives.

CASE HISTORY 4: a clinical psychologist with severe stress problems where dental intervention had probably increased the effects

A 29-year-old clinical psychologist from Los Angeles attended a UK dental hospital. He was referred to the periodontal department primarily because his problems involved occlusion and hypermobility. The immediate cause of his attendance was that tooth 23, bearing a jacket crown abutment off which a pontic for 22 was cantilevered, had fractured horizontally at the neck. He had woken in the night to find the bridge loose in his mouth. In addition, several of his posterior teeth felt loose and about half of them were extremely tender to gentle pressure. On examination, oral hygiene was excellent with no visible plaque; the periodontal condition, likewise, was excellent with no bleeding on probing and a 4-mm probing depth only on tooth 14 distal, with 1 mm of attachment loss. All molar teeth and the right-hand premolars had gold inlays with occlusal coverage, and the patient stated that these were placed by his dentist to compensate for marked tooth wear. Fremitus was elicited from the mobile teeth and some occlusal prematurities were apparent. There

were no other significant clinical findings. All teeth except tooth 23 gave positive vitality test responses, and radiographic examination yielded no further information.

DIAGNOSIS

Bruxism, initially caused by personal stress, subsequently exacerbated by occlusal interferences.

MANAGEMENT

On being informed of the psychological stress component of his problems, the patient decided to undertake some measures for 'stress relaxation'. Occlusal equilibration was performed, tooth 23 was root treated and a new bridge was constructed to replace tooth 22 with abutments on teeth 23, 21 and 11 and special attention to occlusal aspects of design. Although there was residual hypermobility in some teeth 3 months later, all the patient's pain symptoms had disappeared within 1 week of equilibration.

COMMENT

Psychology may be a stressful occupation. This patient required minor attention to his occlusion. The major problem was his stress-related tendency to brux, and this was best treated by someone other than a dentist. Once he understood the problem, as a psychologist he knew what to do.

CASE HISTORY 5: a patient in whom marked hypermobility without attachment loss was related to child abuse 35 years before

A 43-year-old housewife was referred by her general practitioner with a problem of 3–4 mm labial gingival recession on teeth 31 and 41. On examination, oral hygiene was good, there was no other significant periodontal pathology and it was decided to observe the lesions. One year later, the recession was unchanged but the patient complained of hypermobility in some teeth and a tendency to brux at nights. Several teeth were shown to have increased mobility, despite no attachment loss.

DIAGNOSIS

Bruxism related to personal stress.

MANAGEMENT

The patient was advised to seek counselling in relation to the stresses that had caused her to start bruxing, and an occlusal bite guard was constructed. Three months later, the patient reported that she had discontinued use of the bite guard following a resolution of her bruxing problems, and now felt completely comfortable. During counselling, it had become apparent that the major cause of her stress was an episode of sexual abuse that she had suffered at the age of 8 years. Once she had resolved an irrational but emotionally pressing urge to feel guilty for what she had suffered, the whole matter was successfully dealt with. Two years later, the patient was still free of bruxism and occlusal problems, and reported a 'contented life'.

COMMENT

The dentist feels helpless with bruxists and tries to give symptomatic relief related to the occlusion. A more appropriate treatment may be referral to a counsellor or clinical psychologist for help in coping with life's stresses.

We shall look at bruxism and parafunction again in Chapter 25; for the moment, it is important to note that personal stress may produce effects in the periodontium. Patients with problems of psychological origin need to be treated with the methods of psychology.

BEHAVIOUR-RELATED TREATMENT OBJECTIVES

Without good plaque control, much periodontal treatment is futile. Priority must therefore be given to establishing suitable oral hygiene practices in the patient's life. If we go about this in the wrong way, the result will be frustration. Teaching is not simply a matter of providing information.

Another periodontal adverse behaviour is tobacco smoking. This is stress-related behaviour also, and it carries penalties in patients with periodontitis. Some dentists do not see it as their job to encourage patients to give up smoking, but it is hard to see how we can escape our responsibility. There is also the highly significant matter of preventing oral tumours.

It is therefore clear that the dentist is in the business of education, and also of stress counselling and addiction management in the preliminary phase. These are not easy tasks. A dentist may provide useful, informed encouragement as a health professional, and act as an intermediary with other channels of health education, such as the medical practitioner and the UK Smoking Quitline.

COMMUNICATION AND INFORMATION

The relationship of communication and information may be illustrated by one of the superb wildlife programmes produced by the BBC in the UK, or the National Geographic Society in the USA. As communication of the fascinating world of natural history, these television presentations are without equal. They are put together with considerable attention to continuity. Every programme tells a story. Sometimes a single photograph may do the same (Fig. 16,1)

How much information is actually transmitted in a 50-min programme? Next time

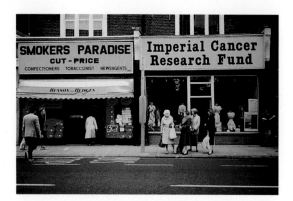

Fig. 16,1

This photograph was taken a few years ago in Palmer's Green, north London. It tells a story about human behaviour. The shop on the left was trying hard to make money whilst incidentally causing cancer; the shop on the right was trying hard to raise money to fight cancer. (Photograph courtesy of Mr Malcolm Lawrence.)

you watch one, wait a few days and see how much new information you can remember. Trying this test with dental students some years ago, the author arrived at a conclusion well-evidenced elsewhere: approximately two pieces of new information may be retained from such a programme by the average viewer.

For communication to be maximal, information needs to be kept minimal. There is an inverse relationship between these two important features of education. If the information is a blitz of facts, hardly any will be learned. If we want our patients to learn, then we must maximize the quality of communication. At the same time, we must refrain from drowning them with information. People want to remember what is pleasant.

EDUCATION AND LEARNING

Two classic series of studies in the literature are a good basis for understanding what constitutes dental education and what its effect may be at a later date. The first study is summarized in Abstracts 16,1 and 16,2: a trial of supervised oral hygiene in children aged

Abstract 16,1 *The effect of supervised oral hygiene on the gingiva of children. Progression and inhibition of gingivitis*

Lindhe J, Koch G, *Journal of Periodontal Research* 1966; **1**: 260–267

In a Swedish school, two randomly selected groups of children originally aged 9–10 years constituted the experimental and control groups in this study. After 3 years in which the experimental group had received daily toothbrushing supervision by a trained dental nurse, both groups were examined for plaque and gingivitis on incisors and first molars. The mean control Plaque Index was 1.62 and the GI was 0.95; respective experimental group scores were 0.7 and 0.24. Both between-group differences were highly significant (P<0.001).

Comment: At the start of this study, the Plaque Index and GI had not been published. It is assumed that with the sample size there were likely to have been baseline similarities, and in the light of the next study this assumption is justified.

9–10 years at the start of the study. After 3 years, there was a substantial difference in plaque and gingivitis scores between the

Abstract 16,2 *The effect of supervised oral hygiene on the gingiva of children. Lack of prolonged effect of supervision*

Lindhe J, Koch G, *Journal of Periodontal Research* 1967; **2**: 215–220

One year after completion of the study in Abstract 16,1, all 64 children were re-examined. During the year, there had been no special toothbrushing supervision of either group. The mean Plaque Index was 1.34 in the control group and 1.36 in the experimental group; respective GI scores were 0.66 and 0.47. Neither between-group difference was significant (P>0.05).

Comment: The apparent improvement in the control scores should be disregarded, because examiner standards may vary from one year to the next. What matters is that the difference apparent a year earlier had now vanished.

Abstract 16,3 *The effect of controlled oral hygiene procedures on the progression of periodontal disease in adults: results after third and final year*

Suomi JD, Greene JC, Vermillion JR, et al., *Journal of Periodontology* 1971; **42**: 152–160

This celebrated study took place in two offices of a large American corporation, and consisted of three control and two experimental groups that were computer-matched in pairs. Initially, there were 560 controls, 452 experimental subjects and the mean age was 31 years. Control subjects were advised to continue with their usual professional care and oral hygiene practices; experimental subjects were given repeated oral hygiene education and professional oral prophylaxis on 11 occasions over a 3-year period. All groups had similar mean scores for all oral parameters at the baseline examination. After drop-out and computer rematching of groups, at the end of 3 years there were 216 experimental subjects and 269 controls. The controls showed significantly more plaque, gingivitis and attachment loss than the experimental subjects. The largest control group lost attachment at an average of 0.1 mm per year.

Comment: This study was large enough to show that controls lost attachment about 3.5 times as fast as the experimental subjects who received treatment. The rate is similar to that of the Norwegian group originally enlisted for comparison in the Sri Lankan study.

Abstract 16,4 *A follow-up study of former participants in a controlled oral hygiene study*

Suomi JD, Leatherwood EC, Chang JJ, *Journal of Periodontology* 1973; **44**: 662–666

Two years and eight months after the study in Abstract 16,3, a full examination was performed for 275 original participants who were traced. A lesser but useful difference in plaque and gingivitis was still present in the experimental group, and they retained their full attachment loss difference with the control group. The authors comment that such persistent preventive efforts may produce beneficial and long-lasting results.

Comment: This is very different from the study in children in Abstract 16,2. The methods in the present study are not appropriate to children in the same way; they tend to relate to their parents in the first decade and later on, in adolescence, to their peer group.

supervised and control groups.

Supervision then ceased. One year later, the effect had disappeared. In contrast, the much larger study in adults shown in Abstracts 16,3 and 16,4 was a deliberate attempt to educate. This study also included a professional prophylaxis in addition to OHI at the frequent maintenance visits during the 3 years. However, all attention was discontinued subsequently until the follow-up examination. This showed a persistent difference between groups and could be interpreted reasonably as evidence of an improvement in plaque control behaviour in the experimental group. Education may have a lasting effect but it takes careful planning and significant effort.

KAB AND HEALTH BELIEF MODELS

Over the past 30 years, our understanding of health-related behaviour has increased. It is clear that the model of health behaviour underlying many former attempts at education is largely invalid. This is the KAB model – impart Knowledge to change Attitude, which will then improve Behaviour.

Study after study has shown that knowledge does not always ensure appropriate behaviour. Giving knowledge is of little use on its own.

A more complex model of behaviour thought to be more relevant is the 'health beliefs' model. This model is a complex set of beliefs involving lifestyle, hygiene, living practices and priorities at the centre of our oral hygiene. To be more precise, oral hygiene is at the periphery of our health beliefs. For us as dentists, dental health should be near the centre of our lives; for our patients, we can make no such assumption.

The subject is enormous. A typical study exploring patient compliance (Abstract 16,5) identified some related health beliefs, but

Abstract 16,5 *The effect of health beliefs on the compliance of periodontal patients with oral hygiene instructions*

Kühner MK, Raetzke PB, *Journal of Periodontology* 1989; **60**: 51–56

A questionnaire was given to 120 patients at a German dental school who were compliant during the hygiene phase of treatment; 96 completed forms were returned. Demographic variables and some health beliefs (e.g. susceptibility, dentist-patient relationship, experience with therapy) did not relate to compliance measured by gingival bleeding. A number of health beliefs were identified that did correlate, including motivation, seriousness, benefits and experience with affected organ. Combined predictor variables (correlations 0.17–0.32) gave a correlation of 0.59.

Comment: This study illustrates the complexity of health beliefs. There is likely to be no simple predictor of hygiene behaviour.

with low levels of correlation. Another study (see Abstract 14,8) examined a variety of beliefs, including locus of control, but only found a clear correlation (which was low: less than 0.4) with good oral hygiene if the patient expressed an intent to comply.

POSITIVE AND NEGATIVE HEALTH BEHAVIOUR

Although we encourage patients to adopt positive health behaviour, we also need to mention avoidance of negative health behaviour. Good oral hygiene is the most obvious positive behaviour. Smoking tobacco is an example of a negative health behaviour, but it is more than this.

In the 1960s in the USA, tobacco companies knew that nicotine created addiction. Not only that, but in some cases they even tried to make it more addictive: detailed information may be found on many Internet sites, such as that of Action on Smoking and Health (ASH).

Consequently, some of our patients today would dearly like to quit the habit but find it next to impossible.

Our role is partly to inform. We need to ensure that the truth is known, and give patients further angles on why it is a good idea to quit the habit.

The next stage in the dentist's role against smoking is to point the patient in the right direction for advice and help. Most family doctors can help. Quit rates are approximately doubled if treatments such as nicotine patches are employed. The aforementioned Smoking Quitline provides a UK base for those attempting to fight nicotine addiction: 0800 00 22 00.

THE DENTIST AS A ROLE MODEL

When talking of oral hygiene, it is more personal and supportive if we can advise from our own experience. It is certainly a good idea for us not to smoke. Some years ago, a humorous article on personal odour (McCormick, 1993) quoted research suggesting that if a 'standard person' who takes 0.7 baths per day has an odour of 1 'olf', then a person who is smoking rates as 25 olfs and a smoker who is not smoking has about 6 olfs of body odour.

A pleasant, sympathetic manner goes a long way towards ensuring a degree of confidence in our abilities. It also helps if we explain technical matters in simple language. One form of professional insecurity takes refuge in technical language that is unfamiliar to most patients. Many patients still associate us with pain. Smiling and shaking hands helps to reduce the barriers that may separate us from patients.

As dentists, we should foster those aspects of our behaviour that we want to see in our patients. It is questionable whether there is any other professional who comes so close to the client that the latter may study the inside of the professional's nose (in the absence of a mask). Oral hygiene is also of prime importance, particularly from the aspect of avoiding halitosis.

LEARNING AND MOTIVES

The word 'motivation' is widely used to describe a process by which the dentist or hygienist somehow converts the patient from a careless individual into a prodigy who regularly removes every last trembling microbe from every surface of every tooth. In fact, this is a misuse of language. If the patient lacks essential motives, then he or she is probably suffering from clinical depression.

The process described is really one of learning. It makes use of motives that the patient already has, such as the desires to be clean, to have a healthy body and not to spend life's accumulated wealth on acquiring a mouth full of implants and bridgework in old age.

When we link up to patients' existing motives, the learning process becomes relatively straight-forward. With a typical adult, it is wise to assume an intention to co-operate from the beginning. We and the patient are on the same side in a battle against disease, and although it may be necessary gently to correct some misconceptions, the dentist should always have the attitude of a helper and show it in action.

SKILLS CANNOT BE LEARNED FROM THE BACK OF A PACKET

When patients are asked to learn a skill, they need support. Support means more than words. In the next chapter, we shall discuss how best to introduce patients to effective oral hygiene procedures. If this is not performed well, then no lasting effect can be achieved.

Knowledge may be acquired by reading, listening or watching. A skill may only be acquired by practising it. Every patient needs to be led through the procedures of oral hygiene, feeling the sensations and understanding it from the viewpoint of a *participant*. A person with the knowledge and experience of a dentist may be able to learn an oral hygiene procedure without being taught, but that is a severe task to set any patient.

CONCLUSION

To summarize, a full diagnosis should include relevant psychological factors. Dental intervention should not be undertaken without attention to psychological causes; for instance, there are other possible causes of hypermobility besides attachment loss. There may be times too when we should advise the patient that a lifestyle alteration is desirable (such as quitting smoking), and suggest a course of action.

Our patients need various types of help to achieve the targets that we set them. There are corresponding barriers that will impede the process (Table 16,1). We need to cultivate an attitude that asks: 'What is the patient's view of what I am doing?'

Table 16,1: *Factors that may affect oral hygiene education*

Positive factors	Adverse factors
Involve the patient in dialogue: ask for questions and comments	Talking *at* the patient
Ensure the patient is comfortable	A sense of tension: surroundings should not obtrude
Demonstrate the patient's condition	Use of technical jargon
Show causal factors	Failure to use a mirror
Show the remedy: help the patient to practise it	Dentist words without patient action
Encourage and praise	Blaming the patient by inference or by implication
Check subsequently and gently correct	Undue repetition

17

ORAL HYGIENE

- Why are some methods ineffective in plaque control?
- Which hygiene aids may be of use in plaque control?
- What may oral hygiene realistically achieve?

A huge mass of evidence continues to accumulate in support of the well-established fact that bacterial plaque is causally related to periodontal inflammation, attachment loss, recession and most types of gingival enlargement. In large populations, oral cleanliness is associated with the level of periodontal destruction (Chapter 6); if plaque is removed regularly from teeth that have had advanced periodontitis, they subsequently have a greatly reduced likelihood of disease progression (see Abstract 15,3); and if plaque control is improved and maintained, gingivitis and periodontitis levels are also reduced (see Abstracts 16,1–16,4). Provided that plaque is controlled at a level that prevents BOP (see Abstract 5,1), further disease probably can be prevented (Fig. 17,1).

It follows that removal of plaque is the basic treatment for periodontal diseases of many kinds.

If plaque accumulates for up to 21 days in a healthy mouth, it will usually lead to clinically obvious gingivitis, with BOP (see Abstract 2,5). Clearly, this does not mean that we only need to remove plaque every 21 days. Inflammation does not resolve immediately, and the same study showed that it might take as long as 10 days to return the tissues to normal.

FREQUENCY OF PLAQUE CONTROL FOR PERIODONTAL HEALTH

With healthy periodontal tissues, it seems that if you clean the plaque off the teeth every other day, you will maintain that state of health (Abstract 17,1). However, somewhere between 2- and 3-day plaque control intervals there is the dividing line between maintained health and gradually developing disease.

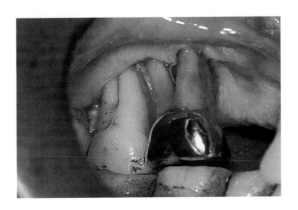

Fig. 17,1

Teeth 16 and 17 have advanced attachment loss but they are maintained without clinical inflammation by the patient's excellent plaque control, and have been healthy without change for 1 year, following rapid attachment loss in a non-insulin-dependent diabetic patient.

Abstract 17,1 *Toothbrushing frequency as it relates to plaque development and gingival health*

Lang NP, Cumming BR, Löe H, *Journal of Periodontology* 1973; **44**: 396–405

Thirty-two dental students with clean teeth and healthy gingiva were randomized to four groups and assessed weekly for 6 weeks. The four groups removed all plaque respectively every 12 h, every 48 h, every 72 h and every 96 h. The 12-h group maintained a Plaque Index of around 0.5–0.8, whereas the other three groups eventually reached a plateau of around 1.5. However, the Gingival Index for both the 12-h and 48-h group reached a plateau of around 0.1–0.2 and stayed there from 4 weeks onwards, whereas the 72-h group steadily climbed to 0.5 at 6 weeks and the 96-h group reached 0.9 at the same point.

Comment: It is interesting that the increased plaque of the 48-h group did not have the same consequences as the similar quantities in the 72-h and 96-h groups; as the authors stated, this points to factors other than quantity having a role in plaque pathogenicity.

How do we best use this finding? Obviously the maximum recommended interval for periodontal plaque control is 2 days, but what other factors enter into the recommendation? First we should note that the regime is sufficient to maintain existing gingival health. If gingival health is not present, it must first be attained, and perhaps pockets full of plaque will mean that we should clean our teeth more frequently.

Secondly, there is the very important matter of habitual human behaviour. If we do something at regular intervals, certain intervals are easier to remember than others. We may change our underwear each day, put out the dustbins each week, pay the credit card bill each month and turn the mattress each quarter day. But what do we do every other day? Not much, and therefore such a habit is harder to remember. For these two reasons, therefore, many periodontists suggest that a thorough plaque removal should be performed on a daily basis.

We should be careful to encourage optimal use of a fluoride toothpaste for caries control, however, so the patient should be advised to apply the dentifrice two or three times per day, once at the thorough periodontally directed session and in a simpler, gentler way on other occasions. It is also important to minimize the risk of adverse effects of oral hygiene on the teeth and gums, and although this seems to be related to dentifrice abrasivity, the physical vigour of oral hygiene procedures may at least be reduced on the other occasions.

REQUIREMENTS FOR PLAQUE CONTROL TECHNIQUES

It is apparent that personal plaque removal techniques should be effective in the task of control, and have minimal adverse effects, i.e. they should be safe. There are two further requirements: they should be simple to learn and economical in time. Some would also add that they should be inexpensive.

In Table 17,1 some common hygiene techniques are compared. Although there are many comparative studies of efficacy in the literature, none relate specific techniques to the issue of safety with regard to dental abrasion and gingival recession. However, there are many case reports of the dangers of toothpicks (Fig. 17,2). These are seriously

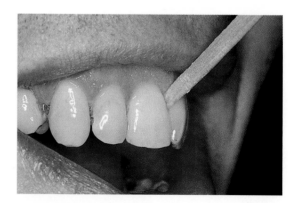

Fig. 17,2

Softwood toothpick in use.

Table 17,1: *Quality of different oral hygiene techniques*

Technique	Effectiveness	Safety (no long term evidence)	Complexity	Economy	
				Time	Cost
Buccal/lingual brushing					
Bass	High		Mid	Mid	Low
Charters	High		Mid	Mid	Low
Roll	Adequate		Mid	Mid	Low
Scrub	High		Low	Low	Low
Proximal					
Woodstick	Mid	Dangers!	Low	Mid	Low
Floss	High		High	Low	Low
Bottle brush	High		Low	Mid	Mid
Concavities					
Bottle brush	High		Low	Low	Mid
Interspace brush	High		Low	Mid	Mid

implicated in adverse effects, frequently through being swallowed.

They have caused perforation of the stomach, duodenum, jejunum, ileum and all parts of the colon, duodenal inflammation, liver abscesses, peritonitis, massive haemorrhage by perforation of the common iliac artery, obstructed a ureter, and even presented as a foreign body in the bladder and foot.

At least three patients have died: one patient was killed by toothpick perforation of the inferior vena cava. A paper in the 1980s estimated that over 8000 toothpick injuries per year occurred in the USA (Budnick, 1984). Children under 5 years were highly susceptible to eye and ear injuries, and the highest injury rate was in those aged 5–14 years.

Because toothpicks are extremely difficult to detect when embedded in tissue and patients do not always realize that they have swallowed them, and because there are other methods of effective and simple oral hygiene, it would seem sensible not to use them in oral hygiene.

TOOTHBRUSHING METHODS

Several methods have been compared in the literature: the popular Bass technique is among them. Bass was a pathologist and the Dean of a US medical school. When his dentist wanted to start removing his teeth because of 'old age', he turned his mind to the problem of periodontitis and its prevention. The result was the Bass method of oral hygiene, which included directing a toothbrush into the gingival crevice, and the use of dental floss to clean proximal surfaces. All this happened in the 1940s, before the explosion of interest in dental plaque in the second half of the 1960s. By the time he died at the age of 100 years in 1975, Bass had seen his method established as a favourite technique of periodontists.

The main problem in comparing the efficacy of oral hygiene techniques is that no one so far has produced a method of studying them in relation to the quantity of subgingival plaque. The nearest we come to a subgingival study is the work of Wærhaug (Abstract 17,2), which examined interdental (bottle) brushes, but this required teeth that were to be extracted.

A typical comparative toothbrushing study is shown in Abstract 17,3. The roll method of brushing has been found less satisfactory than other methods in more than one study. However, no study has shown that a particular method is best.

When patients are instructed in oral hygiene, what toothbrushing method should

Abstract 17,2 *The interdental brush and its place in operative and crown and bridge dentistry*

Wærhaug J, *Journal of Oral Rehabilitation* 1976; **3**: 107–113

In 31 teeth, an interdental brush (a bottle brush) was used prior to extraction to assess its immediate effect. Another 36 teeth were extracted after regular use of the brush for several years. The brush removed plaque in the area under the contact point and the adjacent embrasures. The bristles penetrated up to 2.5 mm subgingivally. Apart from its periodontal effect, this means that subgingival restorative margins may also be cleaned, possibly with a caries preventive effect.

Comment: Another study making maximum use of extracted teeth, from the master of tooth extraction studies. There are few studies as original in concept as some of those by Wærhaug. Several other studies have confirmed a greater effect of interdental brushes on proximal plaque.

Abstract 17,3 *Plaque removal by the Bass and Roll brushing techniques*

Gibson JA, Wade AB, *Journal of Periodontology* 1977; **48**: 456–459

A cross-over study in 38 dental students compared the two techniques. Subjects were asked to avoid dental treatment for the study duration. First, existing plaque was scored, and then fully removed by a hygienist. Subjects were randomly allocated to Bass or Roll twice daily, in each case using a brush suited to the technique. The technique was practised until satisfactory. After 2 weeks, the same procedure was repeated, except that the other technique was then used. The whole 4 weeks was then repeated, using two other suitable brushes. In overall effectiveness, there was no difference between the two techniques in plaque removal; however, when the facial and lingual plaque scores alone were considered, the Bass technique was significantly better. All subjects completed the study.

Comment: This is a small difference and might have made no difference to gingival health, if that had been measured. No proximal hygiene technique was used.

be employed? If the existing method is achieving good plaque control, then it obviously should not be changed. At the outset, the teeth should be disclosed, and the patient shown the findings in a mirror. The significance of the proximal areas should be indicated: they are harder to reach, and they have more disease. If toothbrushing is inadequate, a change of method may be appropriate, and the present author's choice is the Bass technique because it is directed subgingivally (Figs 17,3–17,7).

PROXIMAL CLEANING METHODS

The main choice is between bottle brushes and dental floss. Several studies have shown the former implement to be more effective in removal of supragingival plaque, and we also have the evidence of Wærhaug that the bottle

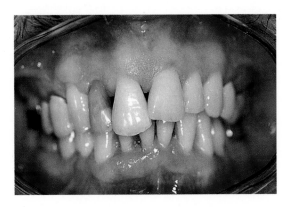

Fig. 17,3

Prior to use of disclosing fluid, this patient's teeth seem well brushed, on the buccal aspect.

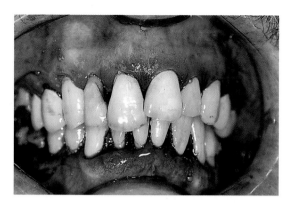

Fig. 17,4

Disclosing fluid now shows proximal plaque deposits. There are also many lingual deposits.

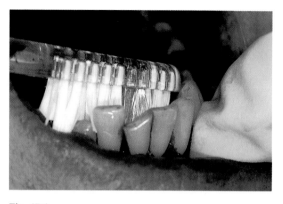

Fig. 17,6

Bass technique: lingual of same teeth. Despite crowding, the brush can reach the crevices.

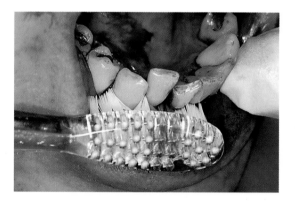

Fig. 17,5

Bass brushing technique: labial of lower anterior teeth. The brush is wriggled, to let the bristles agitate the plaque.

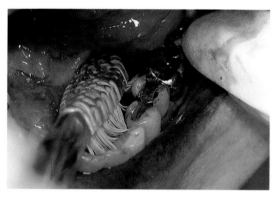

Fig. 17,7

Bass technique: a steep angle for lower posterior lingual surfaces.

brush may remove subgingival plaque also (Abstract 17,2).

However, this implement requires careful use. The bottle brush should be as large as possible, and should not be used where it does not need to be forced between the teeth (Figs 17,8 and 17,9). If it is loose in an interdental gap, there is little chance that it will remove the plaque at the margin. In addition, floss will clean the distal-most surface in the arch and the surfaces of teeth adjacent to saddle areas, but the bottle brush cannot do this because it is flexible and will not press sufficiently hard against the tooth.

Floss may also have an advantage in that once it is learned, it can be used very quickly, and the choice between the two methods is a matter of personal preference. However, for concave surfaces, floss is plainly inadequate (Fig. 17,10).

ONE WAY TO TEACH FLOSSING

The main drawback of floss is that it requires a degree of manual dexterity. Nevertheless, children as young as 8 years of age have been

Table 17,2: *Leading a patient through the steps of learning small-loop flossing*

Showing the application of floss to the lower central incisors
- The patient holds a mirror to view the mouth
- The floss is held by the operator in any convenient way and taken between the teeth, down into the proximal gingival crevice of one of them
- The floss is then moved coronally with firm pressure against the tooth, lifted over the gingival papilla, and used in the same way on the other tooth before being taken out of the gap
- The manoeuvre may be repeated

Showing how to hold the floss
- The patient is invited to break off a length of floss about 1.5 times the size of his or her handspan
- The operator ties a similar length in a loop, using a double knot so that it will not come undone. The patient is asked to do the same
- The operator demonstrates how to hold the loop, and the patient follows suit. In essence the thumbs and first fingers of each hand are kept free to manipulate floss, and the distal three fingers of both hands are used to anchor the loop

Helping the patient to repeat the operator's cleaning manoeuvre
- The patient is guided through the same steps on the lower central incisors
- When the patient has repeated it suffiently to demonstrate the skill, he or she may be asked to clean the next embrasure, and continue to the end of the arch
- At this point the patient is asked to return to the central incisors, and to clean the other quadrant in the same way. Most patients will realize that the hand positions need to be reversed, but if not they may be guided
- After cleaning the lower arch, a similar procedure is employed in the upper arch, again starting from the central incisors

Remember
- The patient needs to see in the mirror
- Patients do not normally work using mirrors, as dentists do. They need guidance
- Praise is given for every achievement of the patient

Instructions for the patient after flossing for the first time
- Do this once per day, and make yourself comfortable in an armchair, with a mirror conveniently placed. The first time will be long, perhaps 20–25 min, so put on some pleasant music to play
- Your target is to floss your teeth in 5 min within 2 weeks. Then you are more likely to keep it up for life
- Two possible problems – sensitivity of teeth in 3–4 days: persevere, and it will go within another 3–4 days; and bleeding: at first this is because the gums are inflamed, but they should stop bleeding within 1 week; after that, it is usually because of nipping the gum (papilla) against the teeth, and the technique needs adjusting

---

taught to floss, although it is doubtful whether they actually needed to. A simple way of teaching the patient is shown in Table 17,2 (Figs 17,11–17,21). It is important that the floss in question should not be one of the new types of slippery floss, because it will be extremely difficult to tie the knot without it coming undone. If the patient is to learn any new oral hygiene method, it will take time. There is no substitute for careful, methodical instruction, leading to the acquisition of a skill to protect the gums for life. It is a mistake to

undertake this important educational task in any way that is not thorough.

CONCAVE SURFACES AND MODERATE POCKETS

There are two ways of entering a concavity on a tooth surface. Where the space is confined, a bottle brush is appropriate, but when the concavity is not in such a space (e.g. facing a saddle area), an interspace brush is better.

The interspace brush is also of use in entering small residual pockets, often on proximal surfaces (Figs 17,22–17,24). A pocket of 5 mm or even more may be maintained in a non-inflamed state by this method.

SELF-ACHIEVED FURCATION TUNNELS (SAFTS)

Some patients with Grade III furcation involvement (Chapter 22) are able to use a bottle brush of suitable size through the lesion without surgical tunnel preparation. The brush is curved to the approximate shape of the tunnel, and firmly pushed through to the other side. The inflammation resolves, the tissues become firm, and the patient is happy at avoiding a possible surgical procedure (Figs 17,25–17,27).

When the tissues have become firm and healthy, they will have shrunk. A larger size of bottle brush may then be needed, and the furcation, like any other, should be explored for attachment loss on the adjacent root surfaces.

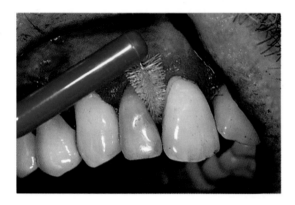

Fig. 17,8

This tapered bottle brush is large enough to fit tightly between the teeth.

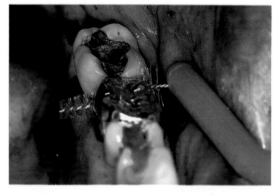

Fig. 17,10

Tapered bottle brush used in a tight posterior interdental gap with concave proximal root surfaces. To ensure full embrasure cleaning, it should also be used from the lingual aspect.

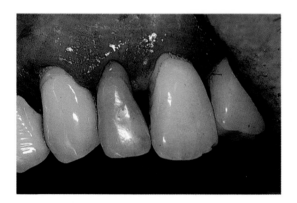

Fig. 17,9

When the brush is removed, it can be seen that the papilla is also clean of disclosing stain.

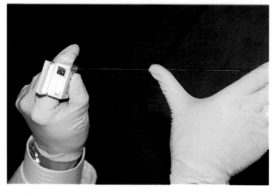

Fig. 17,11

Showing patients how to floss. First, take a piece of floss one-and-a-half times the hand span.

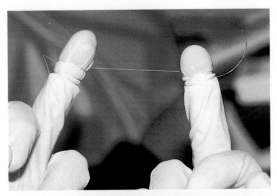

Fig. 17,12

Do not wind floss around the fingers, except for the operator to demonstrate floss in the patient's mouth. We want the patient to learn comfortably.

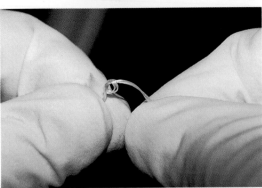

Fig. 17,13

Tie the ends of the floss together with a double knot. If waxed floss is used, scrape off most wax with the thumbnail first. If slippery floss is used, knot-tying becomes an Olympic feat.

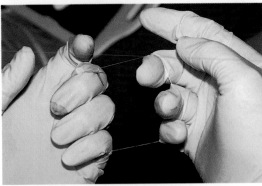

Fig. 17,14

The floss is anchored on the distal three digits of each hand.

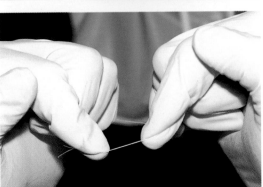

Fig. 17,15

In the lower jaw, forefingers are usually best to guide floss down the teeth.

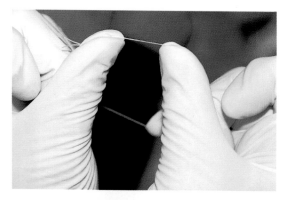

Fig. 17,16

In the upper jaw, thumbs are often preferred, but one may be combined with the fore-finger of the other hand.

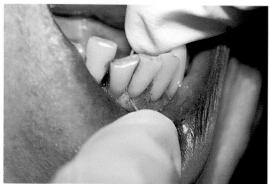

Fig. 17,17

Floss is guided by the operator down the mesial of tooth 31, then taken up and over the interdental papilla.

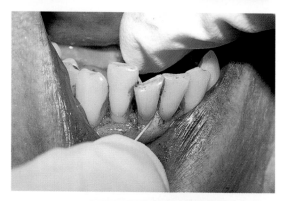

Fig. 17,18

It then reaches the mesial of tooth 41. Note how in each case, the floss curves round the tooth from buccal to lingual without cutting into the papilla.

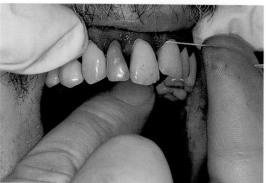

Fig. 17,19

Now the patient is guided, and shown how to take the floss as high (or low) on the lingual aspect as on the buccal aspect.

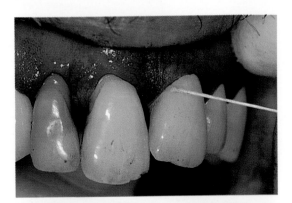

Fig. 17,20

Correctly used, floss does not harm the papilla.

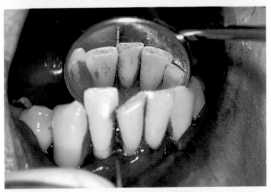

Fig. 17,21

Incorrect use: the floss is beginning to nip the papilla against the distal of tooth 41.

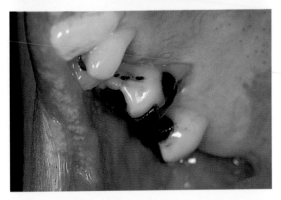

Fig. 17,22

Tooth 15 is missing, and there is a concavity with a 5 mm PD on the mesial of tooth 16.

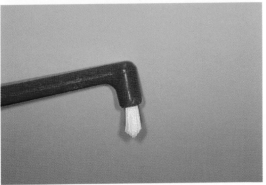

Fig. 17,23

An interspace brush with a pointed end is the best implement to maintain a concavity or a small pocket.

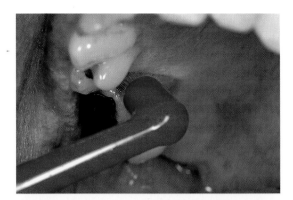

Fig. 17,24

The brush is inserted firmly into the pocket by sliding it up the tooth.

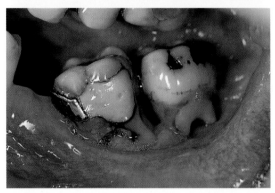

Fig. 17,25

Mirror view of a SAFT. A glass ionomer has been used to restore the tooth after root caries. Note the healthy gingiva just visible in the furcation.

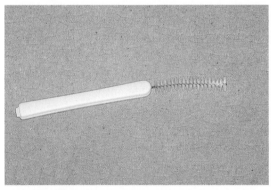

Fig. 17,26

A suitable bottle brush. It should be used with a fluoride toothpaste to resist root caries. Stronger fluoride gels also may be applied according to manufacturers' instructions.

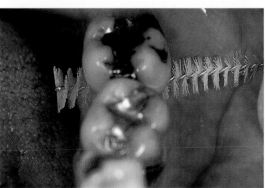

Fig. 17,27

The brush is larger than the SAFT. A few back-and-forth movements are applied each time.

AIDS AND GADGETRY IN ORAL HYGIENE

Oral hygiene is a field in which aids and gadgets have become legion. The main evaluation rule for these devices is the same pragmatic requirement list of effectiveness, safety and ease of use as applies to the various devices and utensils that we have discussed already. However, there is one additional point that should be borne in mind: for some people, an electric device is an object of fascination that almost compels them to use it. Although the disadvantage of cost is obvious with electric toothbrushes, the fun of using them may far outweigh this for many people.

As long as the objective need for plaque removal is satisfied (and a variety of electric brushes have been shown to do this), and the device poses no additional adverse effect, patients who ask about purchasing such devices should be given an appropriate response by the dentist.

In evaluating the vast number of oral hygiene aids, it is clear that the effectiveness requirement must be answered first. Some devices have not been shown to remove plaque, and others are patently unable to do so. An example of the latter is a type of flossing device in the form of a plastic stick with two projections at one end, with floss fixed across the projections. In some cases, the projections are too short to reach the gingival crevice on most teeth, with the plastic stick impacting on the marginal ridges of the posterior dentition. Other floss holders may be more effective, but there is often a flexibility that makes the floss harder to control. In the manual method described above, the active part of the floss may be kept very short and well controlled.

Pulsating water jet devices have not been shown to remove plaque. They reduce debris and were studied as wound-cleansing devices during the US military involvement in Vietnam. However, in recent years their use has been modified to deliver antimicrobial agents such as chlorhexidine into the gingival crevice (Chapter 24).

EFFECTS OF IMPROVED ORAL HYGIENE

The contribution of thorough control of supragingival plaque to periodontal health is twofold. First, there is the direct effect of removing toxic substances from the gingival margin. This reduces inflammation and therefore gingival bleeding, but it also permits the marginal tissue to heal and reduce in size, mainly as a result of collagen deposition and maturation. Thus, there will be an element of recession where oral hygiene is effective (Abstract 17,4).

Secondly, the removal of a large reservoir of plaque, and maintenance of this condition by the patient, permits effective treatment of deeper problems by the operator. Without this control, other methods of periodontal treatment may have an initial effect, but within a comparatively short time it will be lost.

Abstract 17,4 *Effects of oral hygiene with and without root planing in treating patients with chronic periodontitis*

Turner Y, Ashley FP, Wilson RF, *British Dental Journal* 1994; **177**: 367–371

Ten patients with moderate periodontitis were given repeated subgingivally-directed OHI until less than 20% of the sites had plaque present. At this point, half the mouth was root planed. Patients were examined with a constant force-probe before OHI and 6 and 12 weeks after root planing. One patient dropped out. In both groups, plaque reduced from around 75% to 10% at 6 and 12 weeks. Bleeding on probing reduced from 55% to 25% at 6 weeks, and then the root-planed sites reduced further to about 10%. In both groups, probing depth reduced by just over 0.5 mm, an effect almost entirely due to recession. The root planing had a modest additional effect, reducing the number of deeper sites at 12 weeks.

Comment: This study shows what may occur in all patients who improve their oral hygiene procedures.

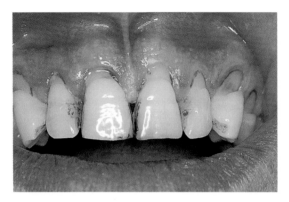

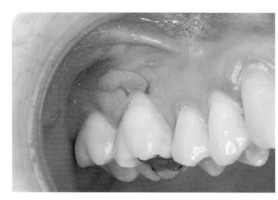

Fig. 17,28

Moderate recession in a well-brushed mouth. There are abrasion cavities present that may benefit from glass ionomer restorations. Although such restorations will wear away in 3–5 years, they are easily replaced and they prevent further physical weakening of the tooth by accumulating abrasion.

Fig. 17,29

Severe toothbrushing ulceration on tooth 16.

In patients with deep pockets, the effects of gingival healing after institution of good oral hygiene may be quite marked. Patients should be advised of the two main side-effects of all successful periodontal treat-ment: gingival recession (Fig. 17,28) and, because the root surface may be exposed, dentine hypersensitivity. Only excessive brushing is likely to produce ulceration (Fig. 17,29).

18

SCALING AND ROOT PLANING

- Do we need to remove all calculus?
- How can planing be made methodical?
- What are the results of root planing?

Scaling is the removal of hard and soft deposits from the root surface by an operator. Root planing is, by definition, the production of a smooth root surface. Much periodontal treatment time is spent in these two occupations, and it is important that the justification for this is clear.

AIMS AND OBJECTIVES

It was mentioned in Chapter 13 that calculus may do two things – impede oral hygiene, and retain plaque against the gingiva. The role of scaling is therefore to remove deposits so as to improve patient plaque control, and also to reduce plaque retention subgingivally.

With root planing, the aim is clear but the justification is less obvious: why take off good tooth substance when only the plaque needs to be removed?

First, there is a mechanical justification for root planing. By producing a smooth surface, we ensure that everything possible has been done to remove the plaque.

Secondly, some have suggested a biological justification for root planing. In this view, there is a significant amount of bacterial endotoxin retained on and in the cementum.

The matter of endotoxin has been explored at length. As an example, one of the studies is given in Abstract 18,1. In passing, this study shows that it is not essential to remove calculus if we are after substances like endotoxin.

Abstract 18,1 *Assessment of ultrasonic debridement of calculus-associated periodontally-involved root surfaces by the limulus amoebocyte lysate assay*

Chiew SY, Wilson M, Davies EH, et al., *Journal of Clinical Periodontology* 1991; **18**: 240–244

From 21 patients, 34 single-rooted teeth were extracted, with chronic periodontitis and at least 30% loss of radiographic bone support. In addition, five totally unerupted impacted wisdom teeth were used as controls for the method of endotoxin assessment. The diseased surfaces of 24 teeth were instrumented ultrasonically without deliberate removal of calculus and then stripped of a further 1 mm of substance, and endotoxin was assessed in this tissue. On the other 10 teeth that were not planed, the surface tissue likewise was removed and assessed for endotoxin. Findings ranged from 0.08–22 ng of endotoxin in ultrasonically-instrumented root surfaces; 15–28 ng in unerupted wisdom teeth and 1900–29 000 ng in the uninstrumented diseased controls.

Comment: As the authors say, the endotoxin was probably in a superficial location, and it is the plaque rather than the calculus that needs to be removed. This study agrees with earlier studies on endotoxin removal with ultrasonic instrumentation.

Better assays of endotoxin and carefully designed investigations still suggest that some minute quantities of endotoxin remain on root surfaces, no matter how thoroughly they are planed. Because root planing often seems effective both in the short and long term, a

Table 18,1: *Objectives of root planing*

Immediately
No detectable plaque or calculus (shown by a smooth surface)

After 6–8 weeks
Improvement in gingival health (less BOP)
Reduction of probing depth (1–2 mm in PD 5+ mm)
Improved probing attachment level (in deeper PD)

more pragmatic approach to the endotoxin question is warranted.

The objectives of root planing are listed in Table 18,1. With most patients, oral hygiene requires further encouragement after the initial education session, and it is convenient to combine it with root planing so that the best use is made of time. Furthermore, because calculus may impede oral hygiene, there is a positive case for thorough scaling and root planing as soon as possible, so that the results of oral hygiene may be maximized.

PRINCIPLES OF INSTRUMENT USE

On the one hand, studies indicate that thorough root debridement is essential to provide a satisfactory environment for the healing of adjacent soft tissues (see Abstract 19,1), but there is a question over what constitutes thoroughness. Do we need to repeat root planing to increase its effect? Apparently not (see Abstract 21,4). Does it matter how much time we spend root planing? Likewise, probably not much (Abstract 18,2).

How, then, do we ensure that we have removed sufficient plaque without taking away excessive root surface tissue? The time-honoured principle of planing still holds sway: it is an indicator of a smooth surface that is probably not contaminated with any significant amount of plaque. Therefore it is still a good idea to use root planing but without overdoing it.

Abstract 18,2 *Effect of non-surgical periodontal therapy (IV). Operator variability*

Badersten A, Nilveus R, Egelberg J., *Journal of Clinical Periodontology* 1985; **12**: 190–200

In 20 patients with advanced periodontitis, following thorough OHI that was subsequently reinforced, one specialist periodontist operator (author R.N.) was assigned at random to debride incisors, canines and premolars on one side of the jaw (528 sites), and one of five hygienists was assigned to debride these teeth on the other side (also a total of 528 sites). The hygienists were all in the Swedish public health services and their experience varied from 3–14 years. The periodontist took an average of 9.1 min per tooth; the hygienists varied from 8.7–12.2 min. Over 3 months post-instrumentation, the PD dropped from a mean of 5.4 mm to 3.5 mm, with minimal gains in PAL. There were only minor differences between operators.

Comment: This study has quite a difference in times and little difference in outcome. Experience apparently has minimal effects on the outcome of root planing.

What is the most effective way of root planing? A sharp instrument should be drawn obliquely across the root surface, maintaining as much surface contact as possible. The operator needs a knowledge of root anatomy and the skill of applying the instrument to a root surface that is sensed largely through tactile stimuli. It is a good idea to practise on the root surfaces of extracted teeth (Figs 18,1–18,3).

Many periodontists appreciate the design of Gracey curettes (Fig. 18,4). On all Gracey pattern instruments, the blade is angled with respect to the shank: the sharp edge is further away from the shank, and the nearer edge is blunt to limit tissue damage (Fig. 18,5).

Often the curve of the Gracey cutting edge fits the rounded angle of a tooth well; on some occasions it may be necessary to lean the instrument buccally or lingually to obtain the best fit of instrument to tooth.

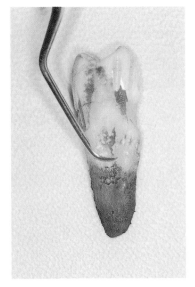

Fig. 18,1

A long-shanked, small-headed Gracey 3/4 curette, showing how the small head fits a premolar up to its root concavity. This tooth has markings on it because it was removed as part of a research study.

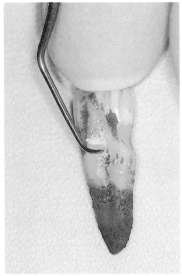

Fig. 18,2

One side of the root is being planed to remove all disclosed plaque and leave a smooth surface.

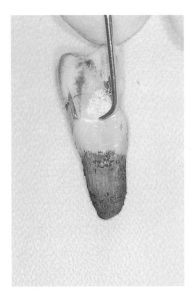

Fig. 18,3

Both sides have been planed. This is a useful practice exercise to carry out on extracted teeth.

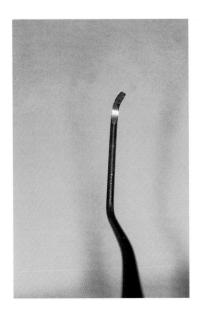

Fig. 18,4

A long-shanked, small-headed Gracey pattern curette. The sharp edge is the offset side, to the left.

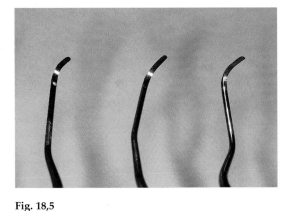

Fig. 18,5

A simple set of three Gracey curettes that will deal with most problems: 1/2 small-headed long-shanked; 11/12 long-shanked; 13/14 long-shanked. The cutting edges are all to the left.

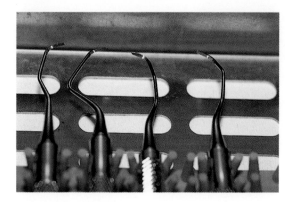

Fig. 18,6

Basic pattern Gracey curettes: 1/2, 9/10, 11/12 and 13/14.

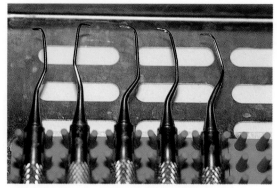

Fig. 18,8

Long-shanked Gracey curettes for deeper pockets.

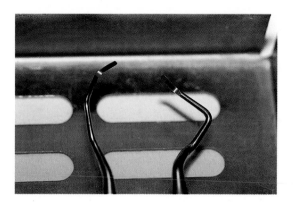

Fig. 18,7

Gracey curettes for difficult access posterior teeth: 15/16 for mesial surfaces, and a specially rigid 17/18 for distal surfaces.

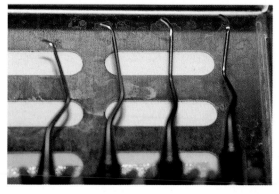

Fig. 18,9

Long-shanked small-headed Gracey curettes for deep, narrow pockets, or for roots with concavities or grooves.

The shank is straight on patterns 1–10, but with varying approach angles. On patterns 11/12 the angle is to fit mesial surfaces of posterior teeth, and a greater angle is permitted on patterns 15/16. On patterns 13/14 the angle is to fit distal surfaces, with a greater angle on patterns 17/18.

Two further pattern modifications are available. First, the quite long cutting edge of a standard Gracey head is reduced on the 'mini' design to about half the length; this helps, for instance, in fitting root surfaces on teeth such as premolars. Secondly, the 'after 5' design is a special long-shanked version, more suited to deeper pockets.

Since much periodontal treatment time is spent in planing teeth, it is a sensible investment to obtain comfortable instruments with balanced handles that are easy to use. Most periodontists and many general practitioners choose a favourite set of instruments with which they can plane virtually all surfaces (Figs 18,6–18,9).

In basic Gracey curettes, for instance, the present author chooses 1/2, 3/4, 11/12 and 13/14 patterns. It is useful also to have a

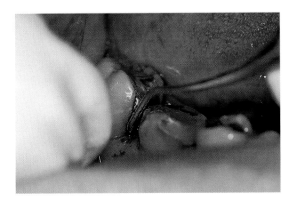

Fig. 18,10

The 15/16 curette with a greater angle for difficult mesial surfaces.

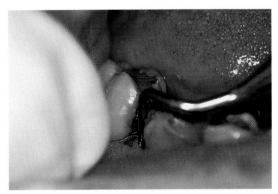

Fig. 18,11

The rigid 17/18 curette for difficult distal surfaces.

similar set in the 'mini' and 'mini-5' designs, and a 15/16 and specially reinforced 17/18 for special occasions (Figs 18,10 and 18,11).

When planing each surface, it is helpful to wipe the instrument on gauze to show what has been removed. When plaque and calculus no longer appear, the surface feels smooth and the instrument appears clean except for a trace of blood, it is time to move to the next surface (Figs 18,12–18,14).

It is also helpful and time-saving to use a systematic method in planing a quadrant of teeth. For instance, if proximal pockets only are present, the present author may use a 1/2

pattern Gracey from the incisors to the canine or first premolar, and then an 11/12 for the mesial surfaces of the remaining teeth; finally, a 13/14 is used on their distal surfaces (Figs 18,15–18,18). Special care and firm application of the instrument may be required to reach the depth of narrow pockets (Figs 18,19–18,22).

With each curette, a series of surfaces is planed on all the teeth; for instance, approaching the incisors and canine first from the mesiobuccal aspect, next from the distobuccal, next from the mesio-lingual, and finally from the distolingual.

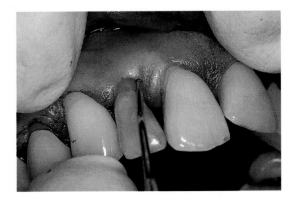

Fig. 18,12

A long-shanked Gracey curette 1/2 planing the mesial of tooth 12.

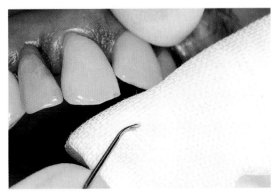

Fig. 18,13

The instrument is wiped on a gauze swab to show any plaque or calculus removed.

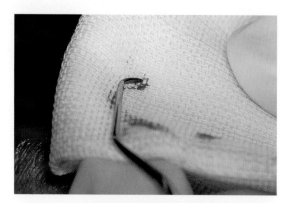

Fig. 18,14

Several planing strokes have removed plaque and calculus; when none is visible, only blood, it is time to move to the next surface.

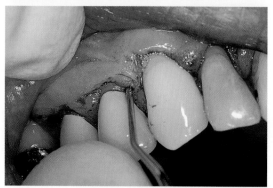

Fig. 18,15

Making the most of time. Here, with a Gracey 11/12, the mesiobuccal aspect of tooth 14 is planed.

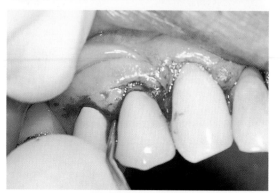

Fig. 18,16

The mesiobuccal aspect of tooth 15 is then planed.

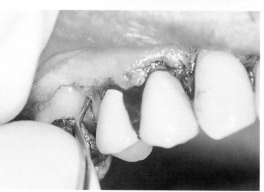

Fig. 18,17

Next in line, the mesiobuccal aspect of tooth 16 is planed.

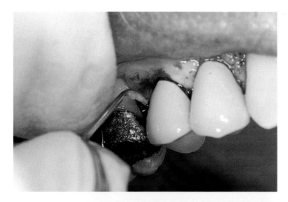

Fig. 18,18

We then change to a Gracey 13/14, and go back along these teeth. There was plenty of plaque removed from the distal surface of 15.

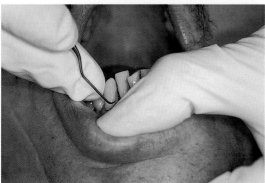

Fig. 18,19

Some deep areas require special care to insert the curettes deep enough. First, the jaw is supported with the operator's non-working hand.

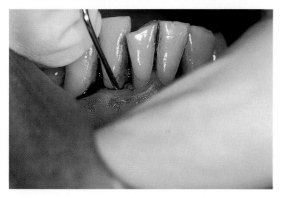

Fig. 18,20

The long-shanked short-headed 3/4 curette is then placed on the mesio-buccal of tooth 42 and slid vertically into the pocket.

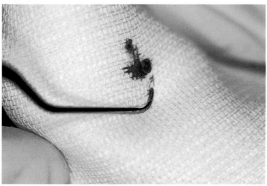

Fig. 18,21

The curette removes plenty of calculus on the upstroke.

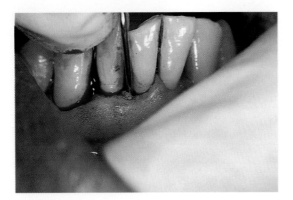

Fig. 18,22

An example of a similar deep pocket on tooth 41.

It should be apparent from Abstracts 18,1, 18,3 and 18,4 that ultrasonic instrumentation is an effective and acceptable alternative to hand instruments in scaling and root planing. Some operators (including this author) use both types of instrument in the procedure, and some express a preference for one mode only. The limitations of ultrasonic scalers and similar instruments are: first, they should be avoided with patients who wear pacemakers, for fear of interference; and secondly, the aerosol may carry infectious microorganisms into the air, so hand instruments may be preferred in patients who pose a known risk of infection.

EFFECTS ON TISSUES

A number of investigators have produced studies of root planing, sometimes in comparison with another treatment such as a modified Widman flap. One particularly well-thought-out series of investigations (largely on single-rooted teeth) was performed by Badersten and co-workers and published from 1981 to 1987. Two from this series have been mentioned already (see Abstracts 21,4 and 18,2); two more will give an idea of typical results in both moderate and severe periodontitis (Abstracts 18,3 and 18,4). In moderate pockets of 5–6 mm, we may expect

Abstract 18,3 *Effect of non-surgical periodontal therapy (I). Moderately advanced periodontitis*

Badersten A, Nilveus R, Egelberg J, *Journal of Clinical Periodontology* 1981; **8**: 57–72

Fifteen patients with a mean PD of 4.1–4.5 mm were given thorough OHI over a 1-month period (4–5 visits). The mean PD reduced by 0.3–0.7 mm by the end of the month. Plaque scores reduced from >60% to <12% and remained there for the rest of the study. At 1 month, the teeth were instrumented with sides randomly allocated to ultrasonic or hand instrumentation. One operator treated seven patients, and the other, the remainder. A third clinician, blind to the type of instrumentation, made all the measurements. Subsequently, each operator decided whether to perform reinstrumentation for individual patients on two occasions after monthly follow-up examinations. By 5 months, the mean PD had reduced by a total of 1.3–1.7 mm from baseline scores. Maintenance continued to 13 months, with little further improvement. The mean BOP reduced from > 75% to 8–16% during the study. Most recession took place within the first 3 months (mean score 1.4–1.6 mm at 13 months). The PAL hardly changed during the period of the study. There were no differences according to operator or type of instrumentation.

Comment: This study was essentially an experimental trial, but with a longitudinal dimension. A constant-force probe would therefore have been an advantage but such instruments were not commercially available at the start of this study; however, the results agree with other studies and the clinical experience of many periodontists. In pockets of this depth, therefore, an average reduction of 0.5 mm may be expected from oral hygiene and a further 1.0 mm from subgingival instrumentation of either sort. As long as the operator is experienced and satisfied that the work has been properly executed, instrument choice appears to be a matter of personal preference.

an average reduction of 1.5 mm as the result of oral hygiene and root planing; in deeper pockets of 8–9 mm, the reduction may be 2.0–3.0 mm.

Abstract 18,4 *Effect of non-surgical periodontal therapy (II). Severely advanced periodontitis*

Badersten A, Nilveus R, Egelberg J, *Journal of Clinical Periodontology* 1984; **11**: 63–76

In 16 patients with an initial mean PD of 5.5–5.8 mm (up to 12 mm pockets), a study was performed with the same basic design as in Abstract 18,3, but with instrumentation at 3 months and follow-up continued to 24 months. Hand or ultrasonic instruments were used randomly for each half of the mouth by two operators. Again, there were marked reductions in plaque and BOP, similar to those of the previous study. Oral hygiene reduced the mean PD to 5.1–5.3 mm by 3 months, and by 12 months the result of instrumentation was a further reduction to 3.6–3.9 mm, which remained to the end of the study. Recession was minimal in the first 3 months, but reached 1.6–1.8 mm at 12 months. By 24 months, there was a mean gain in PAL of 0.1–0.3 mm. The pattern of clinical attachment level gain or loss agreed with the critical PD findings (Abstract 19,6). Again, there were no differences according to operator or mode of instrumentation.

Comment: A further study on non-molar teeth, in agreement with others, and one that periodontists find reflects their experience in practice. On these patients with deeper PD, a mean reduction of 1.5 mm was produced by subgingival instrumentation. Again, a constant-force probe was not used, but the examiner force was measured at the end of the study and found to be relatively high (0.5–0.75 N; about 2–3 times the usual force used in many clinical studies).

FACTORS AFFECTING RESULTS

As mentioned in the last chapter, the two main side-effects of all successful periodontal treatment are recession and hypersensitivity. These may both have an effect on the patient's efforts in plaque control.

If the patient is scared of recession, the toothbrush may not penetrate subgingivally, or may even 'miss' the gingival margin. In some cases of hypersensitivity, patients also reduce their technique to ineffective levels through fear. It is therefore essential that patients are forewarned about these moderate complications, not only from the ethical aspect of avoiding any unnecessary unpleasant surprises but for the very positive reason that they may otherwise reduce their plaque control at a crucial stage of treatment.

Plaque control is one principal factor affecting treatment response after root planing; smoking is another. In the study of Ah et al (see Abstract 14,12), there was about 30% less PD reduction. This averages to about 0.5 mm less for a pocket of 7–8 mm. Compared with plaque control, it is not such an important factor.

Some smokers noticeably attempt to compensate for their unconquerable addiction by maintaining the very highest possible standard of plaque control. An example of this is given in Chapter 30. They certainly need our approval and encouragement. Since smoking exacerbates disease, if the main aetiological factor is controlled, then we may expect an exacerbation of zero to add a zero effect. There may be some effect, however, on the response to treatment.

REASSESSMENT

The earliest time at which the tissues may be healed after root planing is 5–6 weeks (reformation and maturation of collagen, for

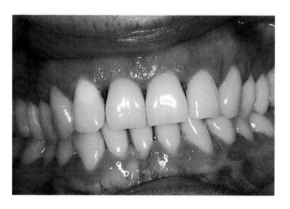

Fig. 18,23

A patient who has had OHI and achieved a plaque score of below 10% now attends for root planing.

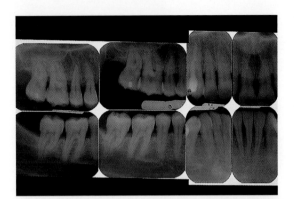

Fig. 18,24

There is moderate bone loss on the right side.

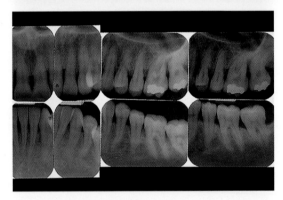

Fig. 18,25

Similarly, there is bone loss on the left side.

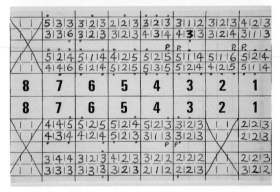

Fig. 18,26

The charts show initial shallow pocketing on the right, despite pus on probing in some places. Almost all pockets of 4–6 mm were reduced 3 months later.

		8	7	6	5	4	3	2	1
\ 1		5 3 3	3 2 3	2 2 3	3 2 3	3 1 1 2	3 2 3	4 2 3	
		3 1 3 6	3 2 3	3 2 3	4 3 1 4	4 **3** 3	3 2 1 4	3 1 1 3	
							P P		P P
/		5 2 4	5 1 1 4	4 2 1 5	5 2 1 5	5 1 1 4	5 1 1 6	5 2 4	
1 1		4 1 4 6	6 1 2 1 4	5 1 2 1 5	5 1 3 1 5	5 1 2 1 4	4 1 2 1 5	5 1 1 4	
		8	**7**	**6**	**5**	**4**	**3**	**2**	**1**
		8	**7**	**6**	**5**	**4**	**3**	**2**	**1**
\		4 1 4 5	5 1 2 1 5	5 1 2 1 4	5 1 2 1 3	3 1 2 1 3	\ 1 1	2 1 2 1 3	
/		4 1 3 1 4	4 1 2 1 4	5 1 2 1 3	3 1 1 1 3	3 1 2 1 3	\	2 1 2 1 3	
						P P			
		3 1 4 1 4	3 1 2 1 3	4 1 2 1 3	3 1 2 1 2	2 1 2 1 2	\	2 1 2 1 3	
/ 1 1		3 1 3 1 3	3 1 3 1 3	3 1 2 1 3	2 1 1 1 2	2 1 2 1 3	/ 1 1	3 1 2 1 2	

Fig. 18,27

A similar condition on the left side. Before treatment, 75 pockets were over 3 mm; afterwards, this had reduced to 28.

	1	2	3	4	5	6	7	8
2 2 4	3 2 3	3 2 3	3 2 4	4 2 4	3 2 5	5 3 4	\ 1 1	
3 1 2 1 4	4 1 2 1 2	3 1 3 1 3	3 1 3 1 4	3 1 2 1 4	3 1 2 1 5	4 1 2 1 3	\ /	
P P P			P . P P		.	. B		
3 1 2 1 5	5 1 2 1 3	3 1 2 1 5	5 1 2 1 5	3 1 2 1 5	5 1 2 1 5	7 1 2 1 3	/ \	
4 1 2 1 5	5 1 2 1 3	2 1 3 1 5	4 1 4 1 5	3 1 2 1 4	3 1 2 1 7	6 1 3 1 4	/ 1 1	
1	**2**	**3**	**4**	**5**	**6**	**7**	**8**	
1	**2**	**3**	**4**	**5**	**6**	**7**	**8**	
4 1 2 1 3	3 1 1 1 3	3 1 2 1 2	3 1 2 1 4	4 1 2 1 4	5 1 3 1 5	4 1 2 1 3	\ 1 /	
2 1 3 1 3	3 1 2 1 4	4 1 2 1 2	2 1 2 1 3	3 1 2 1 3	4 1 2 1 4	4 1 6 1 4	\ /	
. P	P P			.	.			
3 1 2 1 3	2 1 2 1 2	2 1 2 1 2	3 1 2 1 3	3 1 2 1 3	4 1 3 1 4	2 1 2 1 2	/	
2 1 2 1 3	2 1 2 1 3	2 1 / 1 2	2 1 1 1 2	2 1 2 1 3	4 1 2 1 3	4 1 5 1 3	/ 1 1	

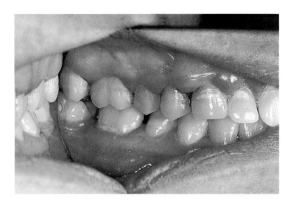

Fig. 18,28

Good oral hygiene with tiny subgingival calculus deposits. The dentist referred this patient with excellent plaque control because he was concerned about a possible blood dyscrasia. Right side, showing marked hyperplastic inflammation adjacent to premolars and anterior teeth.

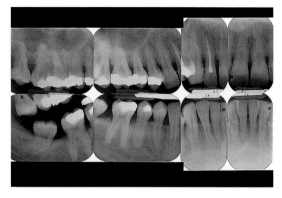

Fig. 18,30

Right-side radiographs show most bone loss in the upper arch.

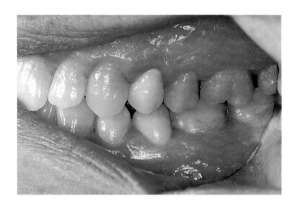

Fig. 18,29

There is less gingival enlargement on the left side.

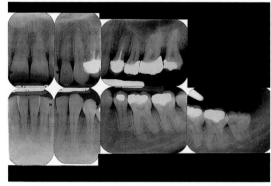

Fig. 18,31

The left side shows a similar condition. Caries on 38 required treatment by dentist.

instance) and it is therefore best not to disturb the deeper tissues until this time, whilst scrupulously removing plaque in the first 2–3 mm of the pocket if required earlier. Figs 18,23–18,27 give an example of the effect of scaling and root planing in a typical patient with moderate periodontitis, 3 months later.

Following reassessment, the response of the tissues to treatment may be evaluated, and informed advice given to the patient. Chapter 30 gives examples of this important decision-making appointment and specimen treatment plans.

ASPECTS OF MAINTENANCE

As we shall see in Chapter 21, there is strong evidence in favour of a frequent and thorough

4|5|4	4|3|3	5|3|4	4|3|4	4|2|3	3|2|4	5|2|3	3|2|2
5|3|5	6|3|3	3|3|3	3|2|4	4|2|5	5|3|3	3|2|3	3|2|2

5|5|6	6|3|6	6|3|6	6|2|5	6|2|5	5|3|6	6|3|7	7|2|3
5|5|6	8|7|6	6|4|6	5|4|8	7|5|8	6|4|7	5|3|5	6|2|3

8	7	6	5	4	3	2	1
8	7	6	5	4	3	2	1

5|4|5		4|3|7	5|2|5	3|3|3	3|2|3	2|2|2	2|2|2
4|3|3	X	4|3|7	5|2|5	3|2|4	3|2|4	4|2|3	4|1|2
5|3|3		3|2|3	3|2|3	3|2|3	3|2|2	2|2|2	1|2|2
3|3|4		2|2|3	3|2|4	3|2|3	3|2|3	3|2|2	2|1|2

Fig. 18,32

Charts show that disease on the right side responded well 3 months after root planing and scaling.

2|2|3	2|2|2	3|2|4	3|2|3	3|2|3	3|2|5	4|2|4	
2|2|3	3|2|3	2|3|3	4|3|4	4|2|3	3|2|5	3|3|6	X

3|3|5	5|2|4	4|2|8	5|2|5	5|2|4	5|3|7	7|3|7	
3|3|5	5|3|4	4|4|5	5|3|7	5|3|4	4|3|7	5|4|8	

1	2	3	4	5	6	7	8
1	2	3	4	5	6	7	8

1|1|2	3|2|2	3|2|3	5|2|3	5|3|5	5|3|5	4|5|5	5|5|5
2|1|3	3|2|3	3|2|3	5|2|3	4|2|4	4|2|4	4|3|7	7|5|5
2|1|2	2|2|2	2|2|2	3|2|2	2|2|3	3|3|3	3|3|3	3|2|5
2|2|2	2|2|3	3|2|3	3|2|3	3|2|4	4|3|5	4|4|5	

Fig. 18,33

The left side also shows a good response. Overall, 102 PDs above 3 mm reduced to just 37, and mean PD reduced from 4.1 to 2.9 mm. Bleeding points reduced in number from 180 to 66.

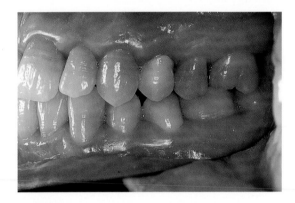

Fig. 18,34

Right-side view at reassessment, 3 months after planing.

Fig. 18,35

Left-side view at reassessment.

follow-up to periodontal surgery in the first 3 months after treatment. However, there is little similar evidence for the situation after root planing. During the four or more appointments of root planing in a typical treatment plan, it is possible to monitor the oral hygiene which the patient maintains, and advise and adjust techniques as necessary. In Figs 18,28–18,37 details are given of a patient who was followed up 4 years after initial root

planing, when a moderate periodontitis was completely resolved.

At every appointment, the percentage of plaque should be scored as a routine, and the patient needs to be shown the problems in a mirror.

If the plaque scores are consistently below 10% of surfaces and the patient appears to be removing the top 1–2 mm of subgingival plaque (test with probe or floss), then after

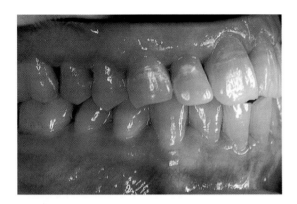

Fig. 18,36

Right side 4 years later, with no PDs anywhere over 4 mm. There has been selective scaling of deeper pockets at maintenance appointments.

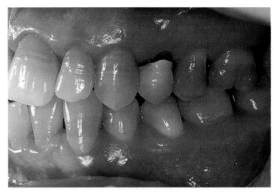

Fig. 18,37

Left-side view. Note the recession of 1–2 mm, compared with initial presentation in both views.

the last planing appointment, 6–8 weeks may be left until reassessment. If there is the slightest doubt about either of these concerns, it is best to have a review at 3–4 weeks.

There is one further long-term assurance of cure after root planing, which occurs often but not always. This is bone repair. Figs 18,38 and 18,39 show examples of this in the same patient 3 years after root planing. The earliest time when this may be seen is 8–12 months after treatment.

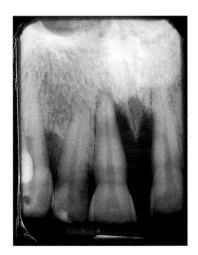

Fig. 18,38

Periodontitis with deep bone loss in mesial of teeth 11 and 21, treated with OHI and root planing. (Reproduced from Watts TLP, Periodontitis for medical practitioners, *BMJ* 1998; **316**: 993–996 by permission of the *British Medical Journal*.)

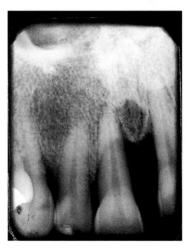

Fig. 18,39

Result after 3 years. With shrinkage, PD had also reduced from 10 to 4 mm, with no BOP. (Reproduced from Watts TLP, Periodontitis for medical practitioners, *BMJ* 1998; **316**: 993–996 by permission of the *British Medical Journal*.)

19 SURGERY FOR PERIODONTAL POCKETS

- When is surgical treatment indicated?
- What are the main philosophies of surgical intervention?
- Are some techniques easier in practice?
- What are the principles of periodontal surgery?
- How do the main techniques compare in their results?

The first serious modern studies of periodontal surgery began in the late 1950s when Ramfjord pioneered a method of measuring the results. Since then, many studies have shown what may be achieved by our surgical interventions and have placed them in perspective.

What, then, is the correct place of periodontal surgery? Why need we use it at all? And what methods are most appropriate if we consider it necessary? To understand some of the answers to these questions, some historical background is required. Earlier periodontists used surgery mainly for two reasons: to remove disease and to restore anatomical form to the tissues. Because the disease was in the gingiva, they reasoned that some gingival tissue needed to be removed; and because the tissues were deformed by disease, it was important to restore them to a functional shape.

Four main techniques were used: subgingival curettage (now defunct in most quarters), gingivectomy, replaced flap (as developed by pioneers like Widman) and pocket elimination (usually the apically positioned flap, often with osseous surgery to eradicate 'reverse gingival architecture' caused by disease).

Because general surgery was used frequently to remove diseased tissue (e.g. appendectomy), and to restore anatomical form (e.g. reducing fractures), its gradual extension into periodontics was a most natural development. However, as periodontal surgery expanded, some researchers were asking disquieting questions about the nature of periodontal diseases and the objectives of treatment. Treatment methods were questioned as never before, and a new biological understanding developed.

REASONS FOR SURGERY

Six main reasons have been advanced for periodontal surgery, and they are listed in Table 19,1. First, lifting a flap may provide better access. In support of this, one of the last papers of the great Norwegian periodontist Jens Wærhaug provided some interesting evidence (Abstract 19,1). The access flap, the

Table 19,1: *Reasons advanced for periodontal surgery*

1. Plaque control access for operator
2. Plaque control enhancement for patient
3. Removal of diseased tissue
4. Access for other forms of dental treatment
5. Regeneration of attachment apparatus
6. Improvement of aesthetics

Abstract 19,1   *Healing of the dento-epithelial junction following subgingival plaque control. II: as observed on extracted teeth*

Author: Wærhaug J, *Journal of Periodontology* 1978; **49**: 119–134

In patients maintaining a high standard of supragingival plaque control, 84 teeth were extracted at various times after thorough subgingival scaling. In 11 cases only, this was combined with flap surgery. On 31 teeth only, scaling was immediately prior to extraction; on the remaining 53, it was 7 days to more than 1 year earlier. After extraction, root surfaces were examined for plaque. On the teeth scaled immediately before extraction, 60% of surfaces were found to have plaque present. On the teeth extracted later: in pockets up to 3 mm deep, 83% of root surfaces were plaque-free; at 3–5 mm, 39%; and >5 mm, only 11%. Where subgingival plaque had been removed and supragingival plaque controlled, healing occurred with a long junctional epithelial attachment. Where subgingival plaque was not completely removed, its reformation took up to 1 year and clinical inflammation did not recur until later in many cases: thus apparent clinical healing was present at earlier stages.

Comment: As the author states, subgingival instrumentation of pockets deeper than 5 mm is more likely to fail; but it is possible to argue with his conclusion that pocket elimination surgery is indicated for pockets deeper than 3 mm that are not resolved by scaling.

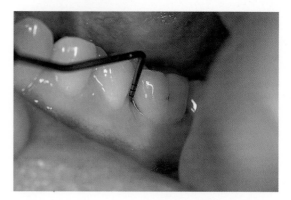

Fig. 19,1

Access flap: after previous thorough root planing, there is still 8 mm PD mesial of tooth 36, with BOP.

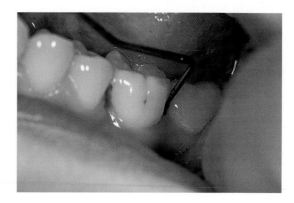

Fig. 19,2

7 mm PD distally, with BOP.

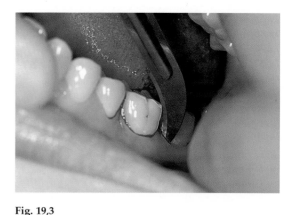

Fig. 19,3

Crevicular incision from tooth 37 mesially to tooth 35 distally with No. 12 scalpel.

simplest of all flap procedures, is shown in Figs 19,1–19,16.

However, this reason for surgery might be questioned. If deeper pockets are less amenable to operator plaque removal, the results of root planing studies still show that pockets may heal as a result (Chapter 18). In other words, total plaque removal is not always essential for a beneficial result.

The second justification advanced for surgery is that the pathological morphology caused by disease needs to be corrected for the patient subsequently to maintain effective plaque control. This, too, was Wærhaug's

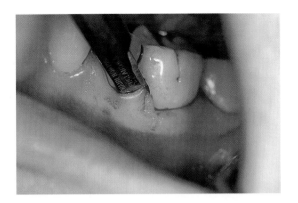

Fig. 19,4

Flap thinned down to bone with No. 15 scalpel from tooth 35 distally to tooth 37 mesially.

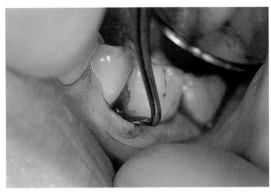

Fig. 19,7

Buck knife undermines proximal tissue.

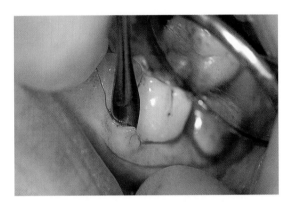

Fig. 19,5

Periosteal elevator turns mesial papilla of tooth 36 off bone.

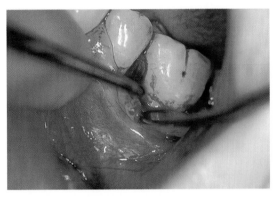

Fig. 19,8

Curette eases up bulk of proximal tissue.

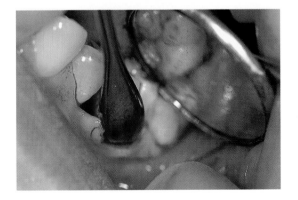

Fig. 19,6

Flap raised to distal papilla.

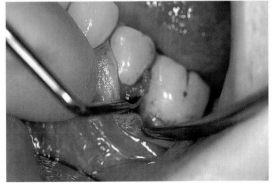

Fig. 19,9

More tissue curetted.

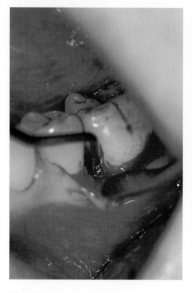

Fig. 19,10

Mesial surface planed: the procedure has been the same on the lingual aspect throughout.

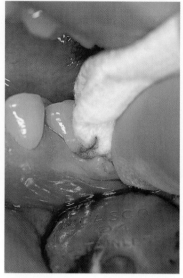

Fig. 19,11

Gauze packed into bony defect.

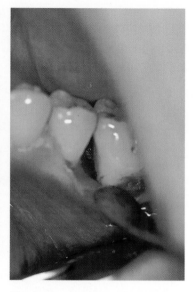

Fig. 19,12

Mesial surface of tooth 36 inspected.

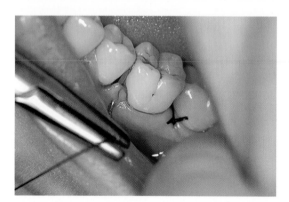

Fig. 19,13

After distal surface of tooth 36 has been treated, sutures are placed.

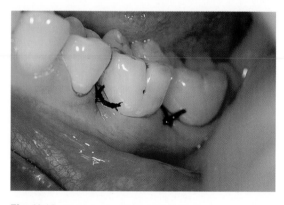

Fig. 19,14

Procedure completed: patient will use chlorhexidine rinse for plaque control in this area.

opinion. In answer, it might be said that the correct anatomical morphology did not help the patient first time round. But a part of all periodontal treatment is to teach the patient effective methods of plaque control, so a case may be argued. However, there are some situations when the patient cannot be taught plaque control until the tissue is reshaped (Figs 19,17–19,22).

The removal of diseased tissue is not a very good argument, as we shall see when comparing surgical and non-surgical periodontal

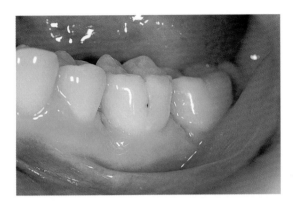

Fig. 19,15

1 week later with sutures removed. Maintenance with scaling every 2 weeks.

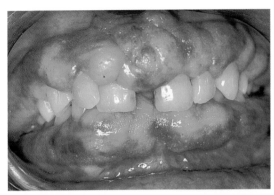

Fig. 19,18

Central view.

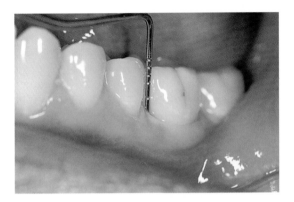

Fig. 19,16

3 months later: PD measures 4 mm without BOP. Note tissue blanching with probe pressure.

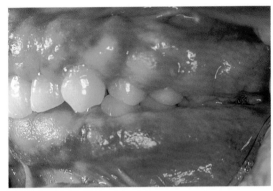

Fig. 19,19

Left mirror view.

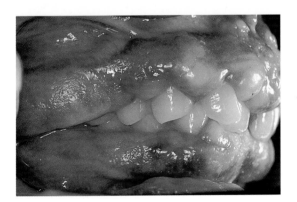

Fig. 19,17

Hereditary gingival fibromatosis in a 23-year-old female: right mirror view.

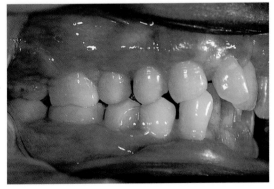

Fig. 19,20

1 year after apically positioned flap surgery: right mirror view.

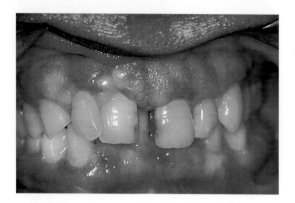

Fig. 19,21

Central view.

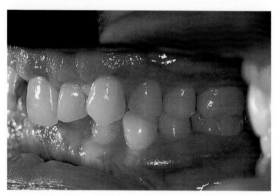

Fig. 19,22

Left mirror view.

treatment. In the 1980s, this old argument was put in a new form by researchers who felt that they had demonstrated microbial invasion of the tissues in advanced adult periodontitis (Abstract 19,2), and again in juvenile periodontitis (Abstract 19,3). However, several studies have shown bacteraemia in healthy patients with good oral hygiene after tooth-brushing, for instance (Abstract 19,4 is an example). If this can occur, then it is clear that organisms may be found at times in the gingival tissues without invasion, because they can gain access and pass through to the blood vessels. The only clearly invasive periodontal diseases are ANUG and NUP, which involve tissue necrosis.

Abstract 19,2 *Bacterial invasion of gingiva in advanced periodontitis in humans*

Saglie R, Newman MG, Carranza FA Jr, et al., *Journal of Periodontology* 1982; **53**: 217–222

In each of four patients with advanced periodontitis, a tooth with advanced periodontitis was extracted with an attached gingival biopsy. In four other cases, gingival biopsies were obtained. After initial fixation for 48 h, specimens were split; in four cases bacteria were found within epithelium, and in one case they had reached connective tissue. The authors used scanning electron microscopy, and their findings agreed with those of earlier authors using transmission microscopy.

Comment: These results are convincing as far as they indicate the presence of microorganisms within tissues: it is not likely that the method introduced what was found. The real problem is the question of invasion.

Abstract 19,3 *Scanning and transmission electron microscopic study of tissue-invading microorganisms in localized juvenile periodontitis*

Carranza FA Jr, Saglie R, Newman MG, et al., *Journal of Periodontology* 1983; **54**: 598–617

An upper molar with extensive juvenile periodontitis was extracted with some gingiva and alveolar bone attached; two further biopsies of gingiva were taken from other molars. Numerous organisms were found within the tissues and some on the surface of the bone. The morphological findings were compatible with the presence of Aa in the tissues and many neutrophils were present, some associated with bacteria. Spirochaetes and *Mycoplasma* were also identified.

Comment: Again, presence of organisms within the tissues does not prove invasion. The neutrophils indicate that the host response is active.

Abstract 19,4 *Toothbrushing and transient bacteremia in patients undergoing orthodontic treatment*

Schlein RA, Kudlick EM, Reindorf CA, et al., *American Journal of Orthodontics and Dentofacial Orthopedics* 1991; **99**: 466–472

In 20 patients aged more than 15 years and receiving orthodontic treatment, blood samples were removed immediately before and 5 min after toothbrushing for 2 min. All the initial blood cultures were negative for microorganisms, but five patients had detectable bacteria afterwards. Both aerobic and anaerobic bacteria were identified. Plaque and GI scores were moderate.

Comment: These patients had little plaque and gingivitis and yet some developed a bacteraemia. To cause the bacteraemia, organisms had to pass through relatively intact periodontal tissues.

Abstract 19,5 *Healing following surgical/non-surgical treatment of periodontal disease. A clinical study*

Lindhe J, Westfelt E, Nyman S, et al., *Journal of Clinical Periodontology* 1982; **9**: 115–128

Following thorough OHI, 15 patients with advanced periodontitis were treated on one quadrant in each jaw (chosen at random) with root planing, and on the contralateral quadrant with modified Widman flap surgery. Maintenance was 2-weekly for 6 months and then 3-monthly for a further 18 months. From baseline to 2 years, the mean probing depth of surgical sites reduced from 4.2 mm to 2.5 mm, and that of non-surgical sites from 4.1 mm to 2.8 mm. Most of this was in the first 6 months, when there was a small difference in favour of surgery; however, the differences were not significant subsequently. There were no significant changes or differences in mean attachment levels.

Comment: The overall result is similar, but there were technique-specific differences that led to further conclusions regarding these treatments.

Access for other forms of dental treatment is mainly in the form of crown-lengthening procedures to facilitate good restorative procedures, but may also include the removal of excess tissue to facilitate orthodontic treatment.

Regeneration is a term that refers to the healing of tissues with reproduction of the full attachment apparatus: this requires special techniques. These procedures mark a significant scientific advance. However, their clinical results are not so different from other procedures (Chapter 20).

Surgical techniques are used in the improvement of aesthetics, usually in the upper anterior and premolar region. These are described and discussed in Chapter 23.

COMPARISONS WITH NON-SURGICAL TREATMENT

Once the main purpose of surgery is established as the removal of subgingival plaque, an important question arises. How do surgical techniques compare with the simpler non-surgical approach? One of the most-quoted studies (although not the first) is given in Abstract 19,5, and showed three main facts which have been borne out by other clinical trials.

First, the overall results of root planing are similar to those for a modified Widman flap (a form of the replaced flap procedure). Secondly, to produce these results with root planing takes longer than with surgery. The authors stated that root planing required more than twice the clinical time. Thirdly, there was a tendency towards greater loss of clinical attachment in shallow pockets, and a greater gain of attachment in deep pockets, with surgery than with root planing. This finding led to the ingenious idea of the 'critical probing depth' (Abstract 19,6).

THE CRITICAL PD CONCEPT

This quantity relates the initial PD for a pocket to the subsequent clinical attachment

Abstract 19,6 *'Critical probing depths' in periodontal therapy*

Lindhe J, Socransky SS, Nyman S, et al., *Journal of Clinical Periodontology* 1982; **9**: 323–336

The initial probing depth and subsequent attachment level change results of the study in Abstract 19,5 were plotted on graphs and regression lines were calculated for the two modes of treatment. The line for surgery was steeper than that for root planing. The critical probing depth at which the attachment level was unchanged after treatment was 2.9 mm for root planing and 4.2 mm for surgery. The two lines crossed when initial probing depth was 5.5 mm, indicating greater attachment gain with surgery for deeper pockets. There was variation with tooth type: molars responded better to surgery than to root planing above 4.5 mm. Poor plaque control by patients in the maintenance phase tended to raise the critical probing depth.

Comment: This is not a manifesto for treatment planning, but it contains some very useful information for decision-making.

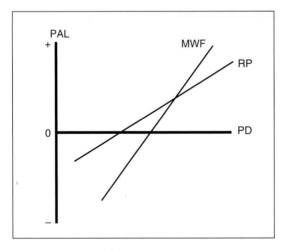

Fig. 19,23

The critical PD diagram. Each line is the best-fit regression line for many points plotting attachment level change against initial PD. Where the line crosses the PAL zero, the PD scale indicates the critical PD for attachment gain or loss. RP = root planing; MWF = modified Widman flap.

gain or loss after a specified therapy. Above the critical PD, there is a predicted gain of attachment; below it, there is a loss. As Fig. 19,23 shows, the mean results for several hundred treated sites may be averaged to give a regression line.

The line may be interpreted to show which therapy is more appropriate for a given pocket, but may not be totally applicable as a guide. For instance, surgical access to proximal sites of over 7 mm PD may necessitate raising a flap over buccal or lingual sites below 3 mm. Nevertheless, the concept has a useful general application in helping to decide treatment for a particular pocket or group of pockets. It also has been used in studies to examine the effect of other factors on periodontal treatment.

PHILOSOPHIES OF SURGERY

Similar effects may be obtained with different approaches to periodontal surgery. It is helpful to consider their underlying principles so that their differences and special indications may be appreciated. A philosophy is a system of thought, and there are at least five approaches to surgery which may be described as philosophies (Table 19,2). These approaches are not all mutually exclusive, but they have their own distinctive features.

POCKET ELIMINATION SURGERY

The positive side of pocket elimination is that it seeks to give the patient a fresh start. The

Table 19,2: *Philosophies of periodontal surgery*

- Pocket elimination (resective techniques)
- Interdental denudation
- Pocket reduction (conservative techniques)
- Bone grafts and substitutes
- Tissue regeneration (new attachment)

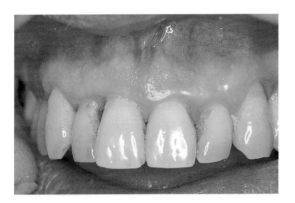

Fig. 19,24

Pocket elimination with interdental denudation: 7–9 mm proximal PD on upper anterior teeth.

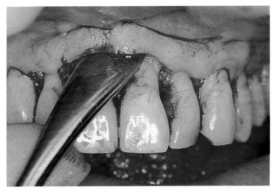

Fig. 19,27

Flap elevation. These procedures are performed also on the palatal aspect.

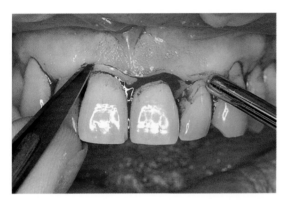

Fig. 19,25

Incision is linear, following the buccal alveolar crest.

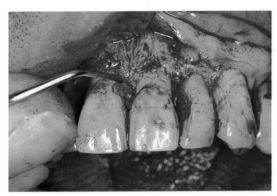

Fig. 19,28

Soft tissue removal.

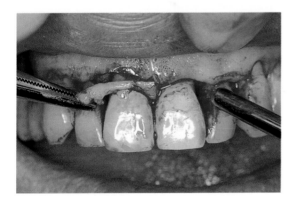

Fig. 19,26

Marginal tissue removal.

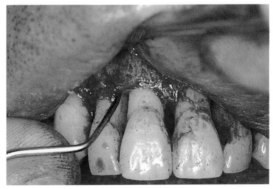

Fig. 19,29

Curetting defects.

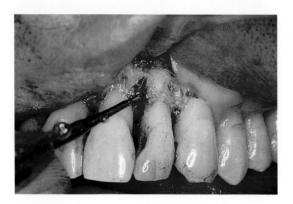

Fig. 19,30

Moderate osteoplasty.

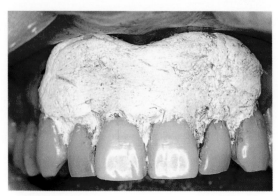

Fig. 19,33

The dressing is placed.

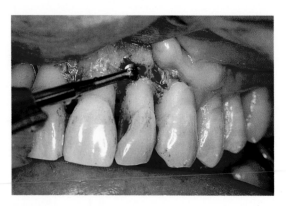

Fig. 19,31

Ostectomy with bur. To avoid damage to root, this is completed with bone chisels.

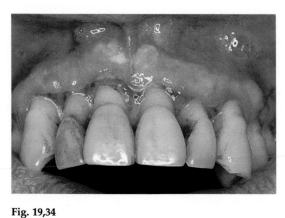

Fig. 19,34

2 weeks later the bone is covered with healing tissues.

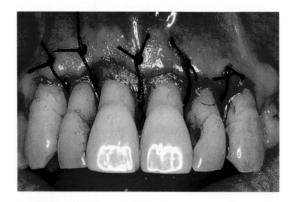

Fig. 19,32

Loose interrupted sutures with an apically displaced flap (apical to the alveolar margin).

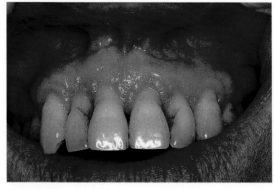

Fig. 19,35

6 months later tissues are well maintained but significantly reduced as a result of the surgical procedure.

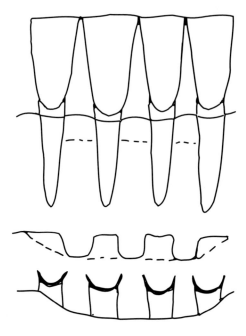

Fig. 19,36

Principles of osseous resection in pocket elimination surgery. In the top diagram, dotted lines represent the base of proximal infrabony craters. Osteoplasty is the removal of non-supporting bone, that is, the buccal or lingual plates between the teeth, leaving the irregular contour in the middle diagram. To give an architecture more amenable to maintenance, some supporting bone is removed from the buccal or lingual aspects of the teeth, leaving them less supported, but in theory more maintainable.

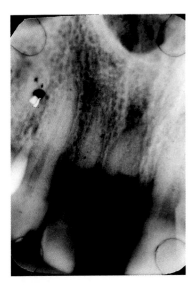

Fig. 19,37

Sequel of pocket elimination with interdental denudation. Teeth 11 and 12 have sustained fracture at the level of the alveolar bone.

patient is educated in thorough methods of plaque control, flaps are raised, roots are planed and tissues are restored to anatomical contour so that they can be maintained in that state. The negative side of this philosophy is that actual support may be lost in the pursuit of anatomical form.

An example of classical pocket elimination surgery which in fact was combined with interdental denudation (see below), is given in Figs 19,24–19,35. In this procedure, the palatal flap was resected to bone level, the buccal flap was positioned apically to the bone margin (apically displaced: see Fig. 19,32), and the two procedures of osteoplasty and ostectomy were performed. In osseous reduction surgery

(Fig. 19,36), 'osteoplasty' refers to the contouring of alveolar bone which does not provide direct support to the tooth via the periodontal ligament. 'Ostectomy' is the removal of such supporting bone to establish anatomical contour.

In the case shown, pocket elimination surgery led to a further sequel 2 years later. The patient sustained trauma and two incisors fractured at the bone margin (Fig. 19,37). Another possible traumatic complication is luxation of teeth from sockets. Patients undergoing pocket elimination surgery should be warned of such potential complications. Where there is a known predisposing factor to trauma, such as body contact sports, a suitable mouthguard should be advised.

INTERDENTAL DENUDATION

This procedure was developed by the influential Texan periodontist John Prichard in the 1950s. Prichard achieved predictable bone fill of intrabony defects (which he defined as three-walled infrabony defects) using linear incisions for flaps and exposing the proximal bone for healing of the gingival tissues by secondary intention. An example of the technique is shown in Figs 19,24–19,35.

At the time when interdental denudation was developed, the main concern of periodontists centred on alveolar bone, and its restoration was viewed as the ultimate goal of therapy. Prichard's view was that epithelial tissues should be surgically moved or removed from the intrabony defect, and that the blood clot should be held in place with a periodontal dressing that should not be allowed to enter the bony defect. We shall consider epithelial retardation in the next chapter, but for the moment let us note that regeneration of alveolar bone does not mean that the periodontal ligament and cementum have also regenerated.

The benefit of interdental denudation is that some bone usually does regenerate, but it is not clear whether there is any difference between this and more conservative procedures. Where denudation is performed by gingivectomy, however, more bone is lost than where proximal bone is covered (see Abstract 19,14).

POCKET REDUCTION SURGERY

As opposed to elimination of pockets by resective techniques, pocket reduction surgery seeks to maintain the tissues and to use surgical access for a thorough process of debridement with the aim of a long junctional epithelial attachment to a clean tooth surface. Foremost among these techniques is the modified Widman flap (Table 19,3) (Figs 19,38–19,50).

Other forms of replaced flap also have been described, but undoubtedly the most adaptable flap technique is that described by Kieser (Table 19,4). Depending on the circumstances encountered, this technique may be adjusted to fit virtually any clinical situation (Figs 19,51–19,73).

The 'secret' of Kieser's approach is that it aims primarily at the correct form of flap from the outset, with an outline incision to match

Table 19,3: *Modified Widman flap surgery*

1. Essentially a form of replaced flap
2. Three incisions and minimal flap reflection:
    Vertical incision close to teeth, with exaggerated scalloping on palatal side
    Crevicular incision
    Flap reflected just beyond alveolar crest
    Horizontal incision to undermine and remove collar of tissue round teeth
3. Very conservative debridement with frequent sterile saline irrigation:
    Removal of all plaque and calculus
    Preservation of root surface
    Preservation of proximal bone surface (not curetted)
4. Exact flap adaptation with full coverage of bone
5. Suturing aimed at primary union of proximal flap projections

Two features often omitted today
1. Use of antibiotic ointment over sutures
2. Placement of periodontal dressing
Instead the patient is commonly advised not to disturb the surgical area, and to use a chlorhexidine mouthrinse 12-hourly for maintenance of plaque control

After Ramfjord SP & Nissle RR (1974) The modified Widman flap. *Journal of Periodontology* **45**: 601–607.

Table 19,4: *An adaptable flap technique*

1. Outline incision
2. Thinning incision, concentrating on the form of the flap
3. With thick tissues, as in some posterior palatal regions, a crevicular incision is made first, and the flap raised for accurate outline and thinning incisions
4. Flap raised preferably 2–3 mm only
5. Cervical wedge is removed, and roots are planed
6. Flap is adapted, or raised further if apical positioning is indicated
7. Suturing, and dressing if indicated

After Kieser JB (1974) An approach to periodontal pocket elimination. *British Journal of Oral Surgery* **12**: 177–195.

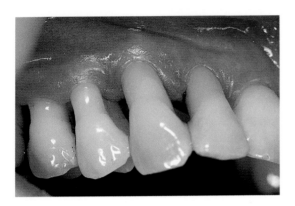

Fig. 19,38

Modified Widman flap: teeth 12–15 have lost some support, and have a 6–9 mm PD after a reasonable response to root planing.

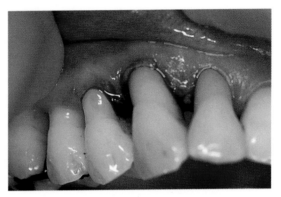

Fig. 19,40

Crevicular and inverse bevel incisions.

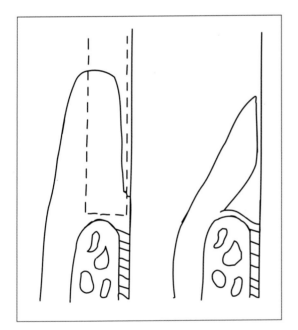

Fig. 19,39

The collar of tissue is removed, leaving access for debridement, and the flap is replaced as near to the same place as possible.

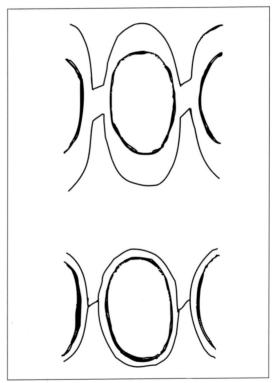

Fig. 19,41

Proximally, the tissues are more easily cut at a slight angle.

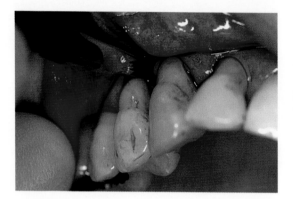

Fig. 19,42

The horizontal incision is made after deflecting the flap labially.

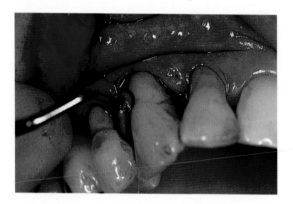

Fig. 19,43

The curette is used always *away* from the bone.

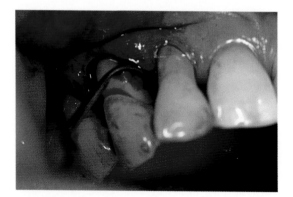

Fig. 19,44

Remaining soft tissue is curetted carefully, but the bone is left covered.

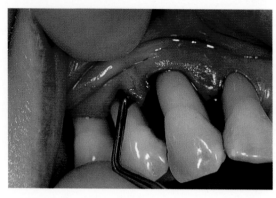

Fig. 19,45

Root planing is performed, but not too close to the bone, to leave supracrestal attachment undisturbed.

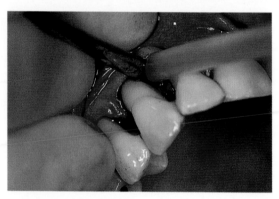

Fig. 19,46

The tissues are frequently bathed with physiological saline.

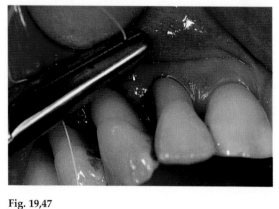

Fig. 19,47

Sutures are placed with an attempt to achieve primary union of the buccal and lingual proximal projections.

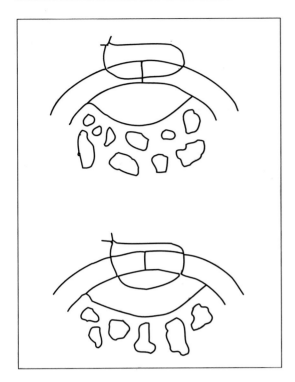

Fig. 19,48

The upper diagram shows where the suture should go. The lower diagram is a simple interrupted suture.

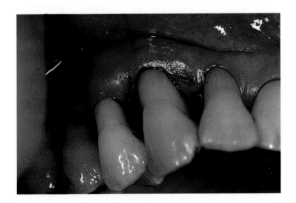

Fig. 19,49

Suturing is complete. Chlorhexidine mouthrinse is prescribed for one week, for oral hygiene.

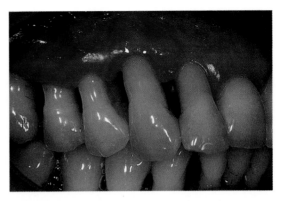

Fig. 19,50

Healing at 3 months.

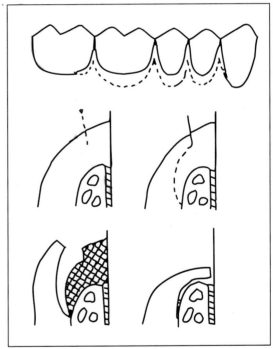

Fig. 19,51

Kieser technique: first an outline incision is made, then a thinning incision to produce an adaptable flap. The flap is elevated, and all the remaining tissue is removed, allowing the flap to be sutured neatly in position.

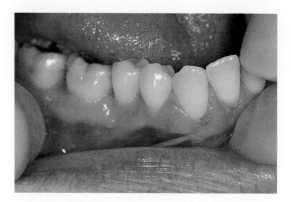

Fig. 19,52

Following thorough root planing, there are still pockets of 6–8 mm present from the distal surface of tooth 45 to the distal surface of tooth 42.

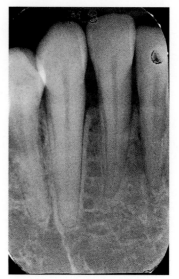

Fig. 19,55

Radiograph of teeth 41 to 44.

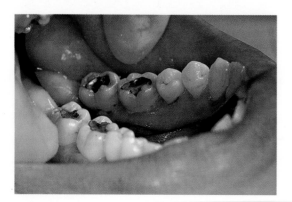

Fig. 19,53

Mirror view.

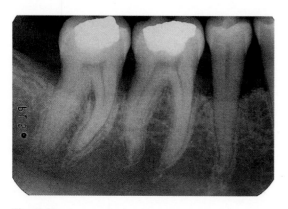

Fig. 19,54

Radiograph of teeth 44 to 47.

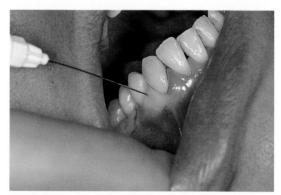

Fig. 19,56

Following local anaesthesia, papillae are injected to reduce bleeding. Blanching is produced in each papilla.

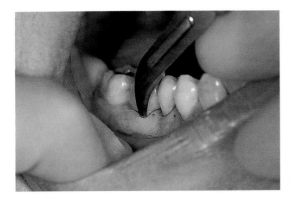

Fig. 19,57

The outline incision is started in the gingival crevice near the mesial line angle of tooth 46 (No. 12 scalpel)

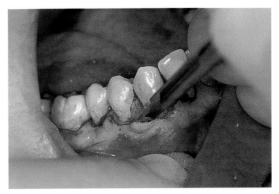

Fig. 19,60

A filleting procedure is used at the papillae.

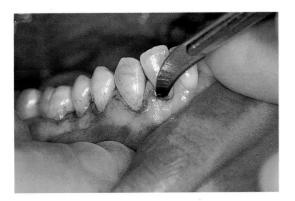

Fig. 19,58

The incision is continued and neatly ended near the distal line angle of tooth 42.

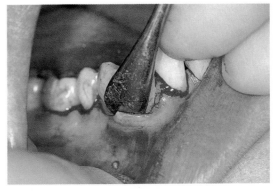

Fig. 19,61

The flap is raised with a periosteal elevator. All these procedures are also performed on the lingual aspect, usually before the labial aspect.

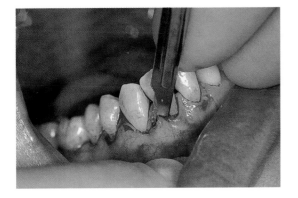

Fig. 19,59

In the reverse direction, a No. 15 scalpel is used to thin the flap and extend the incision down to the bone.

the tooth contours and a thinning incision to ensure a thin and pliable flap. Non-flap tissue is then simply removed, roots are planed, osseous adjustment is performed if necessary and any final flap adjustments are performed easily prior to suturing.

Pocket reduction provides a useful alternative to pocket elimination simply because it does not consign much tissue to the doom of excision. In the upper anterior region, this technique nowadays is used often with a crevicular incision only on the labial aspect, so as to replace the flap as close as possible to its original position.

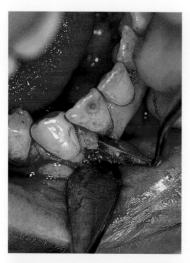

Fig. 19,62

Proximal
tissues are
undermined.

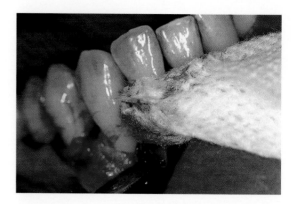

Fig. 19,65

Gauze is used briefly to dry each proximal defect.

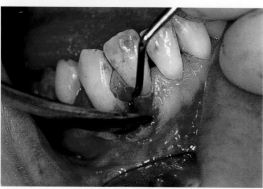

Fig. 19,63

A large curette is used to remove tissue.

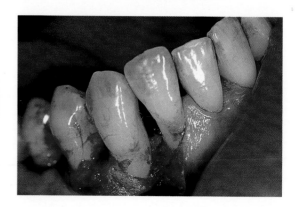

Fig. 19,66

Inspection shows remaining calculus.

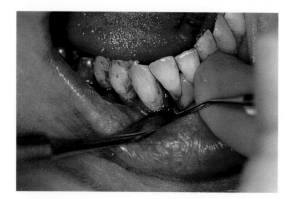

Fig. 19,64

Roots are planed.

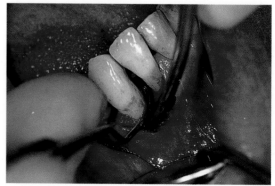

Fig. 19,67

Further planing is performed.

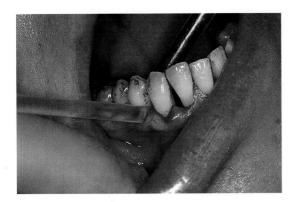

Fig. 19,68

Tissues are washed frequently with saline.

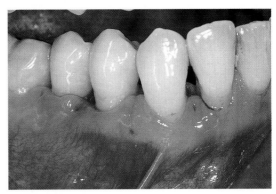

Fig. 19,71

After 1 week, sutures are removed.

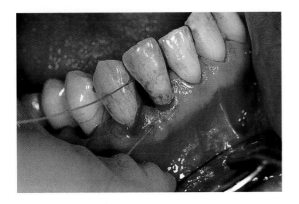

Fig. 19,69

Interrupted sutures are placed (continuous sutures are also an option).

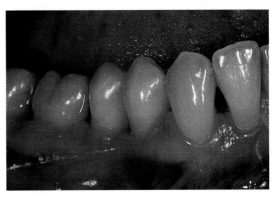

Fig. 19,72

Result after 4 months.

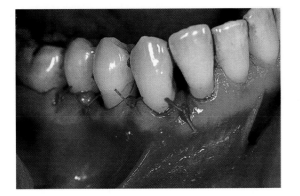

Fig. 19,70

The sutured apically positioned flap. Chlorhexidine mouthrinse is prescribed.

	6	5	4	3	2
1	7│3│8	7│5│8	7│3│5	4│3│7	6│3│5
	7│2│7	8│5│7	6│2│6	5│4│7	6│3│5
2	5│2│4	5│5│8	7│5│5	4│2│7	5│2│3
	5│3│4	7│7│8	6│2│6	4│2│7	6│2│2
3	4│2│3	4│3│5	4│2│3	3│1│4	4│2│2
	5│2│4	4│3│3	3│2│3	3│2│3	4│3│3

Fig. 19,73

Probing charts. Line 1 is initial assessment; line 2 is 3 months after root planing; line 3 is 4 months post-surgery. At the last assessment no BOP occurred, and the tissues appeared well maintained.

BONE GRAFTS AND SUBSTITUTES

In the 1960s and 1970s there was considerable interest in cancellous bone grafts into periodontal bony defects. At least two reasons may be given for this. First, periodontitis was viewed in many quarters as a disease of bone: if this was so, then attention should be given to restoring this tissue. Secondly, several researchers into this technique considered that bone grafting could induce restitution of the attachment.

With regard to the first reason why bone grafting was used, bone is more a bystander in periodontitis, rather than the centre of the disease. The bone simply recedes before the advance of inflammation. Inflammation in turn progresses with attachment loss, which is the real centre of periodontitis.

If the restitution of lost bone is considered, then there is evidence that bone grafting is no more successful than conservative flap surgery, which also results in bone fill of defects. Consider Abstracts 19,7 and 19,8. The first is one of the best grafting studies in the literature, and suggested a mean 0.7 mm overfill in zero-, one- and two-walled defects of 2.1 mm mean depth. The second study showed a mean bone regeneration of 2.5 mm in large two- or three-walled pockets after replaced flap surgery with no osseous adjustments. In this context, grafts do not seem to offer any advantage. A further significant side-effect sometimes has been reported: root resorption and ankylosis (see Chapter 20).

Considering the need for removal of donor bone from another site, and the possibility of root resorption, it is not surprising that workers in this field turned to bone substitutes. These are not grafts, but relatively inert substances. Grafts are specifically living tissues. An early study of one such substance showed similar results to autogenous bone grafts (Abstract 19,9), and one recent study showed moderately better results with a bioactive glass (Abstract 19,10).

Abstract 19,7 *A clinical and histological evaluation of autogenous iliac crest bone grafts in humans: Part I. Wound healing 2 to 8 months*

Dragoo MR, Sullivan HC, *Journal of Periodontology* 1973; **44**: 599–613

In four volunteers with proximal zero-, one- or two-walled bone defects, 12 teeth were subjected to flap surgery with 1.5 mm supercrestal overfill by cancellous bone grafts from the iliac crest of the pelvis, and a total of 21 experimental and adjacent teeth were removed with the attached proximal tissues at 2, 3, 4, 6 and 8 months after surgery. In nine other patients, grafts were placed without subsequent removal of the tissues. A high standard of plaque control was maintained throughout the study. The histological specimens showed a mean 0.7 mm of supercrestal bone fill in a defect of 2.1 mm mean depth. Above this, there was an average 1 mm of connective tissue attachment and 1.3 mm of long epithelial attachment. In the other subjects, the mean alveolar bone height increased by 3.8 mm from the base of defects varying from 1.5 to 7.5 mm.

Comment: This is a good study of the validity of bone grafting as a technique, in a technically exacting situation, albeit without controls. The authors felt that a longer study might have shown more bone, but this is debatable. Remodelling might have reduced it a little. This is not the same as bone fill generated without grafts.

Abstract 19,8 *Osseous repair in infrabony periodontal defects*

Polson AM, Heijl LC, *Journal of Clinical Periodontology* 1978; **5**: 13–23

Apically positioned flaps were performed on 15 teeth with large infrabony defects in nine patients with adult periodontitis. A programme of thorough plaque control was continued throughout. Re-entry 6–8 months later showed total resolution of 11 defects and reduction of mean defect depth from 3.5 mm to 1 mm. From multiple measurements, resolution was accounted for by 77% bone regeneration and 18% crestal resorption.

Comment: This study shows a predictable level of bone repair after flap surgery. Half of the defects extended round three surfaces of a tooth.

Abstract 19,9 *Kielbone in new attachment attempts in humans*

Nielsen IM, Ellegaard B, Karring T, *Journal of Periodontology* 1981; **52**: 723–728

In 55 patients, 46 infrabony defects (mean depth 4.6 mm) were treated with autogenous bone grafts from edentulous areas of the jaws, and 46 (5.0 mm) with a bone substitute made from de-antigenized bovine bone. In each case, the surgery included coverage by a free mucosal graft (epithelial retardation – see Chapter 20) and perforation of the defect with a bur to encourage marrow proliferation. After 6 months, mean probing depths had reduced from 7.6 mm to 2.5 mm for the bone substitute and from 7.7 mm to 2.1 mm for the grafts. The difference between treatments was not significant.

Comment: This study showed that bone substitutes were capable of producing similar clinical results to living bone grafts, with obvious benefits in not needing a donor site in the patient.

Abstract 19,10 *Comparison of bioactive glass synthetic bone graft particles and open debridement in the treatment of human periodontal defects. A clinical study*

Froum SJ, Weinberg MA, Tarnow D, *Journal of Periodontology* 1998; **69**: 698–709

In 16 healthy patients 1–3 months after OHI and root planing, 59 selected infrabony defects were treated by flap surgery, either alone (27 sites) or with the addition of a glass particle bone substitute (32 sites) that appears to have the potential for incorporation within healing bone. After 12 months, the mean changes in recession, attachment level and probing depth were more favourable in the bone substitute sites (1.26, 2.96 and 4.26 mm) than in the control flap surgery sites (1.87, 1.54 and 3.44 mm).

Comment: Surgery soon after non-surgical treatment may take place in a healing environment and produce better results. This study as published does not appear free from potential operator bias (see Chapter 15) but the bone fill in control sites is similar to some other studies. However, it shows results comparable to those of other bone substitute studies, with a mean gain over flap surgery of 1.4 mm in clinical attachment.

Any material placed in a periodontal bony defect should have a regenerative potential. In Abstract 19,7 autogenous bone grafts were shown to result in 1–2 mm of new connective tissue attachment in human beings. However, block dissections of teeth with surrounding alveolar bone and tissue were needed to show these results; these are rarely performed. The results were certainly interesting but probably of little clinical significance.

There is a further reason that may be advanced against placing bone grafts or substitutes in osseous defects. Clinically, the return of bone after other kinds of periodontal treatment is a sensitive indicator of success. Bone will only return after the eradication of inflammation, which means that further attachment loss is unlikely.

Abstract 19,11 *Evaluation of guided tissue regeneration in the treatment of paired periodontal defects*

Pritlove-Carson S, Palmer RM, Floyd PD, *British Dental Journal* 1995; **179**: 388–394

In nine subjects aged 27–47 years, 20 within-subject pairs of proximal defects were selected for an intra-pair comparison of flap surgery, using a crevicular incision, with GTR, using the original non-resorbable type of polytetrafluorethylene membrane. Defects were paired on the basis of marked similarity. At surgery, full site preparation was completed prior to the operator being informed as to which site was to receive the membrane. Mean probing depths measured with an automated probe reduced from 5.83 mm at baseline to 3.16 mm 12 months later in the test group and from 5.28 mm to 3.84 mm in the controls. Corresponding attachment level gains were 0.55 mm in the test group and 0.53 mm in the controls. The difference in probing depth reduction was statistically significant.

Comment: This is apparently the first published randomized controlled trial comparing GTR with conventional surgery in osseous defects, over 10 years after the technique was published. It also may be one of very few trials to incorporate a simple safeguard against operator bias (see Chapter 15), in addition to examiner blinding. The similarity in PAL gains suggests little clinical benefit of the sort that might be expected from GTR.

TISSUE REGENERATION (NEW ATTACHMENT)

By the late 1970s, evidence was accumulating that regeneration of the periodontal ligament and cementum rarely occurred to any significant degree. In the next chapter, we shall consider the scientific basis for regenerative procedures. The results of two representative clinical trials of this new form of therapy are presented in Abstracts 19,11 and 19,12.

There is no doubt that this philosophy has captured the imagination of many outside periodontology. However, it would be wise not to exaggerate the potential of what has been achieved. Scientifically, regenerative procedures are impressive. In clinical terms, however, they may be no better than other forms of treatment. Consider, for instance, the result in Figs 19,74 and 19,75. An apparently 'hopeless' second premolar, treated with root

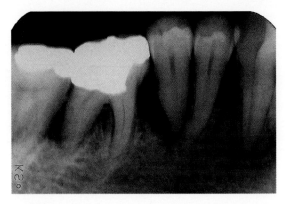

Fig. 19,74

Advanced periodontitis in a 55-year-old female. At presentation, tooth 45 was vital with a distal 9 mm PD, but tooth 46 was non-vital. Treatment of tooth 45 was with OHI and root planing only. The distal root was later resected on tooth 46.

Abstract 19,12 *Enamel matrix derivative in the treatment of intrabony periodontal defects*

Heijl L, Heden G, Svärdström G, et al., *Journal of Clinical Periodontology* 1997; **24**: 705–714

Enamel matrix proteins appear essential to the development of cementum on a root surface. This is the first clinical trial of a preparation derived from these proteins, with the aim of promoting regeneration of connective tissue attachment. An experimental trial was conducted with 34 pairs of sites chosen for limited repair potential in 33 subjects. Modified Widman flap surgery was performed, with thorough cleaning of proteinaceous debris from root surfaces, and test (EMD) or control (vehicle only) preparations were applied. After 3 years, the mean PD reduced from 7.8 mm in both groups to 4.6 mm in test sites and to 5.2 mm in controls; attachment level gains were, respectively, 2.2 mm and 1.7 mm. More than one-third of the bone previously lost was regained in test sites only. All these differences were significant.

Comment: This is a good trial, with results that show some additional potential for the technique. Although modest, EMD gains appear to be long-lasting in comparison to flap surgery alone

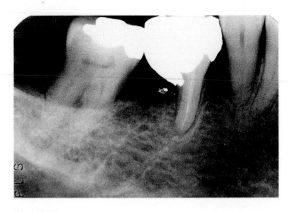

Fig. 19,75

Healing response on teeth 45 and 46 maintained 9 years after root planing. The distal of 45 now has a 3 mm PD without BOP. Tooth 48 was removed for unrelated reasons.

planing only, was vital and healthy 9 years later. Such unexpected events occur occasionally with all types of periodontal treatment.

Longer follow-up studies of GTR so far suggest no great clinical advantage over other modes of treatment (Abstract 19,13). The question to be answered for any clinical adjunctive treatment of periodontitis is whether there are situations in which it could

Abstract 19,13 *Long-term stability of clinical attachment following guided tissue regeneration and conventional therapy*

Cortellini P, Pini Prato GP, Tonetti MS, *Journal of Clinical Periodontology* 1996; **23**: 106–111

In each of 44 patients treated with root planing for severe periodontitis, one infrabony defect was treated with GTR. One year later, each GTR site was matched by PAL to one root planing site. Five years after treatment, there was a further mean attachment loss of 1.2 mm in GTR sites and 1.3 mm in root planing sites. However, two-thirds of all sites remained stable. The 23 patients in whom both sites were stable had continued good oral hygiene, complied with the recall programme and did not smoke; these characteristics were reversed in 10 patients in whom both sites lost probing attachment.

Comment: As with other types of periodontal therapy, GTR depends on maintenance. In patients in whom this is lacking, deterioration is comparable with that of healed root planing sites.

make the difference between keeping and losing a tooth.

A GUIDE TO TECHNIQUES

Surgical technique, like any skill, can be learnt only by doing it. Practice makes perfect, as the saying goes. Nevertheless, each operator develops ways of making the task easier, thorough and perhaps more predictable in outcome. There is no point in struggling to remove a piece of tissue, for instance, when more attention to the incision will make the task simple. Likewise, there are simple ways of thinning flaps, shaping tuberosities and removing bone.

LOCAL ANAESTHESIA AND BLEEDING CONTROL

When anaesthetizing a quadrant for surgery (or even root planing), there are ways of making it more pleasant for the patient. In the lower quadrant, an inferior alveolar nerve block may be given virtually painlessly if the tissues are initially stretched and a drop of solution is expressed in advance of the needle as it travels. Cross-over of lower nerves at the midline is best dealt with by waiting for lingual and mental nerve anaesthesia, and then adding small infiltrations next to the incisors on the same side.

In the upper jaw, a horizontally-angled buccal infiltration that is progressively injected with a long needle may cover several teeth. A quadrant may be covered by three or even two such injections. If the two central incisors are covered, then it is easy to make the incisive nerve block comfortable by injecting slowly and progressively through the central papilla to blanch the incisive papilla. Even a greater palatine nerve block may be made comfortable if a sharp needle (not blunted elsewhere on bone) is *gently* introduced submucosally and the injection is made *slowly*.

The role of a vasoconstrictor in periodontal surgery is sometimes overlooked. Tissue to be removed may be rendered almost haemorrhage-free by epinephrine in the local anaesthetic. A steeply-angled intra-papillary injection usually will produce the desired effect.

INCISIONS

Incisions define the boundary between tissue to be moved or removed and tissue to remain in place. Consequently, they must have a clear beginning and end. A scalloped inverse bevel incision starts and ends within the gingival crevice unless it continues into a further procedure such as a tuberosity resection.

Kieser (Table 19,4) describes two stages in the incision: an outline, which extends 1–2 mm into the tissue; and a thinning incision, which undermines the flap and connects with alveolar bone. When the flap is fully delineated in this way, it may be raised quite easily from the underlying bone with a periosteal elevator.

For the most part, vertical relieving incisions are not needed for flaps raised for access to pockets and root surfaces. On a very small flap, involving one papilla only, it may be necessary. Superfluous incisions allow the possibility of more movement after the procedure is completed.

The essence of an external bevel gingivectomy is the incision, although there are other significant aspects in its execution (Figs 19,76–19,93). The incision is best made with a

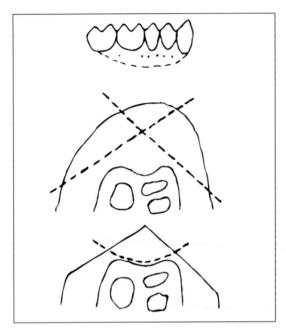

Fig. 19,76

External bevel gingivectomy. (Top): A linear incision is made after marking the extent of pockets on the mucosa. (Middle): Buccal and lingual incisions made. (Bottom): Where bony defects are present, the proximal tissue is curetted.

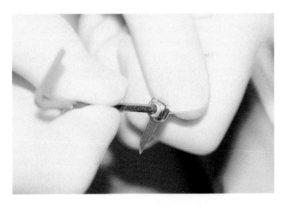

Fig. 19,77

The Blake knife blade is firmly secured with the Allan key.

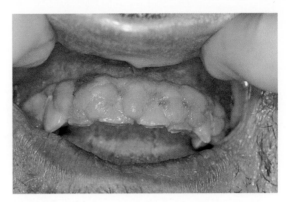

Fig. 19,78

A patient with gingival enlargement from cyclosporin and nifedipine relating to a renal transplant.

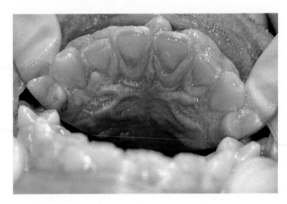

Fig. 19,79

Palatal view.

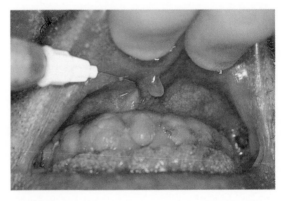

Fig. 19,80

Local anaesthetic is injected over several teeth in a row.

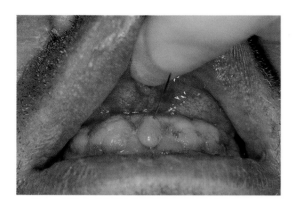

Fig. 19,81

Incisive block is given through the anaesthetized labial papilla.

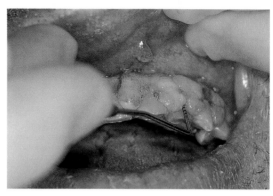

Fig. 19,84

Marking the pocket base: probe in pocket.

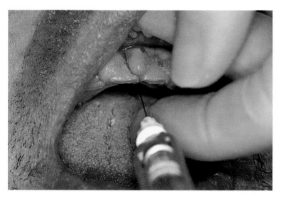

Fig. 19,82

Block is reinforced when incisive papilla is anaesthetized.

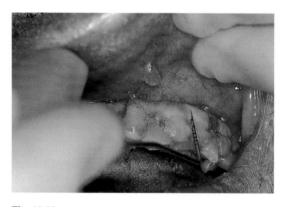

Fig. 19,85

Marking the pocket base: probe is in the same position on surface of gingiva.

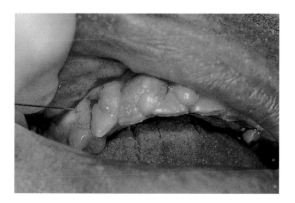

Fig. 19,83

Other papillae are injected for haemostatic control.

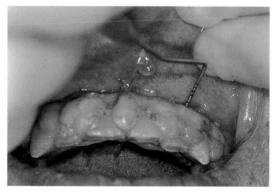

Fig. 19,86

Marking the pocket base: probe is turned at right angle to mark the point.

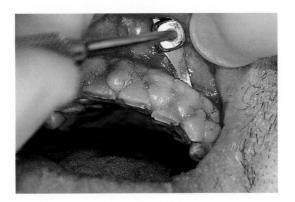

Fig. 19,87

No. 15 blade is drawn along from mesial line angle of tooth 24 to make initial incision.

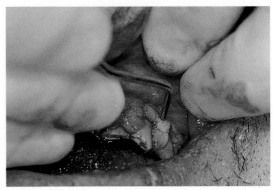

Fig. 19,90

Tissue loosened with curette.

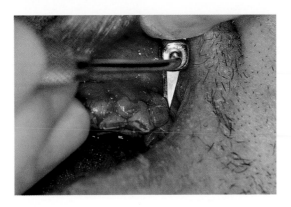

Fig. 19,88

Incision retraced with No. 11 blade to penetrate to the teeth.

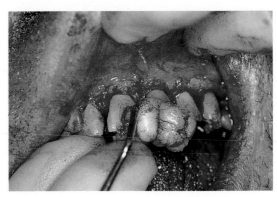

Fig. 19,91

Tissue gradually removed.

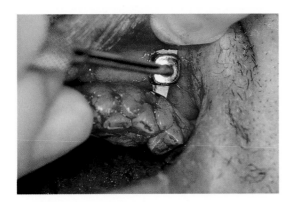

Fig. 19,89

No. 11 blade deep in a papillary region. Similar incisions are made first on the palatal aspect.

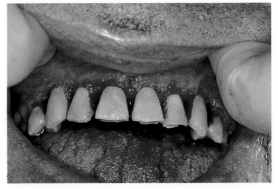

Fig. 19,92

Tissue removed (cf. Fig. 19,78). When haemostasis was achieved, patient was prescribed chlorhexidine mouthrinse.

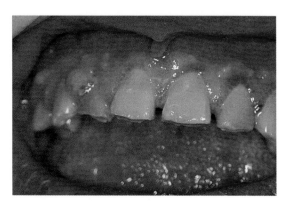

Fig. 19,93

After 4 months, it is apparent that the patient is not maintaining satisfactory hygiene, and enlargement is beginning to recur. Because of this possibility, where the gingiva prevents initial practice of good hygiene it is best only to perform a trial portion of surgery in the most accessible area of the mouth, as here. No further surgery was performed for this patient.

marked guide to its proposed apical extent on the teeth. A measuring probe may be used to indicate the base of the pockets. The incision should be linear, not scalloped. Its 45° angle will ensure a neat anatomical result round the teeth, and it should start mid-dentally adjacent to a papilla. The Blake knife should be drawn across the tissue, using a No. 15 blade, to make an initial incision. This should be followed up with a No. 11 blade in a Blake holder, or perhaps a No. 12 scalpel, to extend the incision into the embrasures and make it complete.

Where the thickness of the gingival tissue is in doubt, such as on the palatal aspect of some upper molar teeth, a crevicular incision should be used first to reflect a full thickness flap, and it will often be possible to judge the correct position for the outline incision.

Soft tissue removal

After completing incisions, the flap may be eased 1–2 mm off the marginal bone. Any difficulty at this stage is due usually to an incomplete incision. When the flap has been raised, the remaining tissue around the teeth is removed.

There may be some difficulty if curettes are the only instruments used, and it is usually time-saving and neater to undermine this tissue with a suitable knife or scalpel. For a modified Widman flap this is mandatory in order to leave the supracrestal connective tissue.

After removal of obvious pieces of tissue, each area should be dried with the corner of a gauze swab. When this is removed, vision is better and further tissue tags may be seen and removed.

There is one further action that may enhance the results of an external bevel gingivectomy. A curette is used to perform interdental denudation. With this modification, gingivectomy may be used to treat infrabony pockets. This is called 'Scandinavian style gingivectomy' and it has been compared with other periodontal surgical procedures in clinical trials.

Root surfaces

Following soft tissue removal, the roots are thoroughly planed. A universal pattern curette is appropriate for this procedure, and thorough inspection may be performed after drying the area with a gauze swab as above.

On occasion, the root surface may need some alteration, such as when a furcationplasty or tunnel preparation is performed to facilitate subsequent oral hygiene (Chapter 22).

Bone decisions

On the whole, it is best to minimize any removal of bone. Sometimes, moderate osteoplasty to remove anatomical or reactive bone will assist flap adaptation. Ostectomy, however, is rarely performed today. A tiny amount of such bone may be removed occasionally where the contour of the healing tissues is thereby enhanced.

As with root surfaces, furcation surgery (Chapter 22) sometimes may involve osseous reduction to produce satisfactory postoperative contours, or for purposes such as tunnel preparation.

Augmentation of bone with substitutes is a decision best made when the shape of the defect is apparent. Bearing in mind the results of flap surgery alone (Abstract 19,8) and the possibilities of GTR, such augmentation often will not be needed.

TUBEROSITY (AND RETROMOLAR) RESECTION

A simple and adaptable extension of the Kieser technique to deal with these areas is shown, along with thinning of a palatal flap and palatal osteoplasty in Figs 19,94–19,111. The sides of a tuberosity are undermined with two incisions that appear parallel on the surface but follow the slopes of the external surfaces. The palatal flap is reflected so that a further horizontal incision can be made to separate the fibrous tuberosity tissue from the bone. Further tissue then may be removed more easily, and bone if necessary. Finally the flaps are brought together, trimmed and sutured into position.

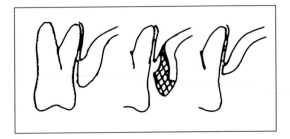

Fig. 19,94

Palatal thinning: a thick palatal mucoperiosteal flap is raised, and following inspection, the initial and thinning incisions are made. The flap is trimmed if necessary and positioned for suturing.

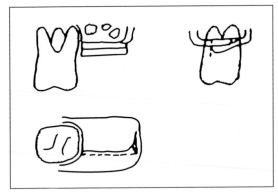

Fig. 19,96

After removal of the wedge, the flaps are brought down, and trimmed if necessary.

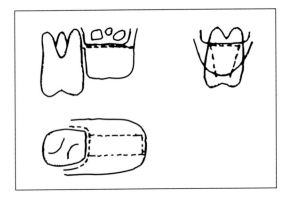

Fig. 19,95

Tuberosity resection: parallel incisions are made, diverging as they undermine the two flaps. A flap is reflected, and the residual wedge is undermined with a horizontal incision.

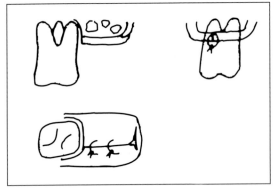

Fig. 19,97

Finally the flaps are sutured together.

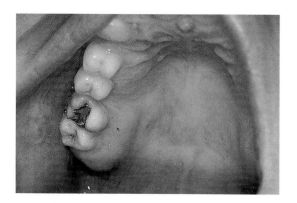

Fig. 19,98

Tuberosity resection and palatal thinning: teeth 16 and 17 have 5–6 mm palatal pockets extending round distal of tooth 17.

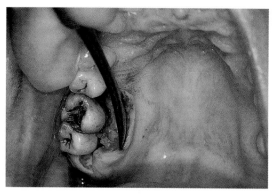

Fig. 19,101

Flap reflected. A minimal buccal flap was also raised.

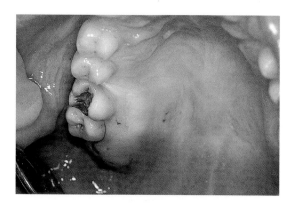

Fig. 19,99

Parallel tuberosity incisions.

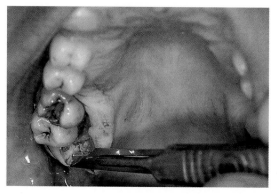

Fig. 19,102

Horizontal incision commenced under tuberosity wedge.

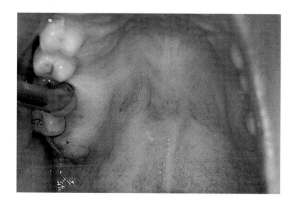

Fig. 19,100

Crevicular incision.

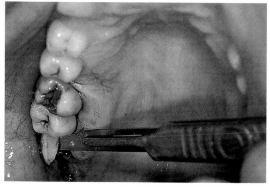

Fig. 19,103

Wedge resected.

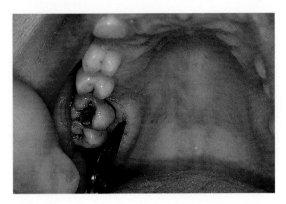

Fig. 19,104

After inspection, outline incision is made on palatal flap.

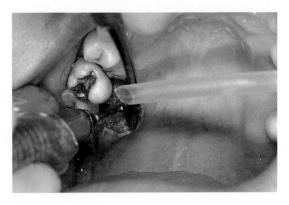

Fig. 19,106

There is a large bony ridge which is reduced for a better contour.

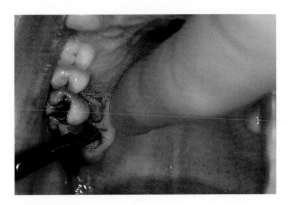

Fig. 19,105

The flap is thinned.

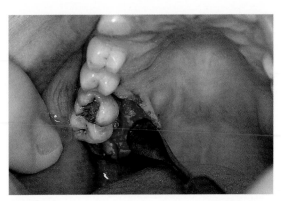

Fig. 19,107

Excisions are complete and the flap is ready to suture.

FLAP POSITIONING

Returning to the ordinary flap procedure, a decision is made on where the flap should be placed for optimum healing. If it is replaced at its former position, no further adjustment is required, but for apical positioning the flap must be undermined beyond the mucogingival junction.

To maintain the flap in its position after suturing while a fibrin clot forms, firm pressure for 4 min. with a saline-dampened swab is helpful.

SUTURING

A variety of suturing techniques have been suggested for different reasons. The simple interrupted suture is effective for most circumstances, but is recommended with a specific

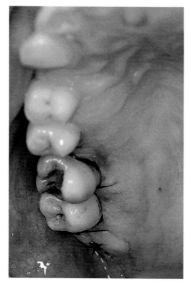

Fig. 19,108

Suturing is complete. Chlorhexidine mouthrinse is prescribed for 1 week.

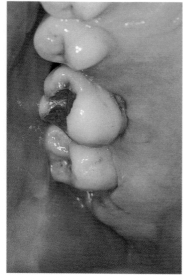

Fig. 19,109

After suture removal 1 week later.

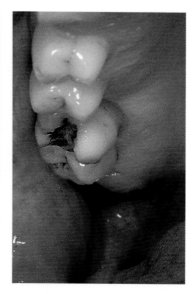

Fig. 19,110

3 months post-surgery.

Fig. 19,111

(1): PDs before surgery; (2): PDs at 3 months.

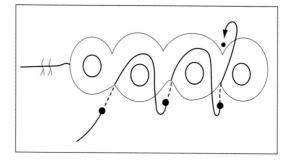

Fig. 19,112

Diagram of continuous suture. On the return journey, the suture will hold the upper flap in the picture, looping round the teeth before ending with a knot to the loose end of the suture.

variation for the modified Widman flap, where one aim is to achieve primary union between buccal and lingual papillary projections.

The continuous suture (Fig. 19,112) is thought by some to be a simpler technique and to allow better adjustment of tension, but studies have shown no advantage over the interrupted suture.

Where increased tension is required, to hold the flap in a specific position, an inverse mattress suture may provide this (Figs 19,113 and 19,114). The horizontally retained form should be employed, because the vertical form provides no more tension than an interrupted suture before it begins to tear the tissue (Fig. 19,115).

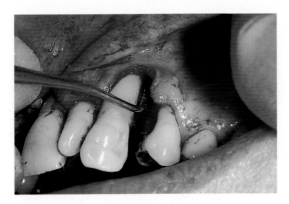

Fig. 19,113

The flap requires some tension distal to tooth 23.

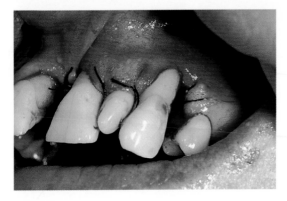

Fig. 19,114

Horizontal external mattress suture providing tension.

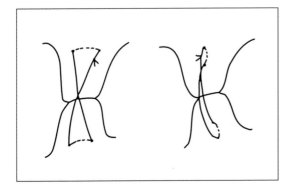

Fig. 19,115

Horizontal (left) and vertical forms of external mattress suture.

DRESSINGS

A dressing or pack should be used only where it has a specific indication. Haemostasis should be achieved before, and not by, the application of a dressing. The only clear indication for a dressing is to achieve tissue stasis, such as with a free mucosal graft, or to protect a clot over bone in the interdental denudation technique.

Dressings have had several reported adverse effects: allergenicity, plaque retention, discomfort and a tendency to fall off. It is better, certainly for routine flap surgery, to place no dressing and use a 0.2% chlorhexidine mouthrinse 12-hourly to prevent plaque development on the clean post-surgical tooth surfaces until normal mechanical hygiene can be resumed (Chapters 21 and 24).

Following an external bevel gingivectomy, many operators will place a dressing almost without considering other possibilities. However, this is not essential, and saline packs may be used to encourage haemostasis before use of the mouthrinse as an alternative.

INSTRUCTIONS

As with any surgical procedure in the mouth, the main advice concerns possible haemorrhage and discomfort. Neither is likely with well-executed flap surgery, and the patient should be observed for 10 min after suturing to ensure that haemostasis is achieved. As a reassurance, gauze swabs may be given to the patient, with advice on soaking them in salty water, squeezing and using them with firm pressure for a sufficient length of time.

Activities likely to promote bleeding should be avoided: vigorous exercise or horizontal resting for the remainder of the day; smoking or alcoholic beverages for 3 days.

Anticipated discomfort may be dealt with by immediate post-operative analgesics, although it is wise to avoid those that affect clotting, such as aspirin. If given before local anaesthesia wears off, these are more likely to be effective. Analgesics should not be a routine, but should be given where the surgery has involved some event that might

Abstract 19,14 *The healing potential of the periodontal tissues following different techniques of periodontal surgery in plaque-free dentitions. A 2-year clinical study*

Rosling B, Nyman S, Lindhe J, et al., *Journal of Clinical Periodontology* 1976; **3**: 233–250

Following thorough presurgical treatment, 50 patients were allocated randomly to five types of surgery for advanced periodontitis. Ten patients each received: apically positioned flaps; Widman flaps; apically positioned flaps with bone removal; Widman flaps with bone removal; gingivectomy with curettage of bone defects but no bone removal. All types of surgery resulted in a satisfactory clinical condition when assessed up to 24 months later. Patients were seen every 2 weeks for maintenance. The principal variations between techniques were: gingivectomy had greater proximal bone loss (mean 2.7 mm) than either flap with bone removal (mean 1.8–1.9 mm); the greatest gain of probing attachment occurred with the Widman flap without bone removal; all two- and three-walled bony defects regenerated to some extent, except for 23% of those in the gingivectomy group; the best bone fill occurred in the Widman flap without bone removal.

Comment: This study occurred under excellent maintenance conditions, and most of the improvements were seen by 6 months, after which there was little change. The findings for gingivectomy may be extrapolated reasonably to interdental denudation, which has not been studied in a similar trial.

Abstract 19,15 *Results of periodontal treatment related to pocket depth and attachment level. Eight years*

Knowles JW, Burgett FG, Nissle RR, et al., *Journal of Periodontology* 1979; **50**: 225–233

Following initial non-surgical treatment, 78 patients with periodontitis were randomly assigned to have each half of the mouth treated with one of three procedures: subgingival curettage; modified Widman flap surgery; pocket elimination surgery. At 5 years, six patients had dropped out of the study, but by 8 years the figure was 35. Results were statistically similar for all three methods. Pockets of <3 mm lost attachment on the whole by 1 year; those of >4 mm gained it proportionately. There was a tendency for further pocket reduction and attachment loss in all depths of site over the next 4 years; little change occurred after 5 years. Most maintenance intervals were of 3 months.

Comment: Although there were minimal differences between results for the three techniques, trends were observed for better PD and PAL outcome with a modified Widman flap in deep pockets (7–12 mm). This large, well-executed study also supports the 'critical probing depth' concept, although not by that name.

give rise to discomfort, such as significant osseous surgery.

If a dressing falls off after 3 days, it is unlikely to be a problem. Loose sutures may need checking or removal. The patient must be encouraged to contact the operator if there is any apparent complication.

FOLLOW-UP AND REASSESSMENT

The very important subject of post-surgical maintenance is dealt with in Chapter 21.

Three months after surgery is a convenient time for reassessment, but there will be further less-marked changes beyond that point.

COMPARATIVE SURGICAL STUDIES

We looked earlier at the various philosophies of periodontal surgery. In conclusion, it is appropriate to consider two of the many studies that have compared different sorts of procedure. These are representative of researchers in Gothenburg (Abstract 19,14) and Michigan (Abstract 19,15).

The overall message of these studies is that clinically effective results may be obtained by a wide variety of surgical approaches. However, the individual differences between them may suggest a preference in specified circumstances. For instance, a Widman flap (modified or not) may be preferred where aesthetic results are important, as in the upper anterior and premolar region of the mouth.

The hidden message of both studies is that thorough maintenance is essential to achieve success. We shall see more of this in Chapter 21.

20

PERIODONTAL WOUND HEALING

- How do periodontal surgical wounds heal?
- What is the importance of the relative speeds with which different tissues heal?
- How much can healing be enhanced by new techniques?

The periodontium is an amazing structure, designed specially to support the tooth in its socket, and composed partly of tissues found nowhere else in the body.

The story of how some of the mysteries of periodontal healing were unravelled is fascinating in itself; even more interesting is the story of how this led to the development of regenerative technology, so that it became possible to reconstruct at least a part of the lost periodontal attachment as it originally was.

First, we shall go back to before those events and see the simpler discoveries concerning simpler types of surgery. A number of studies examined, for instance, what happened to tissues after gingivectomy. One of the most thorough explorations of this subject was a series of studies by Stahl and colleagues, and one very important study is given in Abstract 20,1. In this study, we see that the scene is dominated by epithelium.

THE EARLY SEQUENCE OF EVENTS

When a knife is drawn through the skin, healing begins almost at once. Two sequences of events – protection and repair – are set speedily in motion. The same events are initiated in gingivectomy healing.

A blood clot quickly forms and is a highly active form of defence, utilizing the wonder-

Abstract 20,1 *Gingival healing II. Clinical and histologic repair sequences following gingivectomy*

Stahl SS, Witkin GJ, Cantor M, et al., *Journal of Periodontology* 1968; **39**: 109–118

In 128 otherwise healthy patients with periodontitis, 218 suprabony pockets were subjected to gingivectomy. Subsequently, postsurgical biopsies were taken from all these sites at intervals of 1, 7, 14, 21 and 28 days. At 1 day, inflammation was less in most cases than in the corresponding gingivectomy specimen, and there was mobilization of energy in the form of glycogen at the epithelial edge. At 7 days, epithelium was partly reformed, and at 14 days, a complete layer was present. Vascularization was reducing, after an earlier increase at 7 days. At 21 days, crevicular epithelialization was also complete. At 28 days, it appeared that connective tissue repair was not completed. The authors considered the most striking findings to be the absence of any variations on account of age, gender and pocket location, and the fact that connective tissue was still active at 28 days but epithelialization was complete by 14 days.

Comment: This early study clearly shows how quick is the epithelial response to surgery, whereas other tissues react more slowly. It also demonstrates that healing is a fundamental biological phenomenon that is similar in different places, despite its complexity.

ful powers of neutrophils to defend the body. The meshwork of fibrin fibres in a clot is a guide to the cells that engage in a search-and-destroy mission against any intruding bacteria.

While the phagocyte defence is under way, the repair process begins. There is speedy mitotic activity in the epithelium and the vascular endothelial tissues proliferate underneath. Slowly, the connective tissues increase their activity, which reaches its conclusion long after the epithelium has resumed a more leisurely pace of life.

This initial development of the protective and repair response is common to all skin and mucosal wounds and provides a cloistered scene for the later, concluding phases of the healing process.

THE FOUR PERIODONTAL HEALING TISSUES

In addition to the epithelium, there are at least four other components of the periodontal healing process. Two of them act together, or at least have not been separated out in the events. These are the cementum and periodontal ligament.

Then there is the bone, which may be slow in returning but provides an excellent indicator that inflammation has resolved.

Finally, there is a large quantity of soft gingival connective tissue. This has a resilience and rigidity that contributes strength and protection to the healed periodontium and supports tissues that are important but physically weak, e.g. the long junctional epithelium.

The fate of the blood clot depends on its position. If wholly enclosed in the tissues, it becomes organized and replaced with healthy granulation tissue and eventually with ordinary connective tissue or bone; if it is superficial, it provides a protection for epithelial repair.

THE EARLY DEVELOPMENT OF KNOWLEDGE ABOUT PERIODONTAL HEALING

One early question that was given considerable attention was the role of the epithelium in healing. To many who studied the results of

healing, the epithelium appeared to interfere with the establishment of a satisfactory 'reattachment' after surgery. It seemed that before the periodontal ligament and cementum could re-form, the epithelium had proliferated and raced over the connective tissues separating them from the tooth.

An early clinical contributor to this discussion was Prichard, who believed that he could do something about the epithelium by surgically keeping it as far from the healing periodontal attachment as possible with his interdental denudation technique (Chapter 19). Consequently, he used linear inverse bevel incisions and apically displaced flaps, so that there would be no epithelium near the proximal intrabony defects. An apically displaced flap is one that is positioned 2–3 mm apically to the alveolar bone margin.

It is instructive to see that many clinicians then shared a common view that bone fill in osseous defects resulted from reconstruction of the bone along with cementum and the ligament. Prichard linked these ideas to his technique, and promoted the concept that the interdental denudation procedure led to predictable bone fill. That this is not the reason for bone fill is apparent from studies such as that of Polson and Heijl (see Abstract 19,8), where it occurred with conventionally contoured flaps. Nor is the other idea correct: bone may form without any significant regeneration of the ligament.

It was apparent in the study of Dragoo and Sullivan (see Abstract 19,7) that the grafting of cancellous iliac crest bone into periodontal bony defects was accompanied by a small amount of ligament regeneration. Early animal studies suggested that regeneration was a significant part of healing after periodontal surgery. It was natural for investigators in this field to take matters a step further. In Abstract 20,2 we see the ultimate in restriction of the epithelium, combined with bone grafting.

The scene was ready for a break-through and it happened within 5 years. Before we see the remarkable developments, it is important to discuss two terms that emerged in the literature, and have a bearing on our understanding of the way in which the periodontium heals.

Abstract 20,2 *New periodontal attachment procedure based on retardation of epithelial migration*

Ellegaard B, Karring T, Löe H, *Journal of Clinical Periodontology* 1974; **1**: 75–88

In 88 subjects, the area about 1–2 cm all round an intrabony defect (on facial and lingual surfaces of the gingiva) was cleared of epithelium, and the defect was filled with fresh autogenous bone graft. A free mucosal graft was then placed over the denuded area and graft, and sutured in place. Subsequent clinical and radiographic examination indicated that 60% of defects were completely regenerated, with only 10% resulting in residual pockets of >3 mm. This compared with respective 40% and 60% rates when flap surgery was employed.

Comment: At this time, many investigators assumed that bony regeneration on the radiograph (which was evident in this study) also meant that the attachment had regenerated. Because the free mucosal graft was deprived of its blood supply, the epithelium died but the connective tissue portion survived and subsequently was re-populated by epithelial cells from the surrounding mucosa.

RE-ATTACHMENT AND NEW ATTACHMENT

In the older periodontal literature, the term 're-attachment' referred to the idea that after a surgical procedure the gingiva (which was separated from the tooth by a pocket) re-attached as a result. However, Ellegaard (Abstract 20,2) and others were part of a new generation of experimenters who used the term 'new attachment' to refer to a root surface that became diseased with periodontitis, was treated with surgery and then healed with regeneration of some cementum and periodontal ligament attachment.

We are going to examine selected pieces of research that highlight certain aspects of the new periodontal landscape.

Many researchers believed that regeneration of bone was the sign of a regenerated attachment. Because bone fill is accompanied by the formation of a *lamina dura* parallel to

Abstract 20,3 *Healing following implantation of periodontitis affected roots into bone tissue*

Karring T, Nyman S, Lindhe J, *Journal of Clinical Periodontology* 1980; **7**: 96–105

Periodontitis was induced with floss ligatures on 12 teeth in three beagle dogs. Crowns were removed, separate roots filled, and the diseased root surfaces were thoroughly planed. At the apical limit of the planing, a notch was made round the root surface. Recipient sites had been made 3–4 months earlier by extraction of other teeth: flaps were raised, the roots were gently placed in sockets and flaps were then sutured in place. At each of 1, 2 and 3 months, eight roots and adjacent tissue were recovered. Most of the apical portion of the roots showed functional periodontal ligament with fibres inserted into bone and cementum. The planed coronal portions showed root resorption and ankylosis.

Comment: The epithelium was totally excluded from the healing around the roots. This study is part of the evidence that epithelium has a significant role in healing after periodontal flap surgery. Without it, there might be root resorption and ankylosis. One very significant finding was identified in some of the notches: from the intact apical cementum and ligament, a tiny amount of these tissues had proliferated into the apical part of the cavity. This showed clearly that new attachment had to come from existing attachment on a tooth root.

the root surface, it is easy to see how this idea took root, to coin a phrase. Those who believed this interpretation of events had a number of pieces of evidence, such as that in Dragoo and Sullivan's bone graft study (see Abstract 19,7). However, other studies soon cast a very different light on matters.

THE RELEVANCE OF EPITHELIUM, SOFT CONNECTIVE TISSUE AND BONE TO PERIODONTAL HEALING

The year of 1980 was good for regenerative papers and we shall consider three of them (Abstracts 20,3–20,5).

Abstract 20,4 *Healing following implantation of periodontitis-affected roots into gingival connective tissue*

Nyman S, Karring T, Lindhe J, et al., *Journal of Clinical Periodontology* 1980; **7**: 394–401

In two monkeys and one beagle dog, 48 roots were treated as in Abstract 20,3 but with the difference that they were not placed in healing extraction sockets, but on their sides in shallow bone grooves under mucoperiosteal flaps. Half of the roots and surrounding tissues were recovered at 2 months, and half at 3 months. Planed surfaces adjacent to bone showed resorption and ankylosis; next to soft connective tissue, they showed frequent resorption, and collagen fibres were orientated parallel to the root surface. On the unplaned apical surfaces normal ligament predominated, with attachment to either bone or soft connective tissue.

Comment: The study highlights the importance of the root surface. If it is unplaned and epithelium is kept away, normal attachment is present except where traumatic damage has occurred. If it is root planed after periodontitis, then keeping out the epithelium results in root resorption and, where there is bone, ankylosis.

The two Scandinavian experimental studies eliminated epithelium by making the scene of action underneath mucoperiosteal flaps. At the same time, any interference by bacteria was also excluded. The result clearly showed that a clean tooth root is not something that the adjacent gingival connective tissue and bone find congenial (Fig. 20,1). Instead, they treat it as a foreign body and try to resorb it. In the presence of bone, tooth root resorption is usually accompanied by ankylosis, and that was the case in these studies.

One of the main researchers in these studies, Sture Nyman, also worked with two well-known American colleagues on the next study (Abstract 20,5). This was part of a histological investigation of healing after various surgical procedures in suitable experimental animals. The result was a clear victory for epithelium, thanks to which the roots were not resorbed or ankylosed.

Abstract 20,5 *Histometric evaluation of periodontal surgery II. Connective tissue attachment levels after four regenerative procedures*

Caton J, Nyman S, Zander H, *Journal of Clinical Periodontology* 1980; **7**: 224–231

Symmetrical experimental periodontitis was produced in eight Rhesus monkeys; 3 months later all teeth were scaled. For 3 weeks strict plaque control was maintained, and half of the mouth in each monkey was treated with one of the following four surgical techniques: modified Widman flap (MWF); MWF + autogenous bone graft; MWF + bone substitute; periodic scaling with soft tissue curettage. The other half of each mouth was an untreated control. The strict plaque control programme continued and 1 year later the animals were killed and tissues were examined histologically. When the four techniques were assessed histometrically, there was a long junctional epithelium present on all operated root surfaces. The distance from the CEJ to the apical extent of the junctional epithelium was not different from the control measurement for any of the four procedures (around 3–3.5 mm). As added confirmation that the epithelium had migrated to the apical extent of instrumentation, marks from the latter were often apparent on root surfaces.

Comment: The other studies showed that epithelium is a protection for the root surface after planing; this study shows that it extends just as far as the planing, regardless of surgical technique.

GUIDED TISSUE REGENERATION

The next two steps in the story are a study in monkeys followed by the momentous event of testing a new surgical technology in a human volunteer. In the monkey study, a window in the alveolar bone was covered with a membrane that excluded gingival connective tissue after the cementum was removed. At the margins of the window new attachment regenerated, but less in the coronal aspects.

The study in a human volunteer, although a short communication, is one of the great historical landmarks in periodontology (Abstract 20,6). It showed that the four components of the periodontium (epithelium, gingival soft

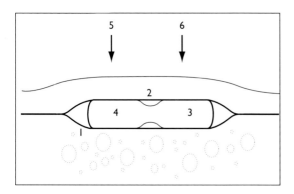

Fig. 20,1

Healing around tooth roots with epithelium excluded (see Abstract 20,4). In a groove in bone (1), a root is placed under a sutured mucosal flap (2). Half of the root is planed (3) and half has natural ligament attached (4). The ligament heals with normal periodontal ligament attachment (5) to both bone and mucosa. The planed surface undergoes resorption next to the mucosa, and resorption and ankylosis (6) next to the bone.

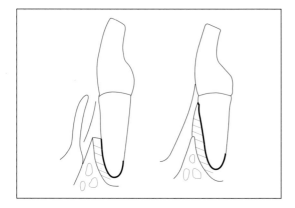

Fig. 20,2

GTR with a membrane. After the root has been planed, a sterile GTR membrane is placed over the root surface and the flap is replaced to cover it. If the membrane is not resorbable, it is removed after 6 weeks. When healing is complete, some regeneration of cementum and ligament has occurred coronally to the existing ligament, and the flap has an epithelial attachment above this.

connective tissue, bone, and cementum with ligament) all had separate potential for regeneration but that time was needed for the attachment to regenerate, during which the other tissues had to be kept from interfering.

The achievement of periodontal regeneration (Fig. 20,2), rather than repair, is a superb technical accomplishment, built on good preceding experimental scientific studies.

A DISQUIETING QUESTION

In the face of this technical achievement, there is one obvious and rather brutal question to be asked. The goal of periodontal regeneration has been achieved, but to what end? Of course, we assumed all along that regeneration is better than repair. The controlled studies mentioned in Chapter 19 show that GTR has a moderate clinical effect that adds nothing after 5 years (see Abstracts 19,11 and

Abstract 20,6 *New attachment following surgical treatment of human periodontal disease*

Nyman S, Lindhe J, Karring T, et al., *Journal of Clinical Periodontology* 1982; **9**: 290–296

Following elevation of mucoperiosteal flaps on the buccal and lingual aspects of a mandibular incisor, granulation tissue was curetted from a buccal angular bony defect and the root was planed. A notch was made on the tooth level with the buccal alveolar margin. A porous filter was placed over the root to 1 mm apical to the buccal alveolar crest, which was 9 mm from the CEJ, and secured to the enamel of the tooth with a composite resin. Flaps were sutured in place. After 3 months, the tooth and buccal periodontium were removed *en bloc*. Epithelium had proliferated on the facial surface of the filter, but under the filter there was new cementum with inserted collagen fibres up to 5 mm coronal to the notch. New bone had formed in the notch but there was no bone coronal to this.

Comment: This is a convincing demonstration of how new attachment may be allowed to form, with epithelium and connective tissue excluded. That the bone had nothing to do with the attachment was shown by the fact that it did not form above the notch marking its coronal margin prior to placing the membrane.

19,13). Other studies have shown apparently greater effects, but without strict controls, particularly in respect of operator bias (Chapter 15).

So is regeneration better than repair? Another study on healing casts some light on this. There is one thing that is even better than regeneration, and that is never losing the attachment in the first place. There is a study that compared this better situation with the long junctional epithelium after conventional flap surgery (Abstract 20,7). In respect of resisting inflammation, at least, it showed no difference between healthy periodontal attachment and long junctional epithelium.

Almost all adjuncts to periodontal treatment have shown gains that are relatively small in absolute terms. When we say that an adjunct improves results by 25–30%, this sounds a worthwhile result, but if we translate it to producing an average of 0.5 mm extra clinical attachment, the immediate question is 'At what cost?'

Newer regenerative therapies are under development and a recent addition is the use of EMD (see Abstract 19,12), which again has a powerful percentage result but at present is expensive. Such biological signalling agents, which organize selected cells into action, are likely to be expensive. But there is one note of encouragement with EMD in the first trial: the effect was present after 3 years.

Abstract 20,7   *A long junctional epithelium – a locus minoris resistentiae in plaque infection?*

Magnusson I, Runstad L, Nyman S, et al., *Journal of Clinical Periodontology* 1983; **10**: 333–340

In each of four monkeys, orthodontic elastics were used round eight teeth to produce periodontitis for 3–4 months, and six control teeth received no treatment. After 1 month without the elastics, the periodontitis was treated with thorough flap surgery, and plaque control was maintained on all teeth for 4 months. Then oral hygiene was abandoned for 6 months, during which four test teeth and three control teeth were ligated with floss to enhance plaque formation. After sacrifice of the animals, the four groups of teeth were compared by histometric examination. In the non-ligated test teeth, plaque-associated inflammation extended to 1.2 mm coronal to the end of the long junctional epithelium. This inflammation was significantly less apically extended than in the other three situations. The authors interpreted this as showing that a long junctional epithelium was not associated with more inflammation, but that such a site had the same defence capacity as normal tissues.

Comment: The length of this study was enough to show a difference in the *Cynomolgus* monkeys used, and the ligated controls lost 0.5 mm attachment.

21

THE VITAL ROLE OF PERIODONTAL MAINTENANCE

- What happens if plaque is not controlled after treatment?
- How frequently should patients be seen?
- What is the importance of plaque control records?

In the 1970s, many periodontists believed that surgery was an ultimate answer to most forms of periodontal disease. The surgical emphasis was such that patients were often treated in this way without much attention being paid to the rationale for the approach. The study of Rosling et al (1976) comparing five types of surgery (see Abstract 19,14) then became the model for a classic trial, often known as the 'plaque-infected dentitions study' (Abstract 21,1).

In this study, treatment was given in a manner that prevailed at the time in many periodontal practices both in Europe and America. Although the importance of bacterial plaque as a cause of periodontal diseases was appreciated, the compulsive manner in which this knowledge needed to be applied was certainly not.

Consequently, patients might receive a session or two to learn oral hygiene and also have some scaling, after which they would have periodontal surgery. They would be seen 1 week after the surgery (to remove sutures and dressings) and then again perhaps 1–3 months later. There might be some encouragement to the patient to maintain good oral hygiene and perhaps some scaling.

We saw in the 1976 comparative surgical study that there was a satisfactory outcome regardless of technique, but that there were some differences in outcome parameters. The plaque-infected dentitions study showed an unsatisfactory outcome regardless of technique; the difference between the two trials was the strict maintenance protocol that went with a satisfactory outcome.

Few other studies could have made a more devastating impact on the view that surgery was the answer to periodontitis. As a result of

Abstract 21,1 *Periodontal surgery in plaque-infected dentitions*

Nyman S, Lindhe J, Rosling B, *Journal of Clinical Periodontology* 1977; **4**: 240–249

Following presurgical treatment in which plaque control instruction was given once only, 25 patients were allocated randomly to five types of surgery for advanced periodontitis. Five patients received: apically positioned flaps; Widman flaps; apically positioned flaps with bone removal; Widman flaps with bone removal; or gingivectomy with curettage of bone defects but no bone removal. Dressings and sutures were removed after 2 weeks' use of a 0.2% chlorhexidine mouthrinse. At 2 months, plaque and gingivitis were much reduced. All types of surgery resulted in unsatisfactory clinical conditions when assessed after 6, 12 and 24 months. Plaque returned to initial scores on all surfaces by 12 months, and probing depths approached original scores within 24 months. Treated surfaces lost 1–2 mm attachment over the follow-up period.

Comment: Surgery without proper maintenance is not merely useless, but contributes to attachment loss. Even in the Sri Lankan study (Abstract 6,3), mean attachment loss was only 0.2–0.3 mm per annum.

Abstract 21,2 *The significance of maintenance care in the treatment of periodontal disease*

Axelsson P, Lindhe J, *Journal of Clinical Periodontology* 1981; **8**: 281–294

Ninety patients were treated for advanced periodontitis in a specialist clinic, and followed up 2-weekly for 2 months. Every third patient was sent back to the referring dentist with detailed instructions for a thorough maintenance programme. All other patients were recalled to the clinic 2-monthly for 2 years and then 3-monthly for the next 4 years for maintenance appointments, including oral hygiene practice and thorough scaling. At 3 and 6 years, examinations showed minimal plaque and gingivitis and virtually unchanged PD and PAL in the clinic patients, and significant continuing deterioration of all these parameters in those patients who returned to their own dentists.

Comment: The point of this study is that the discipline of a recall programme is essential to the success of periodontal surgery. The study overlapped that of Nyman et al (Abstract 21,1), and these two studies confirm the same important fact. It would be unethical today to conduct either of these studies again.

Abstract 21,3 *Significance of frequency of professional tooth cleaning for healing following periodontal surgery*

Westfelt E, Nyman S, Socransky S, et al., *Journal of Clinical Periodontology* 1983; **10**: 148–156

Twenty-four patients who had received periodontal surgery for advanced periodontitis, following appropriate hygiene education, were divided randomly into three groups with post-operative maintenance appointments at intervals of 2, 4 or 12 weeks. At 6 months, patients were reassessed and then recalled 3-monthly up to 24 months. At 6 months, the mean critical PD for clinical attachment gain was 4.4, 4.9 and 5.4 mm, respectively, for the 2-, 4- and 12-week recall groups. Sites with similar plaque scores at that examination had a similar critical PD.

Comment: This is evidence that recall frequency makes a difference to the clinical outcome of surgery.

the knowledge gained in this and similar studies shortly afterwards, it is now considered unethical to treat patients without a proper follow-up programme. One of the other studies is shown in Abstract 21,2.

HOW FREQUENT SHOULD MAINTENANCE APPOINTMENTS BE?

The maintenance programmes resulting in surgical success were labour-intensive, with a 2-week follow-up for 2 years in the study by Rosling et al (Abstract 19,14) but at a lesser level after 2 months in the study by Axelsson and Lindhe (Abstract 21,2). What is a reasonable approach to a maintenance programme, given that resources are not unlimited?

In the first place, these studies show that if a maintenance programme is not possible, then it is better not to do surgery. But what evidence is there about the best maintenance interval at different times after surgery?

Unfortunately, there is very little evidence. One study designed to give an answer to the question is shown in Abstract 21,3. It shows that there is a modest difference in surgical outcome if the interval is 2, 4 or 12 weeks. Perhaps 2–3 weeks is reasonable in the first 3 months, but then we have evidence from the other studies considered, that after 2 months a 2-monthly recall is consistent with satisfactory results. If a surgical reassessment is planned after 3 months, it is reasonable to make this the turning point for a longer interval.

THE MAINTENANCE TREATMENT PLAN

At the surgical reassessment, decisions may involve further treatment, usually non-surgical. However, there appears to be a law of

Abstract 21,4   *Effect of non-surgical periodontal therapy. III. Single versus repeated instrumentation*

Badersten A, Nilveus R, Egelberg J, *Journal of Clinical Periodontology* 1984; **11**: 114–124

In 13 patients, incisors, canines and premolars were treated by patient oral hygiene and thorough supra- and subgingival scaling. On one side of each mouth, this instrumentation was repeated. Over a period of 9 months, periodontal conditions gradually improved, with no further changes over the next 15 months. There were no differences between the single and repeated instrumentation procedures.

Comment: On single-rooted teeth, it is apparent that one thorough debridement will achieve the full healing potential of the tissues. This study did not involve surgical treatment, but may be applied to the post-surgical situation.

diminishing returns at this point. Repeated root planing does not usually achieve much more than one very thorough episode (Abstract 21,4), yet it is apparent in long-term studies (see Abstract 19,15) that further improvement may occur up to about 5 years. How then should we design a post-surgical maintenance treatment plan?

In Table 21,1 an outline is given of an evidence-based approach to this matter. For the first 1–2 weeks, the main concern is the healing of the treated tissues, but plaque quickly takes over the agenda. Because the tissues will shrink, there is a possibility of new hygiene situations developing, and a sharp look-out must be kept for concave surfaces exposed by recession, both proximally and in furcations.

As the tissues remodel, it is important that the patient's brush follows any margins that recede. Although the average recession may be 1 mm after replaced flap surgery, there may be individual sites losing as much as 3 mm.

During the healing and remodelling stages, it is important that the deeper tissues are undisturbed but that the coronal 2–3 mm of each site is cleaned meticulously of plaque (Fig. 21,1).

VARYING RECALL INTERVALS

What are the possibilities of varying the recall schedule if the patient cannot attend at exact intervals? The patient certainly should be seen within 2 weeks of the surgery in all cases. This is to ensure that initial healing has occurred and that the patient is pursuing correct techniques of plaque control for the altered situation.

Table 21,1: *The post-surgical periodontal maintenance treatment plan*

Stage and frequency	Check	Act
Immediate post-surgical stage (weeks 1–2): weekly	Tissue healing and morphology; Plaque deposits, if any; Mechanical oral hygiene	Remove dressings and sutures; Scale up to 3 mm subgingivally; Adjust oral hygiene and add supplementary oral hygiene if needed
Tissue remodelling phase (weeks 2–13): 2-weekly	As above, plus identify areas where healing has created new situation, e.g. furcation entrance	As above, plus new instruction for any new situation
Long-term maintenance phase (beyond 13 weeks): 2–3 monthly in first year, extending to 3-monthly thereafter	Plaque; BOP; PD; Record attachment levels every 1–2 years	As above, plus re-treat any site if appropriate

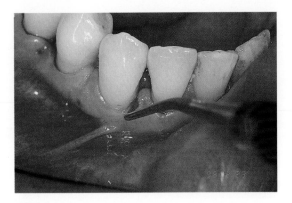

Fig. 21,1

Maintenance during the tissue remodelling phase. A curette is taken 2–3 mm subgingivally to remove early-forming plaque on root surfaces after surgery.

In the tissue remodelling phase, the study in Abstract 21,3 suggests that doubling the interval from 2 to 4 weeks will add 0.5 mm to the critical PD, i.e. clinical attachment will be lost on sites initially 0.5 mm deeper than otherwise. It seems to be a good idea to enhance healing by maintaining a 2-week recall schedule, but never falling as far behind as 4 weeks.

The best evidence on the long-term recall interval comes from the Michigan studies developed by Ramfjord (Abstract 19,15). These comparative surgical studies ran for 8 years, and for the last 7 years subjects were on a 3-monthly recall interval. Once in a while, the 3 months became 6 months, so the occasional lapse may be permissible with an overall favourable outcome.

RETREATMENT DECISIONS AND THE IMPORTANCE OF DOCUMENTATION

During maintenance, because it lasts for ever, there will be an occasional need for decisions about re-treating some areas in a number of patients. Where non-surgical and then surgical treatment have not produced an ideal result, the effect of a 3-monthly maintenance programme often will be to reduce deeper pockets a little. However, if they stay the same depth, the situation is still controlled. If they become definitely deeper (a suitable threshold in treated tissues is 2 mm), then some retreatment may be merited.

The decision depends on the answer to two questions. First, has the patient maintained adequate plaque control? This question can be answered only if the plaque score has been recorded adequately at all maintenance appointments.

However, if the answer is yes – that there has been good patient plaque control, below a level of 10%, say – we need to ask another awkward question: has the treatment given been adequate? Either way, we have a responsibility that involves patient education on the one hand, or our technique on the other. We should not have too low a view of the patient's ability or too high a view of our own. Nobody is perfect, least of all in treating the more difficult periodontal problems.

If patient plaque control has been adequate, then it is likely that our treatment has not. In this case, simple retreatment may be to re-plane the root, or perhaps to perform an access flap for debridement. Paradoxically, re-planing such a surface in the healed tissues may be from a different angle and thus achieve success where the first attempt did not. In any case, it is a low-risk, low-cost possibility of improving the situation, and there is really nothing to lose by re-planing and then reassessing the tissues 2 months later.

Is there anything to gain by using an adjunctive method that was not used first time round? On the whole, adjunctive methods like GTR, EMD and local drug delivery have no more to offer at this point than they would have had in the original definitive treatment plan. The one exception is possibly the use of systemic tetracycline in very resistant or early-onset disease. If it has a useful effect (as in Abstract 11,5), then its cost effectiveness means that it is a reasonable addition to the retreatment armamentarium.

THE IMPORTANCE OF PERIODONTAL MAINTENANCE

It is true that maintenance is a life sentence for the treated periodontal patient. More realistically, it may be viewed as an insurance policy whereby the tissues are kept in a condition of health from which they are less likely to deteriorate and where any reappearance of disease may be detected early, treated thoroughly, and the tissues restored to a state of health. Without a good maintenance programme, treatment is not a worthwhile investment for the patient.

It should not be forgotten that non-surgical treatment may also need good maintenance follow-up. If simple treatment has resulted in good and quick results, and the patient has maintained periodontal health for 1–2 years, a 6-month recall frequency may be more appropriate than the 3-month interval that is advisable for more complicated problems.

There is an art in managing the patient in the maintenance stage of therapy, but it is based on science and the predicted future on the basis of past tissue response and patient adherence to advice. The individual patient may reach a condition where further disease is very unlikely and management may be at less frequent intervals. Nevertheless, maintenance is a subject to be taken seriously for all patients with periodontal problems: see, for instance, the final case presented in Chapter 30, where twice in 8 years there was a definite recurrence of disease in a maintained patient.

22

FURCATION INVOLVEMENT AND MANAGEMENT

- What are the principal difficulties in treating furcations?
- Do all furcation involvements require definitive treatment?
- What are the failure rates associated with furcation treatments?

When periodontitis progresses to where tooth roots divide, it is sometimes the case that attachment loss may continue apically along one or both of the roots concerned. However, when the loss of attachment progresses horizontally into the region between the roots, a new problem of access is created.

In the notable study by Hirschfeld and Wasserman (1978) of 600 patients maintained for 15–50+ years after treatment (see Abstract 4,1), details of furcation involvement were also given (Table 22,1). It is worth noting that a substantial number of furcation-involved teeth was kept in the 'well maintained' group with treatment that was relatively simple and often without surgery.

Immediately following Hirschfeld and Wasserman's study in the Journal of Periodontology, the editors deliberately placed

another long-term cohort study on maxillary furcation involvement (Abstract 22,1). They also wrote a special introduction commending both groups of authors for making the effort to collect these valuable data.

It is clear from these studies that many teeth with furcation involvement have the potential for long-term survival without a substantial investment in treatment (Figs 22,1 and 22,2).

THREE TYPES OF TOOTH

Furcation involvement is essentially a problem related to anatomy. The easiest access to furcations is on lower molars, where they open buccally and lingually. The buccal of an

Table 22,1: *Furcation-involved teeth in the study of Hirschfeld & Wasserman (see Abstract 4,1)*

Group	Well-maintained	Down-hill	Extreme downhill
No. of patients	499	76	25
Average no. of teeth involved	2	3	3.5
Proportion of teeth lost	1/5	2/3	4/5

Abstract 22,1 *A long term study of root retention in the treatment of maxillary molars with furcation involvement*

Ross IF, Thompson RH, *Journal of Periodontology* 1978; **49**: 238–244

This study followed 387 furcation-involved maxillary molars in 100 patients for 5–21 years after treatment. Treatment included OHI, scaling, reduction of occlusal load and soft tissue surgery. There was no osseous surgery or root resection, but tunnels were opened by soft tissue surgery where appropriate. Only 46 teeth (12%) were extracted during follow-up, and half of these survived for 6–18 years. Endodontic therapy was not a significant factor, because only 21 teeth were root treated.

Comment: A conservative treatment approach maintained 9 out of 10 teeth.

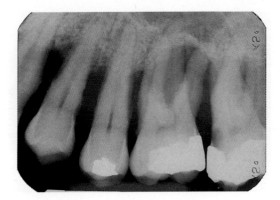

Fig. 22,1

Radiograph showing advanced bone loss on all three roots of upper-left first molar with three-way grade III involvement but vital pulp response. The patient is a male Caucasian aged 50 years. To resect any root would not leave adequate tooth support.

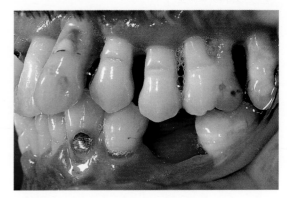

Fig. 22,2

Five years later, thorough oral hygiene and root planing (two courses) have produced massive recession, and a three-way tunnel has emerged without surgery. The patient enthusiastically cleans his 'milking stool' with single-tufted and bottle brushes.

involved upper molar is also easily accessible, but the mesial and distal aspects present more of a problem. Finally, the upper first premolar generally presents the greatest obstacle to furcation access. Its mesial and distal openings may be so placed that the adjacent teeth impede even the passage of a furcation probe.

These features play a part in dictating definitive treatment. The lower molars are easily reached with oral hygiene aids and for complete involvement (grade III) a tunnel preparation may be an appropriate procedure. But where an upper molar, for instance, has a mesial to buccal involvement, difficulty in accessing the mesial aspect may suggest resection of the mesio-buccal root as the preferred treatment. Finally, mesio-distal involvement of an upper first premolar may pose a choice between root resection and extraction.

ASSESSING THE PROBLEM – GRADE, REMAINING SUPPORT AND ROOT FORM

A system of grading furcation involvement was suggested by Hamp et al (1975), and appears to have widespread acceptance (Abstract 22,2). The system classifies horizontal involvement to 3 mm as grade I; an involvement greater than 3 mm but not complete is grade II; and complete through-

Abstract 22,2 *Periodontal treatment of multirooted teeth. Results after 5 years*

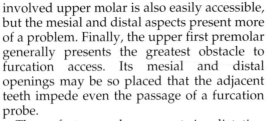

Hamp S-E, Nyman S, Lindhe J, *Journal of Clinical Periodontology* 1975; **2**: 126–136

In 100 patients given full periodontal treatment, 310 furcation involved teeth were treated. Of 81 teeth with grade I involvement, 40% were scaled and planed and 60% had flap surgery with odontoplasty or osteoplasty. Of 229 teeth with grade II or III involvement, 135 were extracted (including most third molars), 87 had roots resected, and 7 had tunnels. During 5 years with good plaque control, caries was detected on three surfaces initially of grade I, on five surfaces following resection and on four surfaces following tunnels. About 10% of teeth had furcation pockets over 3 mm.

Comment: Excellent overall results with a realistic proportion of extractions, but the caries rate appears high in tunnels.

and-through involvement is grade III. These grades correlate approximately with the treatment usually required for resolution of the problem.

Each root needs careful assessment of its remaining support. Radiographs provide some indication of this, but probing is also essential. Particular care must be taken to assess the furca-orientated surfaces of each root in addition to the more usual points for probing. If support is reduced uniformly and markedly, a resection may be ruled out unless the tooth is a bridge abutment or to become one.

The form of roots is of great importance: if they are too close together, access will be impossible without resection; if they are fused, extraction may be indicated; if they are endodontically unfavourable, resection of other roots is undesirable.

There are numerous anomalies in root formation of which the clinician must be aware. Projection of enamel spurs into the furcation is frequent in people of Asian origin and may predispose to periodontal involvement. Additional roots are a common event; lower incisors may have two roots and premolars may even have three, creating an atypical furcation in the event of periodontitis. Molars are also subject to this phenomenon (Fig. 22,3).

Clearly, a decision on the treatment of one furcation-involved tooth cannot be made in isolation, but should be part of a treatment plan for the whole mouth. There may be other reasons why extraction or minimal maintenance is an appropriate treatment.

ENDODONTIC MATTERS

Every tooth with clinical grade II or III furcation involvement should have its vitality assessed because there may be communication with the pulp. Such assessment is not always straightforward, however, because a multirooted tooth may exhibit partial vitality where low-grade infection has been confined to one part of the chamber.

Occasionally there may be a furcation radiolucency in the absence of a furcation that can be clinically probed. This suggests an endodontic lesion, which should be confirmed

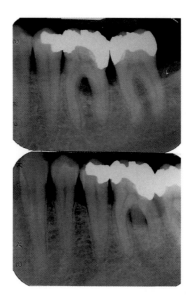

Fig. 22,3

Two radiographs of a lower-left first molar in a male Chinese patient. The first shows an apparently two-rooted tooth with evidence of furcation involvement (also clinically probed). In the second, it is apparent that there are three roots. Although there is radiographic suggestion of previous pulpal exposure, the pulp responded to tests. The patient had two distal roots and it was possible that involvement had commenced from this aspect of the tooth.

by vitality testing and treated speedily to avoid establishment of a permanent periodontal lesion.

Any tooth that has been root-treated loses some of the resilience of its dentine, making it more subject to fracture from lateral forces. If a root has been resected, there is also less support. Fracture risks may be greatly increased in such circumstances. There may be ways of lessening the load on such teeth in order to lower the risk, e.g. by reducing cuspal inclines or by linking the tooth into a fixed prosthesis.

NON-SURGICAL MANAGEMENT

Where there is a grade I involvement of a buccal or lingual furca entrance, access is usually sufficient for brushes and small scalers to control plaque and calculus and to resolve any inflammation.

On proximal entrances, particularly if the furca is penetrable only because of associated inflammation, hygiene and root planing may be sufficient treatment for grade I involvement. If plaque control is inadequate, non-surgical management will become a permanent maintenance routine. The results of the two cohort studies above provide some reassurance that many teeth can be retained.

When is definitive treatment required for furcation involvement? Apart from the desire of patient and clinician to establish the best possible control of plaque, such treatment should be considered for key teeth. These may be teeth that are important for the maintenance of arch integrity or required for support of prostheses. Some may already be abutments.

FLAP SURGERY AND ADJUNCTS

In a grade II furcation involvement, or a grade I where there is an alveolar bone plate impeding access, a mucoperiosteal flap may be raised. In addition to the usual tooth surface debridement and removal of adjacent soft tissue, the procedure of odontoplasty may be employed.

The furcation surface of most teeth is very irregular and is therefore a hindrance to oral hygiene and an encouragement to plaque accumulation, so it may help to smooth it with a finishing bur or similar rotary instrument. All furcation odontoplasty should be moderate because it is only a short distance to the pulp.

There is also evidence that the use of a membrane for GTR has an additional beneficial effect on the healing of non-proximal grade II involvement in respect of several clinical parameters (Abstract 22,3).

TUNNEL PREPARATIONS

The tunnel preparation for a grade III involvement sometimes may be achieved by the patient as part of non-surgical treatment (Fig. 22,2) or may be an extension of flap surgery.

Abstract 22,3 *Guided tissue regeneration in the treatment of degree II furcations in maxillary molars*

Pontoriero R, Lindhe J, *Journal of Clinical Periodontology* 1995; **22**: 756–763

In 28 patients with similar paired bilateral grade II furcation defects (10 mesial, 8 distal, 10 buccal), flap surgery was compared to flap surgery + membrane in each pair with random assignment. In proximal defects, both treatments gave similar improvements after 6 months (PD: approximately 6 mm reduced by 1.5 mm; PAL: 7 mm, no significant change). In buccal defects, membrane gave an advantage (PD: 7 mm, improved by 1.5 mm with flap only but by 2 mm with membrane; PAL: 6 mm improved by 0.5 mm with membrane only). There were associated improvements in buccal recession and horizontal bone probing measurements.

Comment: A small, possibly useful additional clinical benefit, but restricted to buccal involvements.

Abstract 22,4 *The prognosis of tunnel preparations in treatment of class III furcations*

Helldén LB, Elliot A, Steffensen B, et al., *Journal of Periodontology* 1989; **60**: 182–187

Out of 107 patients with 156 tunnel preparations, 102 with 149 preparations were examined 10 months to 9 years later (mean 3 years). Extraction or hemisection had been performed for 12 teeth because of caries and for five other teeth. Root caries was present on 23 other teeth at the re-examination. Thus, root caries was found on 35 of 149 teeth (almost 25%). Root caries developed on no tooth with a zero plaque score at the re-examination (30% of 132 teeth) and on 25% of those with plaque present. Root caries incidence was apparently minimal beyond the first 2 years of follow-up.

Comment: Probably an acceptable risk level of failure with this relatively simple treatment. Good plaque control may also mean good fluoride application.

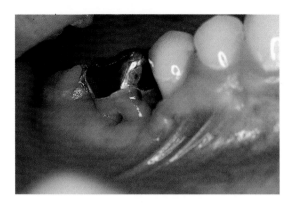

Fig. 22,4

Tunnel preparation on lower-right molar. The brown stain on the mesial surface is arrested caries, and indicates a potential for caries in this patient. There is also plaque on the buccal surface.

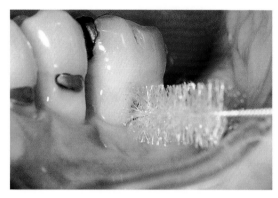

Fig. 22,5

A large-diameter bottle brush in a molar tunnel preparation. This ensures that bristles are pressed into the furca concavities, with the aim of removing plaque adjacent to the gingiva.

Following initial flap raising and debridement, odontoplasty may be performed. If necessary, alveolar bone is reduced. It may be helpful to pass a suture through the involvement to retain the flap at the appropriate position.

Tunnels have had a bad press because of an associated risk of root caries (see Fig. 22,4). In the study summarized in Abstract 22,2, most of a small number of tunnels (4/7) subsequently developed this complication. However, in a larger study much later (Abstract 22,4), the risk appeared less, at around 25%. The use of strong fluoride applications on the brush by the patient may reduce the risk further.

As in other places where they are indicated, bottle brushes for furcation maintenance should be the largest that can be inserted (Fig. 22,5). Although some patients may prefer to use woodsticks (Fig. 22,6) their use here should be discouraged because they cannot conform to the furca anatomy and are therefore unlikely to remove plaque thoroughly.

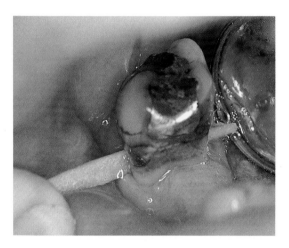

Fig. 22,6

Patient using a woodstick for furca hygiene. The adjacent root surfaces are likely to be concave at this level and a large bottle brush would be a better choice for plaque removal.

ROOT RESECTIONS, HEMISECTION AND PREMOLARIZATION

These are the most complex treatments advocated for furcation involvement. They should be reserved for grade III situations where extraction is unsuitable, because supporting endodontic and perhaps fixed prosthetic treatment is required and there are therefore increased possibilities of failure.

The one situation where resection may be the only alternative to extraction is when an upper first premolar has a grade III involvement and a buccal furcation groove. This frequent anomaly – a groove running the length of the buccal root on the furcation aspect – becomes an impossible plaque trap with a potential for abscess formation (Figs 22,7 and 22,8).

In root resection, virtually the whole of the crown is retained, whereas hemisection means the simultaneous loss of that part of the crown supported by a resected root. A resection may be completed with endodontic treatment only, but hemisection necessarily implies the provision of a restoration (usually a crown) on the altered tooth or its use as a bridge abutment. Premolarization should strictly refer to the retention of two molar roots with the provision of coronal restorations resembling premolars.

Elective root resections should normally have prior endodontic treatment. Instead of root canal obturation, an amalgam restoration is placed in the coronal part of the canal of the root to be removed. This treatment requires the usual flap surgery, followed by careful identification of the furca with a suitable instrument. The root is sectioned from the furca outwards, to avoid the risk of damaging the remaining support. Elevation is usually easy, but may require judicious removal of a small amount of bone over the root. The tooth

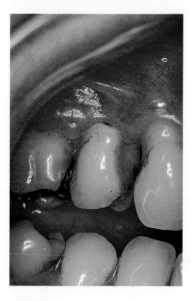

Fig. 22,7

Upper-right first premolar after buccal root resection in patient who originally presented with periodontitis complicated by an acute furcation abscess.

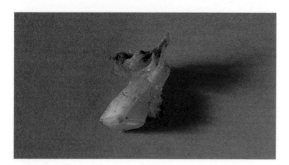

Fig. 22,8

The root removed from the premolar, showing the buccal furcation groove on its palatal aspect. The abscess was trapped within the coronal part of this groove and the tooth was very sensitive to pressure. Fragments of abscess tissue are attached to the root but have been moved partly, to show the groove.

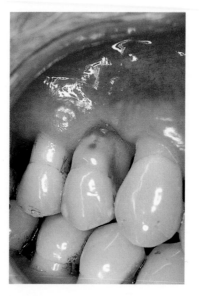

Fig. 22,9

One month after vital buccal root resection of first premolar. At flap surgery, a grade III involvement was identified and the root was resected with a calcium hydroxide dressing and a glass ionomer cement provisional restoration. After 2 months, discomfort led to root canal therapy.

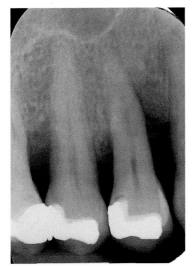

Fig. 22,10

Radiograph prior to surgery.

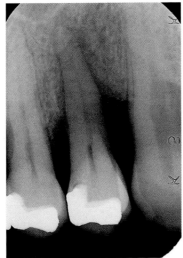

Fig. 22,11

Radiograph at time of discomfort, showing rarefaction adjacent to root.

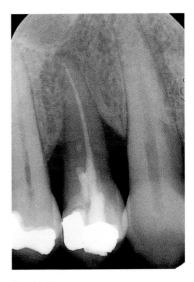

Fig. 22,12

One year after surgery and 10 months after root canal therapy, with good healing of bone.

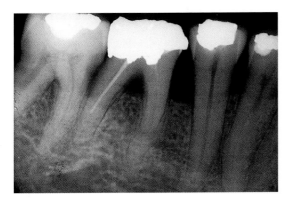

Fig. 22,13

A lower molar treated with mesial root resection in preference to tunnel, because of fear of root caries, showing favourable root anatomy for resection.

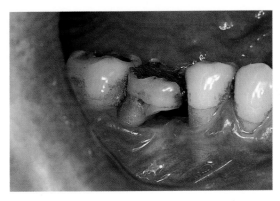

Fig. 22,14

Six months later, the tooth is tilting mesially. Connection to a bridge would have prevented this, but a tunnel might have been more appropriate in the first place.

surface then is contoured gently for ease of subsequent hygiene.

Vital teeth may be treated by resection in certain circumstances. In a few cases, it may not be possible to establish what the root anatomy is until a flap is raised. Rather than perform a second surgical procedure, the root may be resected with the patient's consent, and a calcium hydroxide dressing is placed over the pulp exposure. Some such teeth have remained vital for several years. However, it is more usual to complete the work with endodontic treatment within a few weeks (Figs 22,9–22,12).

Unless the remaining part of the tooth has good support, resection may not be the best treatment. A lower molar, for instance, despite tempting root morphology, may be treated better with a tunnel or hemisection and used as a bridge abutment (Figs 22,13 and 22,14).

There have been few long-term studies of root resection. One of the longest is shown in Abstract 22,5, which shows that thorough treatment may fail because of its complexity. Each aspect of treatment has its own associated risk of failure.

CONCLUSION

With many complex problems, the best treatment is often simple. Non-surgical treatment may be adequate for most furcation involvements.

Abstract 22,5 *Evaluation of root-resected teeth. Results after 10 years*

Bühler H, *Journal of Periodontology* 1988; **59**: 805–810

After 10 years, a series of 28 root resected teeth in 16 patients was re-evaluated. Most had been used as bridge abutments. Failure occurred in nine cases, with endodontic or periodontal-endodontic reasons in five of these. Two cases failed for periodontal reasons and one for technical reasons connected with the restoration. In only one case was failure due to root fracture. As in other studies, most failures occurred after 5 years.

Comment: This 32% failure rate agrees with earlier studies over a 10-year period and the long follow-up may account for its magnitude. Most failures were not primarily periodontal.

23 ATTACHED GINGIVA, MUCOGINGIVAL PROBLEMS AND TREATMENT

- When may mucogingival surgery be used?
- What problems may occur with mucogingival surgery?

The attached gingiva on the buccal aspect of upper and lower dental arches has provoked the fertile imagination of periodontists to develop a large number of interesting and innovative surgical procedures. Patients who had gingival recession became anxious that teeth were going to be lost. Clinicians had their attention focused on attached gingiva, fraena and recession (Fig. 23,1).

Naturally, surgery began to develop. There were apically positioned flaps to conserve attached gingiva, coronally or laterally positioned flaps to cover areas of recession, double papillae flaps where lateral flaps were too narrow to cover a tooth, and partial thickness flaps and free mucosal grafts to increase the attached gingiva. We have seen apical positioning in Chapter 19 and now we shall see some of these other procedures. But first let us clarify one or two questions and objectives.

What is the natural history of the attached gingiva? We have seen that it tends to increase with age (see Abstract 3,1), and that there are connective tissue factors that determine the nature of the epithelium (see Abstract 3,2). But can we say that recession will continue or, conversely, that it is unlikely to progress? Indeed, is there a minimum amount of attached gingiva that is necessary to prevent mucogingival problems?

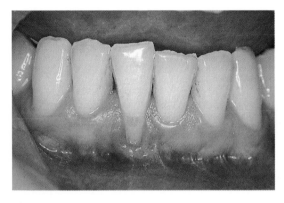

Fig. 23,1

Recession has occurred on tooth 41 adjacent to a lower labial fraenum, but the patient has been shown how to maintain plaque control, and there is no inflammation present.

MINIMUM AMOUNT OF ATTACHED GINGIVA

The first researchers to face this question were Lang and Löe, who published an interesting and sometimes misinterpreted paper in 1972 (Abstract 23,1). This paper was sceptical of the consensus at that time and set a new low figure for the required amount of keratinized gingiva. It has been quoted as indicating a need for surgery where sites have less than 2 mm (equivalent to 1 mm of attached gingiva in healthy sites). This is not a correct interpretation.

Abstract 23,1 *The relationship between the width of keratinized gingiva and gingival health*

Lang NP, Löe H, *Journal of Periodontology* 1972; **43**: 623–627

Oral hygiene was supervised for 6 weeks in 32 dental students with no periodontal pockets. Plaque Index, Gingival Index and width of keratinized gingiva were assessed on all teeth. Of 1406 buccal and lingual surfaces, 83% were plaque-free. Crevicular fluid was also measured on 116 plaque-free surfaces with <2 mm keratinized gingiva and on 118 randomly selected from 371 with 2.5–3.0 mm of this tissue. All gingival surfaces with <2 mm keratinized tissue had Gingival Index scores of 1 or 2. As the width of keratinized gingiva increased, Gingival Index scores decreased. Above 2.0 mm, all were 0 or 1. Crevicular fluid also indicated more inflammation for sites with <2 mm attached gingiva. The authors concluded that less attached gingiva was needed to maintain health than was formerly believed, and pointed out that 2 mm of keratinized gingiva means 1 mm of attached gingiva in a healthy site.

Comment: Very few areas had a GI of 2, meaning bleeding on gentle probing; GI 1 is colour change, and easy to mis-score, particularly if the redder reflected mucosa is very close. Nevertheless, there seemed to be a gradient of the degree of inflammation from the 20% bleeding of 1-mm sites to the GI scores approaching zero for 3 mm and greater. Where the tissues are fragile, of course, inflammation might be a response to toothbrush trauma or even to normal toothbrushing.

Abstract 23,2 *Gingival condition in areas of minimal and appreciable width of keratinized gingiva*

Miyasato M, Crigger M, Egelberg J, *Journal of Clinical Periodontology* 1977; **4**: 200–209

From 250 members of the staff and students of a dental school, 16 subjects were selected. Six had contralateral lower bicuspids where one had ≤1 mm of keratinized gingiva (minimal: M), and the other ≥2 mm (appreciable: A). Fraenal attachments were specifically excluded. Ten other subjects had a pair of such bicuspids on one side of the jaw. The mean amount of crevicular fluid from all 16 pairs of teeth was statistically similar for the M and A groups of teeth; the only trend was towards less fluid for those with minimal keratinized gingiva. An experimental gingivitis for the six pairs of contrasting contralateral teeth showed similar development of plaque and gingival fluid exudate for the M and A groups.

Comment: This is very carefully gathered evidence that supports the view that there is no relationship between inflammation and the amount of attached gingiva, whether or not plaque is present. Consequently, health does not require the provision of a minimum amount of the tissue.

WHAT IS THE PROBLEM – PLAQUE CONTROL OR AESTHETICS?

There may be certain problems that suggest a need for intervention. When plaque is persistently present in an area of recession and the patient is unable to maintain just that one area of the mouth, then treatment may help. The reason may not be fully identifiable; perhaps a fraenum makes toothbrushing difficult, or perhaps the buccal sulcus is not a convenient shape.

Likewise, when there are problems of aesthetics caused by recession, it may be appropriate to cover up the teeth concerned. If this is the problem, it is important not to make it worse by using the wrong technique. For instance, a free mucosal graft from the palate to the lower labial gingiva always carries a different colour with it.

Five years later another study appeared, from California (Abstract 23,2). Starting with a large number of possible subjects, only 16 had a suitable pair of lower premolars (teeth that have less keratinized gingiva than others). This work has helped to alter views on mucogingival surgery to a more conservative approach. We do not need to augment the attached gingiva to a particular level in the absence of any specific problems.

IS SURGERY APPROPRIATE?

Where there is no aesthetic problem and the patient can control plaque (Fig. 23,1), surgery is unnecessary. Recession is managed with plaque control and, if appropriate, treatment of dentine hypersensitivity.

However, in some patients recession means a plaque control problem. Here there may be a need to make space by moving the fraenum apically, and there are two techniques for doing so. One of these is old-fashioned, but still applicable, and the other is nearly as old-fashioned but periodontists seem to prefer doing it.

HOW TO MAKE SOME SPACE FOR HYGIENE

The first technique is the apically positioned partial thickness flap. This builds on the work of Karring and others (see Abstract 3,2). It is a pedicle flap – which therefore maintains its blood supply – and it can be positioned apically by 1 cm or more, carrying with it some connective tissue that maintains keratinized gingiva whilst leaving more of the same connective tissue behind to be covered with new keratinized epithelium (Fig. 23,2). The fraenum is put well out of the way and the patient has space to maintain better oral hygiene.

The technique of the partial thickness flap is really quite simple (Figs 23,3–23,6) and the one point requiring special care is to keep the blade turned towards the bone when dissect-

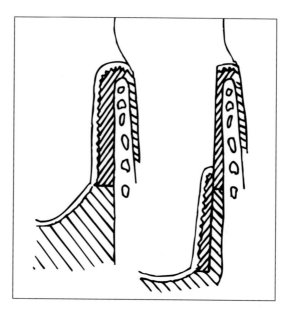

Fig. 23,2

The principle underlying any attempt to increase the attached gingiva. Here, a partial thickness flap is positioned apically, and takes with it some connective tissue that will determine the nature of the epithelium, leaving similar connective tissue covering the bone. Alternatively, a free mucosal graft carries the connective tissue with it, and the epithelium dies and is replaced by the division and migration of cells surrounding the receptor site, a principle mentioned in Abstract 20,2.

ing the flap, so that button-holes are not created.

The partial thickness flap may encourage the phenomenon of coronal creep of the gingival margin when recession has occurred and toothbrushing is uncomfortable (Figs 23,7 and 23,8).

Fig. 23,3

This 45-year-old female patient has moderate periodontitis, but is also having difficulty keeping the lower central incisors free from proximal plaque. The position of the fraenum is likely to be more of an interference when a flap is raised, so in this case the decision has been made to raise a partial-thickness flap and position it apically.

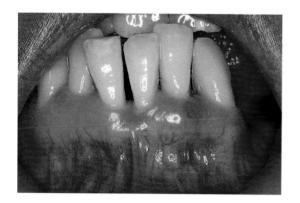

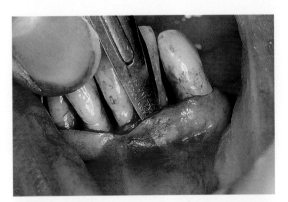

Fig. 23,4

Following removal of marginal tissue, the initial dissection of a partial thickness flap has begun. The blade is kept turned towards the periosteum.

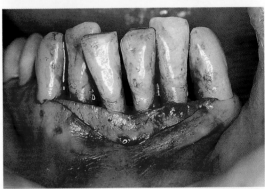

Fig. 23,5

Dissection of the partial thickness flap is complete and the margin is positioned about 5 mm apically to a new resting place. Resorbable sutures are used to hold the flap to the connective tissues. A dressing is placed at this point to prevent discomfort from the suture ends.

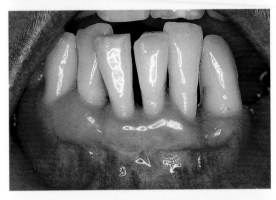

Fig. 23,6

The tissues have healed well with no plaque problems. The fraenum is separated from the gingival margin by 0.5 cm of new attached gingiva.

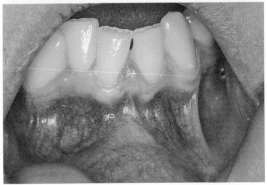

Fig. 23,7

Recently progressing recession on the lower central incisors in a 24-year-old female patient with minimal keratinized gingiva remaining. The plaque is not a problem but the toothbrush trauma probably is.

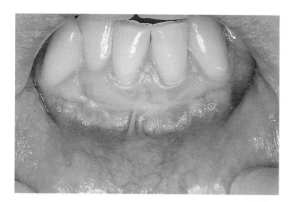

Fig. 23,8

One year after a partial thickness flap, there is a large zone of attached gingiva and evidence of about 1 mm of coronal creep of the gingival margin on the central incisors. This phenomenon is well-recognized, but has no recognized explanation.

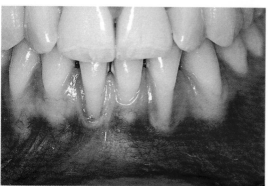

Fig. 23,9

Teeth 32 and 41 have marked recession with a plaque control problem. The fraenum is probably interfering with satisfactory oral hygiene. A free mucosal graft is one way of solving the problem.

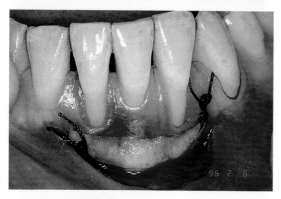

Fig. 23,10

A graft has been taken from the palate and sutured in place. Firm pressure has been applied for 4 min with a gauze saline-soaked swab to press the graft against the receptor site periosteum, from which the reflected mucosa has been dissected.

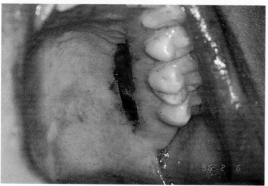

Fig. 23,11

The donor site. Following gentle pressure of a saline-soaked gauze swab by the patient's tongue for 5 min, this site is healing and needs no additional attention other than avoidance of trauma.

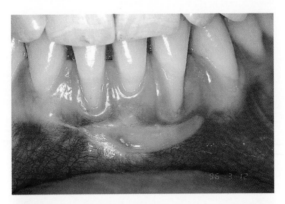

Fig. 23,12

A satisfactory outcome 4 months later. The graft is clearly in evidence and the gingival margins, which formerly had persistent gingival inflammation, are now healthy with no plaque control problem.

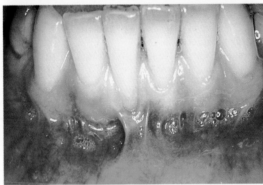

Fig. 23,13

A well-developed fraenum-assisted plaque trap on tooth 41.

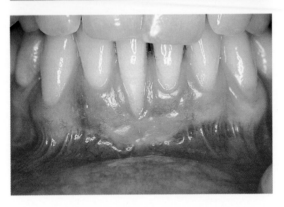

Fig. 23,14

One year after a free mucosal graft, the area is well maintained with no plaque problem. This graft is unusually well colour-matched, but that does not matter in this position.

A FAVOURITE TECHNIQUE

The free mucosal graft (Figs 23,9–23,12) is a useful and easy technique but has certain disadvantages when compared with the simpler apically positioned partial thickness flap.

A free graft needs to establish its new blood supply within 3 days or else it will not survive. Its colour may be different to that of the tissues to which it is transplanted. There is one blunder that may occur, namely that it is transplanted face down. Fortunately, this may be prevented by the simple device of putting a suture through it while it is still not fully removed from the donor site. Finally, there are two sites which need to heal, but the palate is usually no problem.

Having said this, the free graft is versatile and capable of giving excellent results. Some operators may find the dissection of a graft easier than that of a partial thickness flap.

Fraena can be easily displaced (Figs 23,13 and 23,14) and keratinized tissue can be supplied where traumatic toothbrushing has worn it away.

One situation where the free graft is sometimes better than the partial thickness flap is where there is a moderate buccal pocket in conjunction with recession. The lack of any flap tissue to position apically, and the proximity of the reflected mucosa both suggest a need to provide tissue from another donor site.

COVERING UP RECESSION

On the whole, where recession needs to be covered it is best not to use a free mucosal graft. As well as the problem of colour matching, there is also the fundamental question of the blood supply.

The best way of ensuring a blood supply is by using a pedicle flap, of which there are two essential varieties: laterally positioned and coronally positioned. The laterally positioned flap (Fig. 23,15) is usually limited to one tooth at a time and is subject to certain restrictions (Table 23,1). It is usually not possible to cover an upper canine from either the lateral incisor or the first bicuspid, which is why the double papillae flap was invented.

A laterally positioned flap may also be of use to cover tissue where a biopsy has been removed (Figs 23,16 and 23,17). Partial thickness dissection will let the bone remain covered with periosteum and other connective

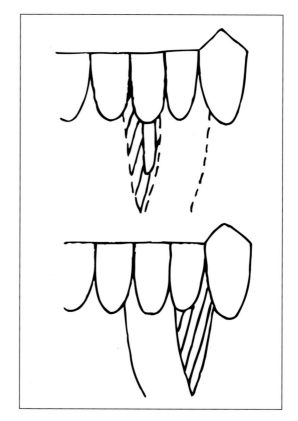

Fig 23,15

The principle of a laterally positioned flap. The recession on tooth 31 is excised and tissue is moved from tooth 32 to cover the recession area. A partial thickness dissection will prevent unpleasant surprises in the form of uncovered dehiscences.

Table 23,1: *Comparison of the restrictions and assets of the main mucogingival surgical techniques*

Restriction/asset	Technique			
	Apically positioned partial thickness flap	Free mucosal graft	Laterally positioned flap	Coronally positioned flap
Teeth need proximal support	No	No	Yes	Yes
Intact blood supply	Yes	No	Yes	Yes
Dehiscences a problem	No	No	Yes	No
Colour-matched	Yes	No	Yes	Yes
Multiple teeth	Yes	Yes	No	Yes
Tooth width is important	No	No	Yes	No
Predictable root coverage	No	No	Yes	Yes

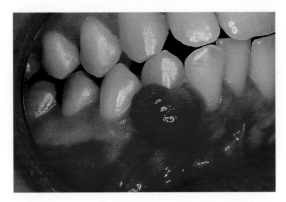

Fig. 23,16

A pyogenic granuloma, unusually placed over the buccal attached gingiva on tooth 43.

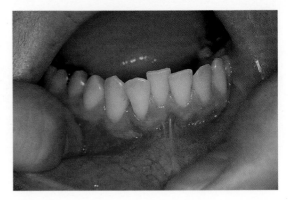

Fig 23,17

Following excision of the granuloma, a laterally positioned flap from tooth 42 was used to cover the buccal bone on tooth 43.

tissue. It may also avoid the problem of uncovering a dehiscence and, in effect, transferring the recession to the donor site, a situation that has appeared without comment in at least one published periodontal paper (no reference will be given, to avoid embarrassment, but it was in 1974).

Coronally positioned flaps are satisfactory ways of covering one or several teeth provided that it is remembered that periosteum is not elastic and must therefore be severed beyond the mucogingival junction under the base of the flap if the latter is to be freed to move coronally. This procedure has been used in conjunction with GTR, and also with free connective tissue grafting from the palate. A recent study (Abstract 23,3) suggests that the latter may be clinically more satisfactory.

COMPLICATIONS OF RECESSION

The exposure of root surface may produce hypersensitive dentine, as well as providing a new location for caries. It is important to provide suitable follow-up for these problems and to prevent them if possible.

In general, hypersensitivity decreases with time provided that good plaque control is maintained. Root caries prevention depends on good diet control and use of topical fluorides. If caries occurs, the best approach is to attempt remineralization with the patient

Abstract 23,3 *Subpedicle connective tissue graft versus guided tissue regeneration with bioabsorbable membrane in the treatment of human gingival recession defects*

Trombelli L, Scabbia A, Tatakis DN, et al., *Journal of Periodontology* 1998; **69**: 1271–1277

In 12 patients, 24 recession defects were treated on teeth with no proximal pockets. In each patient, one tooth was randomized to a coronally positioned flap with resorbable GTR membrane, and the other to a coronally positioned flap with connective tissue graft from a palatal donor site. In the GTR group, after 6 months, recession had reduced by 1.5 mm, PD was the same, keratinized tissue had increased by 0.8 mm and PAL had improved by 1.7 mm. In the connective tissue graft group, comparable figures were 2.5 mm, the same, 1.8 mm and 2.3 mm. Between-technique differences in recession and PD were significant.

Comment: Although GTR increased new attachment, the aesthetic effect of the graft was greater and there was also more keratinized tissue.

using a 0.4% stannous fluoride gel. This is applied in a small quantity each evening after conventional oral hygiene, prior to sleeping, and is not washed out of the mouth.

24

LOCAL AND SYSTEMIC PERIODONTAL DRUG USES

- When is it appropriate to use a locally applied drug?
- When is a systemic drug indicated in periodontal treatment?
- What are the results of periodontal adjunctive drug therapy?

The idea of treating disease with a systemically administered drug has many attractions both for patients and for clinicians. Periodontal diseases are largely caused by bacteria, goes the reasoning; so why not use antibacterial drugs against periodontal diseases? In some patients, the motive may be fear of oral intervention by the dentist: medication is convenient, generally comfortable and involves the patient as little as possible in what is going on.

Other patients may wonder about the cost and inconvenience of a long course of periodontal treatment, and still others may be feeling that there really is such a thing as a 'magic bullet' after reading some enthusiastic but irresponsible piece of journalism or advertising.

Likewise, there may be several scenarios where the dentist might wish to prescribe a drug, e.g. the patient who is very insecure and worried about every aspect of periodontal treatment, yet who thinks that somehow modern dentistry can solve every problem; the patient who is so nervous that the slightest touch causes a sudden movement; and the patient who attempts to lay down requirements and objectives that are impossible to attain. These frequently make the dentist wonder about the placebo or even real effects that might occur with appropriate medication.

SYSTEMIC DRUGS AND DENTAL PLAQUE

For reasons touched on earlier, there is little possibility of satisfying the desires of patients and dentists as far as plaque-directed treatment of chronic periodontitis is concerned. The reasons are twofold: first, periodontitis occurs in a unique anatomical situation (Chapter 9); and, secondly, bacterial dental plaque is a biofilm (Chapter 7).

Therefore, in the gingival tissues, there is a powerful response to bacteria, but because the bacteria colonize the tooth outside these tissues they are placing the defences at a disadvantage, including any systemically administered drugs.

In the second place, we have noted the robust defences that any biofilm has, simply by providing a hostile environment for attackers and a medium that may not be penetrated easily by menacing liquids.

POSSIBLE USES FOR DRUGS IN PERIODONTAL TREATMENT

If the systemic use of antibacterial drugs is of little or no use alone, then what may we consider appropriate periodontal indications for these and other medications? In Table 24,1 some examples are given of uses that have been tested and may be found in the literature.

Broadly speaking, there are three ways in which drugs may be used to provide

Table 24,1: *Examples of modes of drug employment in periodontal treatment*

Target	Systemically administered	Locally delivered	Mouthrinse or dentifrice
Acute infections	Penicillin Metronidazole Aciclovir		
Periodontal microflora	Tetracycline Metronidazole	Chlorhexidine Tetracycline Metronidazole	Chlorhexidine Triclosan Other antiseptics
Host defences	NSAIDs*		
Periodontal structures	Tetracycline	Tetracycline	

*NSAIDs = non-steroidal anti-inflammatory drugs

periodontal treatment. As we have mentioned, they may be given systemically (usually by mouth), but the effect depends upon the target. An acute infection may respond well with the right choice, although appropriate follow-up is needed (Chapter 12).

Where antibacterials are systemically administered against chronic periodontitis, they are adjuncts to conventional treatment, such as root planing (see Abstract 11,5). They have also been dispensed by various local delivery methods, such as placing preparations in pockets after root planing (see Abstracts 15,1 and 15,2). Finally, patients may apply substances in mouthrinses or dentifrices.

In addition to antibacterials, pharmacologically active substances may be used for other purposes. Thus, non-steroidal anti-inflammatory drugs (NSAIDs) have been shown to reduce inflammation slightly in relation to periodontal diseases, and tetracyclines have been used with the aim of reducing collagen breakdown.

PLAQUE SUPPRESSION AND GINGIVITIS

In addition to the problems of antimicrobial drugs mentioned above, there is one further problem that should be mentioned. There are drugs that can reduce plaque without affecting gingivitis. In Abstract 24,1 we see the last

Abstract 24,1 *Studies on the effects of a urea peroxide gel on plaque formation and gingivitis*

Kaslick RS, Shapiro WB, Chasens AI, *Journal of Periodontology* 1975; **46**: 230–232

A trial involving 97 dental students compared an 11% urea peroxide gel applied with Bass technique brushing aimed at subgingival delivery, and two control groups. One control group used a placebo gel applied in the same way and the other control group used their customary brushing methods, with a control dentifrice that was also used by the two gel groups. When groups were compared in pairs, plaque was significantly different in the active and placebo gel groups, but the difference between all three groups did not quite reach significance. However, there was no significant difference in gingivitis between any groups.

Comment: There had been two previous studies, which reached similar conclusions: the first employed a very mixed periodontal population in a 1-month cross-over design trial; and the second used a student population to reduce subject variation, but in randomized groups for 6 months. Both previous studies used the gel in a 'rub-on' manner, and so the present study also included an attempt to deliver the gel subgingivally. All three concluded that plaque was reduced, but not gingivitis.

of a fascinating trio of clinical trials, all of which showed the same result.

Successive trial designs became increasingly fastidious, because the researchers plainly did not believe that an anti-plaque agent would have no effect against gingivitis. In the last trial the plaque effect almost vanished as well.

Other studies have shown the same effect for several substances. As a result of such studies, it was realized that trials had to show gingivitis reduction, because a plaque reduction could not be assumed to have an effect on the tissues.

PLAQUE SUPPRESSION WITH MOUTHRINSES

As a result of the pioneering study of Löe and his colleagues linking plaque formation to the development of gingivitis (see Abstract 2,5), a powerful new experimental design became available: the experimental gingivitis model. All it required was for a group of people with healthy gums to cease oral hygiene, after which some of them were randomly allocated to use some proposed anti-plaque treatment, whilst the others used a placebo. The groups were compared after a time.

Löe himself used the model to explore the potential of chlorhexidine. Later we will examine the properties of chlorhexidine in more detail, but here we will look at one of the studies that has shown it to be an extremely potent plaque inhibitor (Abstract 24,2).

This study featured several items that are part of the routine use of a chlorhexidine rinse today. Starting from no plaque, twice daily use prevented any plaque from accumulating and inhibited the development of gingivitis. The dose is usually 10 ml of 0.2% for 1 min in European countries, but in America a more recent formulation is 0.12%. However, the six rinses used after 17 days have no counterpart in the treatment of our patients today. Where plaque is well established, it requires definite removal before use of a chlorhexidine rinse, but then new plaque will be inhibited.

Other mouthrinses have been marketed, but none has the high activity and substantivity of the biguanides. Quaternary ammonium compounds, such as cetyl pyridinium

Abstract 24,2 *The effect of suppression of the oral microflora upon the development of dental plaque and gingivitis*

Löe H, Rindom Schiøtt C, In: McHugh WD, ed, *Dental Plaque, a symposium* (E & S Livingstone: Edinburgh) 1970, pp 247–256

Oral hygiene was ceased by 13 male dental students for 3 weeks. Plaque and gingivitis developed. Oral hygiene was reinstituted and 5 weeks later all students received scaling and practised thorough oral hygiene until plaque and gingivitis scores approached zero. At this point oral hygiene ceased and the students were divided into three groups. Four students in group A rinsed with 10 ml of 0.2% chlorhexidine for 1 min five times daily for 21 days. Five in group B used the same dose twice daily for 24 days. Four in group C, after a 17-day plaque accumulation, used the rinse six times for 1 min every 10 min and subsequently for 6 days twice daily. During the first period, all groups showed increasing plaque and gingivitis. During the second period groups A and B maintained zero plaque and gingivitis. Group C increased in plaque and gingivitis until day 17, when both returned to zero by 24 days.

Comment: A classic demonstration of the power of chlorhexidine. The repeated rinses in group C must have penetrated the plaque more than the usual single rinse does. Teeth became very stained.

chloride, have been tested. A widely used phenolic, originally marketed more for its halitosis-killing effects, has also been tested. Other substances include hexetidine and povidone iodine.

In general, these all have a lesser effect against plaque, and much less effect against gingivitis. To obtain these limited effects, instead of the 12-hourly regimen for chlorhexidine, other mouthrinses need to be used every 6 h. Unless a patient wishes to use them for other reasons, such as imparting freshness to the breath, there is no periodontal clinical gain in their use. Even chlorhexidine should be recommended only in certain specific clinical situations, as we shall see below.

CHLORHEXIDINE AND ITS LIMITATIONS

The chlorhexidine molecule is strongly cationic, which means that it will attach to most surfaces in the oral cavity. The effect on plaque lasts for 12 h with a 0.2% rinse because it is retained all over the mouth and gradually released (high substantivity). One point to remember is that, with the exception of the study in Abstract 24,2, the best effect of chlorhexidine has been shown on clean tooth surfaces. If the mouthrinse is to be used in normal clinical practice, it must either follow a procedure where the teeth are thoroughly cleaned (e.g. after surgery) or where they can be pronounced clean (as in Case History 3, Chapter 16).

When chlorhexidine is used at this dosage and frequency, it prevents plaque from colonizing the tooth surface and reduces the salivary microflora to about one-fifth of its previous level. Chlorhexidine has been called a cytoplasmic membrane poison, and it has effects against host cells also, including neutrophils.

Because chlorhexidine is adsorbed onto bacterial surfaces, its initial effect is damage to the outer aspects of their cell walls. Because mechanisms for cell membrane defence are damaged, the bacterial walls become more permeable and the chlorhexidine enters. Here the protoplasmic contents are precipitated, and the cells are permanently damaged.

These are profound effects for a mouthrinse, and it is not surprising that there are certain side-effects associated with the use of chlorhexidine. First, the strong adherence to any appropriate molecule is probably the reason for the stain on the teeth and tongue with prolonged use. Dark pigments are retained from tea, coffee, red wine and other substances.

Secondly, chlorhexidine has been reported to cause less frequent adverse effects in use. These include enhancement of calculus formation, desquamative gingivitis and a reversible swelling of the parotid glands. The first two of these are probably linked to the chemical and biological effects mentioned above; because the last apparently occurs only with rinsing and not with dentifrice formulations, it may

Abstract 24,3 *Use of oral irrigators as vehicle for the application of antimicrobial agents in chemical plaque control*

Lang NP, Räber K, *Journal of Clinical Periodontology* 1981; **8**: 177–188

Forty dental students were randomly allocated to one of five groups, ceasing mechanical oral hygiene for 3 weeks, after a phase of thorough oral hygiene with plaque and gingivitis approaching zero. Once daily, the groups used: mouthrinse with 30 ml of placebo; mouthrinse with 30 ml of 0.1% chlorhexidine; fractionated jet irrigator with 600 ml of placebo; monojet irrigator with 600 ml of 0.05% chlorhexidine; fractionated jet irrigator with 600 ml 0.05% chlorhexidine. The highest plaque and gingivitis scores occurred with the placebo mouthrinse, followed by the once-daily chlorhexidine rinse, the placebo irrigator, the monojet chlorhexidine irrigator and the fractionated jet chlorhexidine irrigator. The two chlorhexidine irrigators maintained gingivitis at virtually baseline level, although plaque rose slightly. In the other three groups, both plaque and gingivitis rose steadily with time. One week after the three experimental weeks, plaque and gingivitis were found to be back to baseline levels in all groups. In all chlorhexidine groups, there was significant staining of the teeth.

Comment: Chlorhexidine once daily in an irrigator was better than once daily as a 0.1% mouthrinse, but the latter is not a satisfactory regime.

be related more to the physiological events in using a mouthrinse.

Generally, there are no other clinically significant local side-effects of chlorhexidine, such as emergence of resistant or opportunist organisms, and there are no systemic effects.

Chlorhexidine has been used also in oral irrigation devices to treat gingivitis. One early study is shown in Abstract 24,3. A further study compared different dosages and suggested that a single daily application of 400 ml of 0.02% chlorhexidine solution was the most appropriate level in a fractionated jet irrigator. This amounts to twice the dose needed for regular 12-hourly mouthrinsing.

SYSTEMIC ADJUNCTIVE ANTIMICROBIALS

So far, we have considered total suppression of the plaque microflora, and we shall return to this topic when dentifrices are considered. This is non-specific plaque country, however, and we have yet to consider a huge variety of research that has followed the specific plaque ideal that some bacteria are more essential than others.

The main lines of research have been with tetracyclines and metronidazole, although penicillin, clindamycin and mixtures such as metronidazole and amoxycillin have also been tested. It is fair to say that only the main drugs have any significant use at the present time.

RESISTANCE AND ACQUIRED RESISTANCE

With all antimicrobial chemotherapy, there are possible risks of selecting resistant microbes by killing their competitors. Where resistance is coded on a plasmid (extra-chromosomal DNA molecules in a microorganism), this may be transferred easily to many other bacteria. Acquired resistance is one of the great problems of our time.

Because antibiotics are derived from living organisms and act against other organisms, it is not surprising that acquired resistance is a problem: it is the result of defence mechanisms that operate in the microbial environment. Some antibacterials that are artificial, such as sulphonamides, also suffer from acquired resistance. This is because their action is to interfere in a metabolic chain in the organisms they attack, and the organisms have found a way round it.

However, there are other artificial antibacterials that are not antibiotics and do not have a significant acquired resistance problem. These are the nitroimidazoles, of which metronidazole is the best-known member. The action of these drugs is against bacterial DNA in strict anaerobes, and resistance is very rare. Acquired resistance (transferred from another organism) is virtually unknown.

SYSTEMICALLY ADMINISTERED TETRACYCLINES

Metronidazole and tetracyclines have become the most widely employed systemic antimicrobials used in periodontology. In the case of the tetracyclines, some significant organisms are susceptible, particularly Aa, which is facultative.

This organism has great difficulty in resisting the drug, and because of its more frequent involvement in some early-onset periodontitis, tetracycline has become a favourite for treatment of the disease. In crevicular fluid it may be concentrated up to five times the serum level. Of course, when clinical effects of

Abstract 24,4 *Effect of long-term tetracycline therapy on human periodontal disease*

Lindhe J, Liljenberg B, Adielsson B, *Journal of Clinical Periodontology* 1983; **10**: 590–601

Following thorough OHI, which was reinforced throughout the study, 14 patients participated in a split-mouth study of root planing with double-blind allocation of tetracycline or placebo to seven subjects each. For 2 weeks the dose was 250 mg four times daily, and for the remaining 48 weeks it was 250 mg daily. Two randomly chosen quadrants were scaled and root planed in each subject. By 50 weeks, visible plaque had vanished and gingival marginal bleeding had ceased in all but the sites that were not scaled. By 50 weeks, the mean PD reduced from 7.5 to 4.4 mm in scaled tetracycline sites, from 7.7 to 5.4 mm in scaled control sites, from 6.9 to 5.0 mm in unscaled tetracycline sites and from 7.7 to 6.8 mm in unscaled control sites. The PAL changed by 1.7, 1.4, 0.7 and −0.4 mm, respectively, in these groups. The changes were statistically significant in all scaled sites, and in the case of PD in the unscaled tetracycline sites also. There were substantial reductions in motile rods and spirochaetes in all but the unscaled control sites.

Comment: As the authors say, other studies have shown that the suppression of microbes ends when the drug is stopped. It is undesirable to administer any antibiotic for so long.

the drug are demonstrated (see Abstract 11,5), it is impossible to say whether its effect against any organism is involved or whether the anticollagenolytic effect (see Abstract 2,2) is responsible.

One longer study of tetracycline as an adjunct to root planing is shown in Abstract 24,4. It was apparent in this well-designed study that tetracycline alone had some useful effects, but the marginal plaque was also extremely well controlled.

There is little to gain from administering tetracycline in this way. The long-term effects of tetracycline use include significant bacterial resistance and opportunistic infections such as candidiasis.

SYSTEMIC METRONIDAZOLE AND PERIODONTITIS

The evidence for using metronidazole in the treatment of periodontitis is not very convincing. Where there is significant multiple abscess formation, the drug magically makes the pus disappear. However, although adjunctive effects have been demonstrated, they are similar to the limited effects of tetracycline. One recent large trial showed no advantage to metronidazole, taken systemically or locally delivered (Abstract 24,5).

Some previous studies have shown effects with metronidazole in the short term, but these have not persisted. It is probable that there is a modest effect, but it is not of any clinical significance. Perhaps the greatest use of metronidazole is with multiple abscesses, where pus occurs on probing (see Chapter 30).

LOCALLY DELIVERED CHLORHEXIDINE, TETRACYCLINE AND METRONIDAZOLE

The large study of a locally placed chlorhexidine chip after root planing (shown in Abstract 15,2) is typical of many studies of adjunctive antimicrobials. Is it really worth the clinical time and expense to add 0.2–0.3 mm to the results of thorough root

Abstract 24,5 *Non-surgical periodontal treatment with and without adjunctive metronidazole in smokers and non-smokers*

Palmer RM, Matthews JP, Wilson RF, *Journal of Clinical Periodontology* 1999; **26**: 158–163

In a randomized trial completed by 28 smokers and 56 non-smokers (drop-out rate 7%), three treatments were compared in sites with PD of 5 mm or more: scaling and root planing by a hygienist with an ultrasonic scaler and local anaesthesia (SRP); SRP with 1 week of metronidazole (200 mg three times daily); and SRP with two subgingival applications of metronidazole gel. An automated Florida probe was used to measure the PD and PAL. At 6 months, smokers had significantly less mean reduction in PD (1.23 mm versus 1.92 mm) and there was no difference in mean PAL gains (about 0.55 mm) between groups. Non-smokers also had a significantly greater reduction in the proportion of spirochaetes in subgingival plaque. Multiple linear regression analysis showed that smoking was a significant explanatory factor for a poor outcome, but the use of adjunctive metronidazole was not. There were no differences in outcome between the three treatments.

Comment: Although this paper places its emphasis on the difference between people who smoke and those who do not, it is also clear that the different treatments made little difference in any patients.

planing? In many cases, going by the studies, the addition has to be made two or three times to gain the modest benefit.

The same level of benefit applies to most locally applied antimicrobials. One previous abstract has illustrated the effect of minocycline, a tetracycline given in that study as a subgingival gel after root planing (see Abstract 15,1). On the whole, adjuncts show little long-term effect and about 25% additional improvement in the short term. These gains are not cost effective.

There are other trials in the literature, including some showing similar benefits for 25% metronidazole gel when compared with subgingival scaling. One problem in these studies is that, according to the manufacturers, a placebo formula cannot be produced because metronidazole is essential to make the gel. However, the study in Abstract 24,5 did not show any adjunctive effect of this gel with root planing.

DENTIFRICE EFFECTS

There are few dentifrice studies showing significant antiperiodontitis effects. However, minimal gains have been obtained from chlorhexidine dentifrices, and in recent years certain formulations of triclosan have been shown to produce quite useful long-term effects in maintenance programmes.

In a dentifrice, the additional cost of an active agent is usually very little in comparison to the cost of a locally delivered agent after root planing. If a toothpaste application brings a moderate benefit, then it may be worth having. This is the case with the triclosan-copolymer dentifrice featured in Abstract 24,6. Of course, it is unlikely that this dentifrice really improved the attachment level, but it may well continue to reduce or prevent inflammation during maintenance.

REFRACTORY PERIODONTITIS

The subject of refractory periodontitis, which is resistant to treatment, has cropped up frequently in the literature of the 1980s and 1990s. There are two issues to confirm before this diagnosis may be made. First, is the patient a smoker or otherwise immunosuppressed? Secondly, has the patient maintained good plaque control *and* been well treated by the dentist? If the answer to both questions is favourable, then the diagnosis may be made.

There is no clear consensus in the literature as to how resistant disease should be managed. If the patient's condition does not deteriorate, then that may be viewed as successful treatment, but it may take 5–10 years to show that this is the case. However, many dentists would repeat non-surgical treatment using an adjunctive systemic antimicrobial. According to the type of microflora, this may be either a tetracycline or metronidazole. Both strict and facultative anaerobes may be present, and tetracycline

Abstract 24,6   *The use of a triclosan/copolymer dentifrice may retard the progression of periodontitis*

Rosling B, Wannefors B, Volpe AR, et al., *Journal of Clinical Periodontology* 1997; **24**: 873–880

A randomized double-blind trial compared a dentifrice containing 0.3% triclosan and 2% copolymer with a control dentifrice in 60 subjects who had completed active treatment 3–5 years earlier but had shown signs of recurrent periodontitis during maintenance. Both dentifrices contained fluoride. For a 3-year period no subgingival therapy was given, but subjects were given all necessary instruction in oral hygiene procedures at 3-monthly recalls. The mean test PD reduced from 3.2 to 3.06 mm over the 3 years, compared with the control increase from 3.0 to 3.19 mm. Mean PAL loss was 0.18 mm in the test group, compared with 0.52 mm in the controls.

Comment: Although it is improbable that the test formulation prevented real attachment loss, it almost certainly reduced new or recurrent inflammation. For a dentifrice, these effects are profound, and a difference of 0.2–0.3 mm is worth having at this stage of treatment.

has a greater weight of evidence in the literature. This may be because of antimicrobial or anticollagenolytic effects.

The dose prescribed varies, but many periodontists use doxycycline (a tetracycline) because of the need for only one dose daily, provided that the first is a double dose (200 mg with breakfast on the first day and thereafter 100 mg with breakfast for 13 days). If possible, all the root planing is done on the first day, but if not, it is completed within 1 week.

CONCLUSION

It is clear that there are periodontal uses for a variety of drugs. Most of these are adjunctive to thorough conventional treatment, and for the most part their additional improvements are modest. Nevertheless, there are some definite indications for the use of chlorhexidine, tetracycline and metronidazole.

25

OCCLUSION AND THE PERIODONTIUM

- What are the periodontal effects of occlusal forces?
- How should occlusal trauma be dealt with in periodontal management?
- When does hypermobility matter?
- What are the psychological aspects of occlusal trauma?

To many dentists, occlusion appears as an untidy area of dental knowledge. Some patients have a grossly irregular occlusion but full periodontal health; in other patients the minutest of occlusal interferences seems to trigger a habit of bruxism that creates significant discomfort and tooth hypermobility.

Some periodontists do not view the adjustment of occlusion as part of periodontics; at the other extreme, in the past there have been some who considered occlusal disharmony to be the major cause of periodontitis. Although the former view is held by some today, it is doubtful whether any maintain more than a passing role for occlusal factors in periodontitis in the light of documented research findings.

To understand this complicated area, a simplified overview will help us.

HUMAN NECROPSY EVIDENCE

To start, let us return to the great American periodontist Irving Glickman who introduced the concept of the 'bone factor' in periodontitis, one aspect of host resistance that he felt accounted for the high variability of the disease between patients. Not surprisingly, such views were held by many researchers in the 1960s and 1970s.

Glickman produced evidence for 'co-destruction' from three human necropsy

Abstract 25,1 *Effect of excessive occlusal forces upon the pathway of gingival inflammation in humans*

Glickman I, Smulow JB, *Journal of Periodontology* 1965; **36**: 141–147

In three jaw specimens removed post-mortem from males aged 54 and 59 years, sections were cut to examine selected periodontitis-affected teeth *in situ* in the jaws, after making study models and taking radiographs. In the first specimen, of teeth 24–26 mesiodistally, angular defects were identified that were attributed to factors other than tooth position, such as forces deduced from the position, state and angulation of trans-septal and principal fibres of the ligament. In the second specimen of teeth 43 and 44 mesiodistally and in the third specimen of tooth 47 buccolingually, the authors made similar deductions from similar data. In the last specimen, mesiobuccal facets were identified on a tooth with lingual infrabony pocket. The authors concluded from their findings that the presence of occlusal forces on teeth with pre-existing inflammatory lesions were the cause of the irregular pathway of inflammation into the periodontal tissues and hence that, in this situation only, occlusal trauma combined with inflammatory lesions to cause a co-destructive effect, namely angular bony defects and infrabony pockets.

Comment: Although this was the result of careful study by distinguished investigators, it seems that the association (which was quite well demonstrated, particularly on tooth 47) might be interpreted equally within an opposite causal relationship, i.e. instead of the occlusal trauma causing irregular bone (and attachment) destruction, it might be the result of teeth tending to move away from the site of greater attachment loss. This illustrates the frequent difficulty in identifying causes from an association at a single point in time. There might also be other ways of explaining it.

Abstract 25,2 *The angular bone defect and its relationship to trauma from occlusion and downgrowth of subgingival plaque*

Wærhaug J, *Journal of Clinical Periodontology* 1979; **6**: 61–82

This was a unique study started in 1944–5, when the author believed that occlusal trauma was the principal cause of destructive periodontitis. At that time he collected 64 whole sets of teeth (and jaws) from individuals who had died violently. Prior to dissection, detailed post-mortem occlusal analyses were performed, including an attempt to identify mobility and interferences. Complete records were available only for 31 specimens, and 106 interdental spaces were examined. The most significant findings were: plaque was always related to loss of attachment; to a lesser extent, so was bone loss; angular defects were found equally often adjacent to teeth not subjected to occlusal trauma, as to those where it was apparent; and infrabony defects were always associated with subgingival plaque.

Comment: The key finding was from the control group of teeth, which were not apparently subject to occlusal trauma but had just as many angular defects.

idea of co-destruction. It is important that co-destruction is carefully defined, because Glickman and Wærhaug did not describe exactly the same thing.

We may define co-destruction as an increased loss of periodontal attachment owing to an additional effect of occlusal trauma upon plaque-induced periodontitis. Both Glickman and Wærhaug were of the view that occlusal trauma produced no co-destruction in the absence of bacterial plaque. As we saw in Chapter 2, the effect has certainly been produced in the presence of plaque in some animal studies; whether it ever occurs in human beings is another matter altogether and is still to some extent controversial, as we shall see.

EFFECTS OF OCCLUSAL FORCES

It is frequently evident that occlusal forces have produced both clinically visible and radiographic signs of their presence. Visible signs include facets on the occlusal or incisal surfaces of teeth from bruxism or parafunctional activities (Fig. 25,1), hypermobility or fracture, and drifting or rotation of teeth (Figs 25,2–25,4). It is important to note that tooth

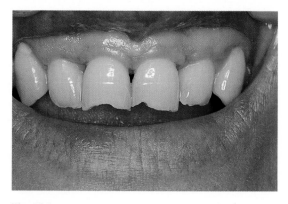

Fig. 25,1

Unusual facetting of upper central incisors in a 30-year-old male, probably caused by bruxism in an eccentric posturing of the mandible in a protrusive lateral excursive movement. Such lesions suggest a combination of obsession and stress-related behaviour.

specimens (Abstract 25,1). Although he certainly considered the state of the fibres of periodontal attachment, his main conclusion concerned bone, particularly the angular defect and the infrabony pocket. It took some time for this view to be challenged on the basis of similar evidence, but 14 years later Wærhaug did so (Abstract 25,2).

By the time of Wærhaug's paper, the periodontal landscape had changed. He therefore gave prominence to the idea that the periodontal attachment fibres were lost in relation to subgingival plaque, and not in relation to occlusal trauma. For good measure, he also cast significant doubt on the link of trauma to angular and infrabony bone defects.

There may be imperfections in necropsy studies, because post-mortem changes could perhaps affect the material, but at the moment Wærhaug's extensive work is a good indication that their evidence does not support the

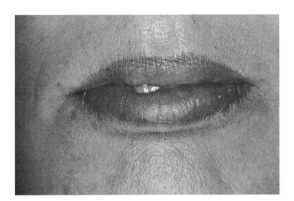

Fig. 25,2

Habitual lip trapping of tooth 11 in a 38-year-old female.

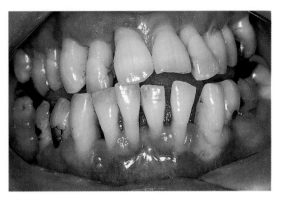

Fig. 25,4

What was not at first apparent was that the patient also had an obsessional behaviour of locking tooth 12 behind the lower teeth, which may have been one reason for its marked hypermobility.

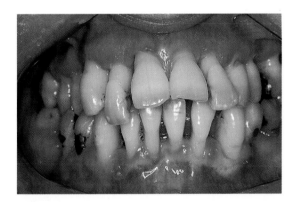

Fig. 25,3

Intercuspal position of the patient. Tooth 12 is over-erupted and the lip obviously helps to accentuate the gap between teeth 12 and 11. The teeth have moved easily because their support has been reduced by periodontitis.

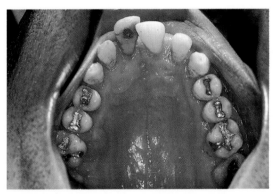

Fig. 25,5

Occlusal view of a dentition in which marked drifting has occurred because of advanced periodontitis. The spacing and drifting of the upper incisors are entirely due to advanced generalized periodontitis with irregular patterns of attachment loss. There are no occlusal factors that have played any part in this.

movement may result from other factors, particularly advanced attachment loss (Fig. 25,5), and also from hidden pathology such as cysts or tumours.

Radiographic signs suggestive of the effects of occlusal forces include widening of the coronal periodontal ligament space, thinning of lamina dura, apical resorption and certain patterns of bone loss termed 'crescentic'. In rare instances cemental tears may be apparent (usually the result of a sharp impact), and even ankylosis.

THE TYPES AND CIRCUMSTANCES OF OCCLUSAL FORCES

Three types of occlusal force can be distinguished. First, there is the impact force: a single blow to the tooth that may cause

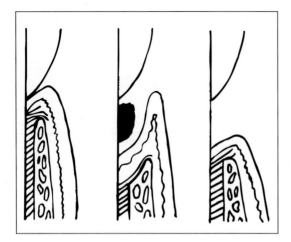

Fig. 25,6

The three periodontal situations to be distinguished in matters of occlusion: health, untreated periodontitis, and restored health with reduced support.

damage. It can cause fracture, death of the pulp, hyalinization of the ligament, resorption, and ankylosis. Secondly, the sustained unidirectional force is well recognized in dentistry because it results in orthodontic tooth movement. We do not need to deal with orthodontic forces here. The third force is jiggling, which has no counterpart in other dental disciplines and consists of a repeated back-and-forth shifting of the tooth, usually caused by occlusal forces in one direction and occlusal or muscular forces in the reverse direction.

Next, we need to consider the circumstances of the forces (Fig. 25,6). Are they applied to well-supported teeth with no attachment loss? Do they concern teeth that have untreated periodontal disease? Do they involve teeth that have previously had disease but now, as a result of treatment, have healthy but reduced support? The first and last conditions relate to 'primary occlusal trauma', but the second has been called 'secondary occlusal trauma'. The significance of this definition is that the condition of untreated disease is singled out for special consideration. Furthermore, teeth can move as a result of disease, which may then induce a condition of occlusal trauma.

TWO ANIMAL MODELS

Most of our knowledge of the effects of jiggling forces comes from two animal models that have been used to investigate the effects of experimental periodontitis and experimental occlusal trauma. The experimental effects have been produced by several different techniques, although periodontitis occurs naturally in the beagle dog.

However, natural beagle periodontitis differs from that produced by plaque in human beings in two respects: recession follows attachment loss, so that PDs rarely increase; and infrabony defects are almost unknown. In the study of Lindhe and Svanberg (see Abstract 2,3) artificial infrabony lesions were produced by drilling away bone on a proximal tooth surface and maintaining the defect with a copper band contoured subgingivally to retain plaque.

Later beagle studies used a ligature, which helped bacterial plaque to accumulate, although the nature of the disease remained dissimilar to periodontitis in human beings. Histological examination suggested that these lesions had much in common with human early-onset periodontitis. Ligatures were advanced apically as pockets occurred.

In the other model, the squirrel monkey, periodontitis was produced with elastic ligatures around teeth to help plaque accumulation. Again, this was not the same as what is found on the rare occasions when human periodontitis is examined under the microscope.

Occlusal trauma was produced in the beagle dog with a premature contact every time the jaw closed, and a spring enabled the tooth to return to its previous position. In the squirrel monkey, orthodontic separators pushed the two teeth adjacent to the experimental septum in one direction, and 48 h later the separator was placed two teeth away to push the teeth in the other direction.

TRAUMA WITH AND WITHOUT PLAQUE CONTROL

In both models, where healthy periodontium was subjected to occlusal trauma, there was a

Table 25,1: *A summary of principal findings in animal studies of occlusal trauma*

Model	Plaque	Occlusal trauma	Remove plaque	Remove trauma	Remove both
Beagle dog	BL; AL[1]	BL only[2]			
	Increased BL and AL[3]				
	Increased BL and AL			AL maintained; little evidence of BL reversal[4]	
	Increased BL and AL				AL maintained; substantial BL reversal[5]
Squirrel monkey	BL; AL[6]	BL only[7]			
	Increased BL; AL as for plaque[8]				
	Increased BL; AL as for plaque		AL maintained; BL substantially reversed[9]		
	Increased BL; AL as for plaque			AL maintained; little evidence of BL reversal[10]	
	Increased BL; AL as for plaque				AL maintained; substantial BL reversal[11]

AL = histological attachment loss; BL = histological bone loss.
Sources: [1]Lindhe et al (1973); [2]Ericsson & Lindhe (1977); [3]Abstract 2,3; Ericsson & Lindhe (1982); [4]Lindhe & Ericsson (1982); [5]Lindhe & Ericsson (1976); [6]Kennedy & Polson (1973); [7]Polson et al (1976a); [8]Abstract 2,4; Polson & Zander (1983); [9]Polson et al (1983); [10]Polson et al (1976b); [11]Kantor et al (1976)

response of bone loss. Bone was lost from the septal crest, and adjacent to marrow spaces in the septum.

When periodontium with untreated and progressing attachment loss was subjected to trauma, the models gave different results. In the beagle dog (see Abstract 2,3) there was definite co-destruction of the attachment, but in the squirrel monkey, there was no further attachment loss (see Abstract 2,4). In both models, occlusal trauma enhanced bone loss.

Table 25,1 summarizes the many studies in both models. An important question is what happens if either the experimental periodontitis or the occlusal trauma is removed. Both series of studies suggested that the control of plaque resulted in profound treatment effects, but the removal of occlusal trauma from a joint plaque-trauma lesion had little effect.

AGREEMENTS AND DISAGREEMENTS IN ANIMAL MODELS

Naturally, there were lively discussions at research meetings about the disagreement of the two animal models. These centred on the differences between the studies: for instance, the squirrel monkey is phylogenetically closer to human beings than the beagle; the teeth were single-rooted in the squirrel monkey and double-rooted in the beagle; the surgical periodontitis in the beagle was even more artificial than the ligature periodontitis in the squirrel monkey; the studies were of much longer duration in the beagle than in the squirrel monkey; and so on.

Where possible, new studies tried to answer the criticisms. However, the results stubbornly refused to change: at the one most interesting point, beagle studies showed co-destruction, and squirrel monkeys did not.

Yet despite the disagreement at this point, the crucial evidence showed quite clearly that plaque was the initiator of periodontitis, and that if it was controlled then occlusal factors had little, if any, effect. Removal of plaque meant that most of the bone returned and attachment loss progressed no further. There was little need to 'treat' the occlusal factors, according to the animal models.

HUMAN EVIDENCE AND EXTRAPOLATION FROM MODELS

There is a limit to what we may learn about the human condition from animal models. Where they disagree, there is an even greater limitation, but certain conclusions may be drawn that do not do violence to the data and give us more than studies in human beings.

In the first place, we may say categorically that occlusal trauma does not initiate lesions of periodontitis, or indeed gingivitis. Both of the animal models agree that only plaque can initiate inflammatory periodontal diseases.

Secondly, although the beagle dog and squirrel monkey models disagree over co-destruction, certain details of the studies suggest that human beings are unlikely to experience this effect. For instance, the forces used in the beagles were considerably in excess of those which human beings might be expected to tolerate.

INDIRECT EVIDENCE FROM HUMAN STUDIES

The overwhelming evidence from studies of periodontal treatment in human beings indicates that total plaque control is the one factor which will stop the progression of attachment loss in all but certain bizarre circumstances. Although some earlier studies incorporated occlusal equilibration as a routine part of periodontal treatment, there

have been many that did not but still achieved an excellent outcome.

The reduced periodontium is not a special risk factor for further attachment loss, despite the plainly increased leverage that might cause a tooth to be extracted or fractured, given sufficient force. The success of Nyman's cross-arch fixed-bridge prostheses (Chapter 28) on periodontally reduced abutments shows clearly that attachment loss was not a problem in these structures, whatever other factors caused the rare failures.

EFFECTS OF OCCLUSAL PROCEDURES

There are a few occlusal matters that do not have a clear explanation. Abstract 25,3 is an account of a trial that showed an interesting difference in respect of occlusal treatment in

Abstract 25,3 *A randomized trial of occlusal adjustment in the treatment of periodontitis patients*

Burgett FG, Ramfjord SP, Nissle RR, et al., *Journal of Clinical Periodontology* 1992; **19**: 381–387

This study compared a randomized split-mouth design trial of modified Widman flap and scaling with root planing in 22 patients who received occlusal adjustment after completing hygiene phase therapy and in 28 patients who received no adjustment. Following occlusal adjustment, both treatments improved the mean PAL by 0.4 mm after 2 years, compared with no change to PAL in patients receiving no adjustment. There was no significant difference in PD between those who did or did not receive occlusal adjustment, but surgery produced a slightly greater improvement than scaling with root planing.

Comment: It is hard to provide any explanation for this effect, and the conditions of the study suggest that it was real. One possible bias factor that was not usually explored in studies at that time would be whether there was an uneven distribution of smokers in the two groups.

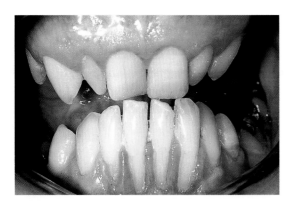

Fig. 25,7

Severe gingival recession caused by direct trauma from opposing incisor teeth. (Photograph courtesy of Professor Richard Palmer.)

human beings. Although unexpected sources of bias are always possible in trials, the difference was quite convincing.

In conclusion, it seems that we should proceed with caution. The evidence suggests little, if any, effect of occlusal trauma on human periodontal disease, and yet there is a suggestion of occlusal adjustment having an effect on treatment outcome.

GINGIVAL TRAUMA FROM OCCLUSION

In some patients there is a severe overbite that permits upper incisors to contact and damage the lower incisor labial gingiva (Fig. 25,7). Occasionally the lower incisors also may contact the upper palatal gingiva. This is essentially a mechanical problem, although sometimes it creates a very difficult situation in the presence of chronic periodontitis.

In many cases, direct occlusion of teeth with the gingiva may produce no problem, and periodontal health may be maintained satisfactorily with good oral hygiene. Where gingival recession is caused, this also may be managed conservatively if the situation is judged static by comparison of study models over 6 months or 1 year.

Other treatment approaches may include bite-raising appliances, orthodontic treatment or orthognathic surgery.

HYPERMOBILITY

Although it is a symptom, hypermobility on its own does not necessarily require treatment. Provided that the periodontium is healthy (although it may be of reduced support), the tooth is not required as a prosthetic abutment and there is no progressing deterioration, then if the patient is content the symptom may be accepted without treatment. Hypermobility is usually either the result of a loss of periodontal support, when simple leverage produces a greater effect, or a consequence of the supporting tissues adapting to forces applied by occlusal irregularities.

In many cases treatment may reduce mobility because it is usually the result either of occlusal forces or of attachment loss. Therefore judicious adjustment of the occlusion or thorough periodontal treatment may contribute to reduction in tooth mobility. Abstract 25,3 suggests that if occlusal adjustment is planned, then it will enhance the outcome if performed before any definitive periodontal therapy.

There is difficulty in assessing mobility. A deviation just greater than physiological (perhaps 0.5–1 mm) may be given a score of 1, and definite hypermobility beyond 1 mm may be given a score of 2. Where there is definite vertical movement of the tooth in the socket, a score of 3 may be given.

OCCLUSAL EQUILIBRATION

The adjustment of occlusion has been the subject of numerous complex and learned texts in the periodontal literature. The present author uses a very simple approach in adjusting occlusion on the rare occasions when it appears to be indicated. This arises partly from the belief that occlusal adjustment does not have much clinical effect in most periodontal treatment and is probably more for the patient's comfort, and partly from the belief that it is not possible to reproduce minutely the details of occlusion on study models mounted on an articulator.

The first rule is that the mouth is the best articulator. Consequently, clinical examination with articulating paper is the basis for any adjustments. Bi-coloured paper with red on one side and blue on the other may be used, first for any excursive movements; and secondly with reversed colours for intercuspal and, if appropriate, retruded contacts. The excursive movements are marked by asking the patient to grind teeth in the appropriate direction, and the intercuspal contacts are marked by requesting a firm tapping of the teeth together.

Before this articulating paper analysis, it may be useful to identify teeth that display fremitus – individual movement when the occluded teeth are moved laterally or protrusively. These teeth may be specially considered, along with others that exhibit hypermobility.

The second and last rule is to maintain intercuspal and retruded contacts when adjusting excursive contacts. If lateral or protrusive prematurities need to be reduced, then in the interests of stability of the dentition the vertical stops of teeth must be protected.

One example of this is the famous BULL rule, which holds that in a normal occlusion only the buccal upper (BU) and lingual lower (LL) cuspal inclines may be ground to correct working side interferences in lateral excursion. This means that the palatal upper and buccal lower contacts maintain the intercuspal and retruded contact positions.

Another example, again in the normal occlusion, is that when correcting protrusive excursive prematurities in the incisor region, only the upper incisors may be ground because the intercuspal and protrusive contacts coincide on the lower incisors.

SPLINTING

A brief note about this subject is appropriate, although the details are more appropriate to works on fixed prosthodontics. There are four situations where a splint may be helpful in the periodontally reduced and treated dentition. These are: for the patient's comfort; where a tooth increases in mobility and appears unstable; to spread the load where teeth have considerably reduced support; and following orthodontic treatment to prevent relapse.

An example of the first situation is given in Figs 25,8 and 25,9. A patient found the residual mobility of a lower central incisor persistently irritating, and requested a solution.

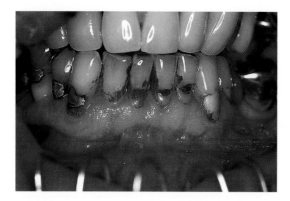

Fig. 25,8

Following treatment of chronic periodontitis, the patient was concerned about the hypermobility of tooth 41.

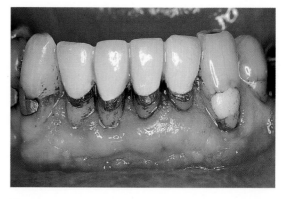

Fig. 25,9

Full coverage splint constructed to immobilize tooth 41. (The bleeding was traumatic, caused by removal of cement with a sharp instrument.) The patient was pleased with the result, although a bridge to replace the tooth was a clinically feasible option. Some patients do not like losing teeth even if they are replaced with a fixed prosthesis.

This was in the form of a full coverage splint. It should be noted that extraction of the tooth and provision of a similar bridge would be an alternative solution.

Other examples of splinting are given in Chapters 26, 28 and 30.

PSYCHOLOGICAL FACTORS AND OCCLUSION

In Chapter 16, two examples were given of the effect of behavioural factors on the occlusion (Case Histories 4 and 5). It is apparent that personal stress and occlusal irregularities, independently or together, may cause various problems. In these cases, the dominant factor is behavioural and should be treated by a professional with appropriate counselling skills.

However, it is of interest that the kindly expressed opinion of a dental professional may also have a useful effect. The study in Abstract 25,4 indicated that reassurance may play a useful part in treatment of the often occlusally-related syndrome of temporomandibular joint dysfunction or myofacial pain dysfunction.

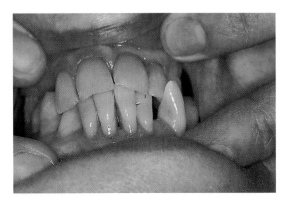

Fig. 25,10

Anterior view of patient with stable and periodontally sound occlusion despite unorthodox appearance.

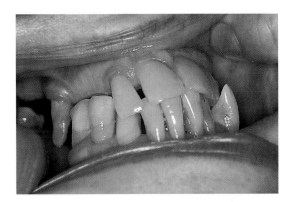

Fig. 25,11

Right-side view of same patient.

Abstract 25,4 *Conservative treatment of temporomandibular joint dysfunction: a comparative study*

Franks AST, *Dental Practitioner* 1965; **15**: 205–210

Three groups, each of 20 patients, were given a graded series of treatment and the response was assessed after 6 weeks. The first group received reassurance, and advice on diet and the careful use of their jaws; the second group received, in addition, restoration of their dentition and replacement of missing teeth; the third group received the same as the first group and the provision of an occlusal night guard. Respective success rates were 41%, 70% and 84%.

Comment: This shows that what amounts to counselling had a beneficial outcome in two out of five cases without further intervention.

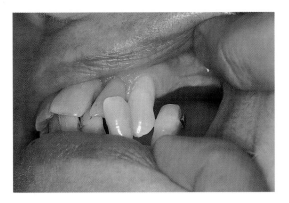

Fig. 25,12

Left-side view of same patient.

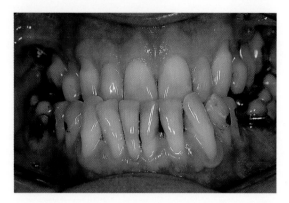

Fig. 25,13

Anterior (habitual occluding position) view of patient with class III dental base relationship and irregular occlusion but no problems, periodontal or otherwise. There was some adaptive hypermobility.

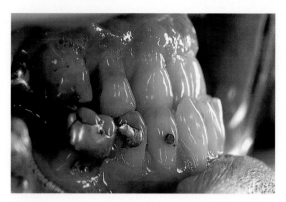

Fig. 25,15

Right-side view of the patient.

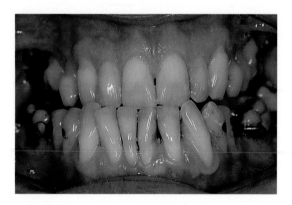

Fig. 25,14

Anterior (attempted edge-to-edge position) view of same patient.

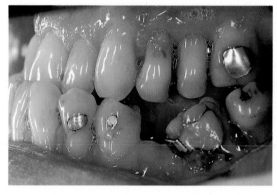

Fig. 25,16

Left-side view of the patient.

A LESSON FROM TWO PATIENTS

Finally, to emphasize that behaviour and attitude are important factors in patients when occlusion is considered, here are two examples showing that extreme conditions may be tolerable to some patients, without any objective need for treatment.

In Figs 25,10–25,12, the condition is illustrated of a 68-year-old lady who was seen many years ago. Nowadays, it is unlikely that any dentist would have let her reach this extreme of occlusion without trying to intervene in some way.

Overeruption, spacing, drifting and rotation are all apparent on various teeth. There is occlusion of teeth 44 and 45 with the opposing edentulous ridge, and the situation on the left hardly seems stable, yet this showed little change from a photograph of the patient about 15 years before. The upper-left edentulous ridge shows marked frictional keratosis, because the patient used it and the other ridges in mastication.

Her periodontal condition was well maintained and satisfactory. Plaque or calculus was present on fewer than 10% of surfaces, there was no BOP, and crevice depths did not exceed 2 mm. The patient was contented with the occlusion, which satisfied her needs and desires in mastication, aesthetics, comfort and speech. No treatment was required, beyond the advice to return for routine examination at 6 monthly intervals, or earlier if desired, with particular reference to the hyperkeratosis.

The second patient is a 55-year-old male who has a class III dental base relationship and a very irregular dentition (Figs 25,13–25,16). Again, the periodontal condition is excellently maintained. All lower molars have grade 2 hypermobility, which is partly from attachment loss through recession and partly from adaptation to the occlusal situation. He had been like this for many years and was content with the situation, which outwardly had acceptable aesthetics.

The lesson is that we should not seek to alter situations that function satisfactorily and have a stable condition. As with oral hygiene, the correct occlusion is one that works. In the case of occlusion, the patient's objectives determine what is satisfactory.

26

ORTHODONTICS AND PERIODONTOLOGY

- When is orthodontic treatment appropriate in periodontitis?
- How may the periodontium be managed during orthodontics?

Among the sequelae of advanced periodontitis are drifting, tilting, spacing, rotating and overeruption of teeth. Orthodontic disturbance in the adult dentition may occur as a result of periodontitis but also through occlusal forces and parafunctional habits. In addition, tooth loss may create a space into which other teeth may deviate.

Where the periodontal support is reduced, teeth may move more easily. It may not take long for noticeable malalignment to be manifest and, conversely, orthodontic treatment may take a shorter time than in the fully supported dentition.

Under such circumstances, there are certain aspects of normal orthodontic practice that may alter. Where movement is much easier, a light force may suffice, but if reduced support is widespread, anchorage may require the involvement of more teeth or extra-oral headgear.

OVERERUPTION, INTRUSION AND STABILITY

A further significant variation of orthodontics in the reduced support dentition is that where teeth have tilted they may also overerupt. This means that the orthodontist has to intrude the tooth for it to regain a satisfactory position. For intrusion to be periodontally successful, plaque control has to be so good that no pocket is formed as a result. The reason why this undesirable effect may occur is that when teeth with or without periodontal attachment loss are moved, the attachment level travels with the tooth. If a clean tooth surface is intruded, a long junctional epithelial attachment is a likely outcome.

A study on intrusion of periodontally involved teeth is shown in Abstract 26,1. Where good gingival health is present, this is appropriate treatment to realign anterior teeth in the periodontally disordered arch. However, the treatment is very likely to require permanent retention with a fixed appliance.

Abstract 26,1 *Intrusion of incisors in adult patients with marginal bone loss*

Melsen B, Agerbaek N, Markenstam G, *American Journal of Orthodontics and Dentofacial Orthopedics* 1989; **96**: 232–241

Incisors were intruded by three different methods in 30 periodontal patients who had a deep overbite, overeruption and spacing. Clinical crown length was reduced by 0.5–1.0 mm, and in 24 cases the marginal bone level was brought close to the CEJ. All cases showed root resorption of 1–3 mm. Total alveolar support was calculated as the area of the alveolar wall, and appeared unaltered or greater in 19 cases. The authors considered that their best results were with low but well-directed forces, healthy gingiva and no interference with perioral function.

Comment: Moderate root resorption appears to be a regular side-effect of intrusion, and that may explain in part any unaltered or lessened alveolar support.

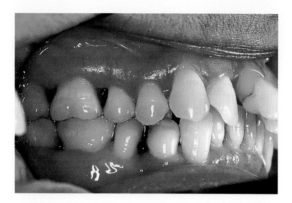

Fig. 26,1

Right-side view of a 36-year-old patient with treated advanced periodontitis. Most crevices are 1–2 mm deep and the maximum PD is 4 mm, but without BOP. Plaque is undetectable. Note the drifting and tilting present in the upper labial segment.

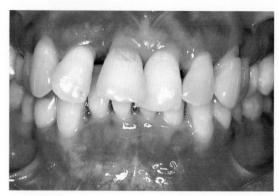

Fig. 26,2

Central view.

Where teeth have moved in other ways because of periodontitis, and then been returned to a suitable position by orthodontic techniques, there is always a possibility of relapse, which implies that fixed retention is needed. For this reason, a careful decision must be made at the outset of periodontal treatment, or as close to it as possible. If the outcome of any aspect of the treatment is in doubt, the alternative of extractions and prosthodontic treatment must be considered.

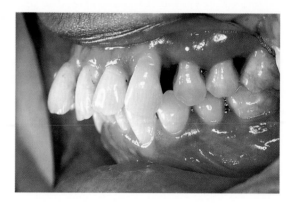

Fig. 26,3

Left-side view.

ANTERIOR SEGMENT REALIGNMENT

This is the commonest situation in which the orthodontist's help is sought for a patient with periodontitis. The aesthetic requirement is obvious, and the most important periodontal contribution is an assessment of prognosis. For this to be realistic, the outcome of a course of non-surgical treatment is a good indicator.

The patient whose dentition is shown in Figs 26,1–26,3 was assessed on the basis of a good response to non-surgical treatment. Subsequently, her treatment was completed and a thorough maintenance programme was instituted. At this stage, orthodontic treatment was started and she continued immaculate oral hygiene throughout.

The result of orthodontic treatment is shown in Figs 26,4–26,6. Maintenance is still outstanding. At this point, it was necessary to provide fixed retention, and this was done with a wire and composite splint (Figs 26,7 and 26,8). Another example of post-orthodontic splinting is shown in Figs 26,9 and 26,10. Orthodontic treatment is inadvisable in the periodontally reduced dentition unless the patient has total control of plaque.

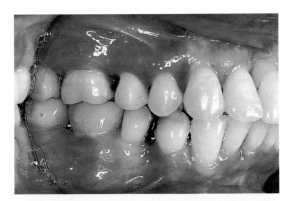

Fig. 26,4

Right-side view 2 years after orthodontic treatment. There has been realignment and some intrusion of the upper anterior teeth, and recession on the mesial surface of tooth 12.

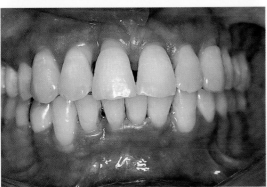

Fig. 26,5

Central view.

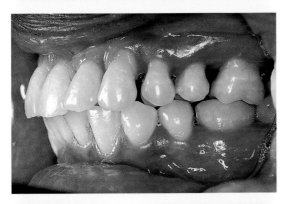

Fig. 26,6

Left-side view.

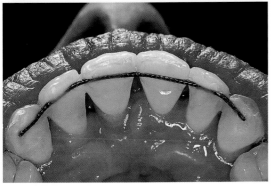

Fig. 26,7

The upper anterior teeth have been placed in long-term retention with a wire and composite splint (treatment courtesy of Dr Ravi Saravanamuttu).

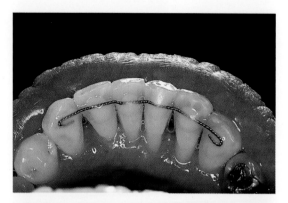

Fig. 26,8

Similar splint on lower teeth (treatment courtesy of Dr R Saravanamuttu).

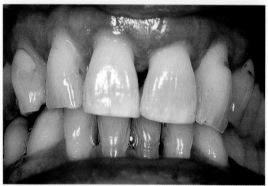

Fig. 26,9

Following periodontal treatment, the upper anterior segment has been realigned and splinted for retention. (Photograph courtesy of Mr B J Smith.)

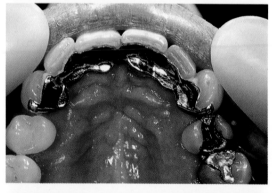

Fig. 26,10

The resin-bonded splint has provision to retain the lower anterior teeth, which were orthodontically intruded. (Photograph courtesy Mr B J Smith.)

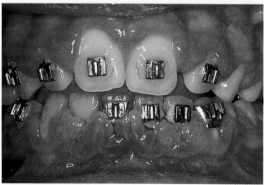

Fig. 26,11

Central view of an adolescent undergoing orthodontic treatment. There is a marked hyperplastic gingivitis, mainly in relation to the bonded attachments.

Abstract 26,2 *The effect of orthodontic therapy on certain types of periodontal defects. I – Clinical findings*

Brown IS, *Journal of Periodontology* 1973; **44**: 742–756

Four patients with a single lower molar tooth (mean mesial PD 8 mm) to be uprighted were compared with a control patient with a similar molar (PD 6 mm) that received repeated root planing. Initial scaling on the teeth to be uprighted produced a mean 0.4 mm-reduction, and subsequent uprighting added a mean 3.1 mm to this. Bone height improved by approximately 1 mm. The control tooth reduced the PD by 1 mm.

Comment: The improvements were followed up for 3 months after 3–4 months of orthodontics. The author added a supplementary argument to the effect that no patient had received any advice on plaque control and that this was therefore not necessary. He also advocated earlier orthodontic treatment in the periodontally involved dentition. Most clinicians today would advise initial periodontal treatment at least before any orthodontics.

MOLAR UPRIGHTING

A useful application of orthodontics in the periodontally involved dentition is the restoration of a suitable inclination to molars that have tilted. This procedure may produce a satisfactory abutment for a prosthesis but there is another important effect that has been studied (Abstract 26,2). In this unusual study, the author contended that orthodontic movement might have a stimulatory effect on the periodontal attachment, and the study showed the ability of molar uprighting to reduce an awkward pocket to about half its depth.

ORTHODONTICS AND ADVERSE PERIODONTAL EFFECTS

The presence of an appliance can markedly interfere with normal oral hygiene practices. Fig. 26,11 shows what may happen in some

Abstract 26,3 *Periodontal considerations in the use of bonds or bands on molars in adolescents and adults*

Boyd RL, Baumrind S, *Angle Orthodontist* 1992; **62**: 117–126

The periodontal condition at the mesiobuccal line angle of teeth 16 and 36 in 20 adults and 40 adolescents was assessed immediately prior to placing fixed appliances, at intervals during active orthodontic treatment up to 18 months and then 3 months after removal of appliances. During treatment, banded molars showed significantly more plaque and gingivitis than bonded molars. Three months after treatment, the formerly banded molars showed significantly more gingivitis and attachment loss than molars that had been bonded. There was also greater maxillary plaque and gingivitis in adolescents than in adults.

Comment: Obviously, this could not be a blind study during treatment but the post-treatment difference was less likely to have this possible source of bias. The message is that bonding is preferable if it is possible. At least one other study has shown a return to pretreatment conditions after appliance removal, but in that study banding and bonding were consistently on the right and left sides of the mouth, hence there is a possibility of bias in the post-treatment examination.

patients if special attention is not given to plaque control during orthodontic treatment.

Patients are sometimes referred for orthodontics without sufficient consideration being given to their periodontal condition. There are two aspects to this. First, patients without satisfactory plaque control run the risk of problems such as those illustrated. Secondly, and of particular significance, teeth may alter position because of unrecognized advanced periodontitis.

Not surprisingly, studies have shown that orthodontic bonding is periodontally better than banding (Abstract 26,3). Unless other constraints apply, it seems preferable to use bonding for fixed appliances.

Abstract 26,4 *Long-term effect of orthodontic treatment on crestal alveolar bone levels*

Polson AM, Reed BE, *Journal of Periodontology* 1984; **55**: 28–34

A comparison was made of the bone level in 104 subjects aged 21–36 years (mean 29 years) who had completed orthodontic treatment at least 10 years earlier (mean 13 years) and in 76 subjects aged 21–36 years (mean 30 years) who had malocclusions but had not received treatment. Bone level was measured and compared in different tooth types and surfaces. On the distal surfaces of molars only, the control group had significantly less bone (1.4 mm from the CEJ versus 1.1 mm), a difference that the authors attributed to intrusion of the treated teeth in the treatment group. No other significant differences were found.

Comment: The overall similarity between groups suggests that orthodontic treatment does not cause bone loss.

Abstract 26,5 *Does orthodontic proclination of lower incisors in children and adolescents cause gingival recession?*

Ruf S, Hansen K, Pancherz H, *American Journal of Orthodontics and Dentofacial Orthopedics* 1998; **114**: 100–106

In 98 children of average age 12.8 years, 392 lower incisors were proclined by 0.5° to 19.5° with Herbst appliance treatment. Comparison of casts and photographs before and after treatment showed that recession levels were unchanged in 97% of teeth. In the remaining 3%, recession developed or increased. In these 12 teeth there was no relationship between the degree of proclination and amount of recession.

Comment: A well-documented study indicating that orthodontic proclination is unlikely to affect recession. Other factors may also account for recession, including variation of oral hygiene practice.

ORTHODONTICS, PERIODONTAL SUPPORT AND GINGIVAL RECESSION

Certain investigators have asked whether orthodontics may adversely affect the periodontal support of teeth. In one large and thorough study (Abstract 26,4), there was no indication of such an effect. Other studies have shown similar results.

Some clinicians have been concerned that gingival recession may be a by-product of labial tilting of teeth. Studies on incisor proclination by both orthodontic (Abstract 26,5) and surgical methods have not confirmed this hypothesis.

Orthodontics therefore appears periodontally safe. There are also indications that it may have a beneficial effect on periodontal health (Abstract 26,6). This may be partly or wholly through a Hawthorne effect, with the appliance helping to concentrate the patient's attention on the mouth.

Abstract 26,6 *The effect of orthodontic treatment on plaque and gingivitis*

Davies TM, Shaw WC, Worthington HV, et al., *American Journal of Orthodontics and Dentofacial Orthopedics* 1991; **99**: 155–161

In a cohort of 1015 children, 417 were found to have significant malocclusion and 114 received orthodontic treatment. Three years after the baseline examination, both treated and untreated children had reduced plaque and gingivitis on all tooth surfaces. There was a greater improvement in the treated group, but this did not appear to relate to improvement of dental alignment.

Comment: The experience of orthodontic treatment, with continual focusing on oral health, may be the reason for the greater improvement in this group.

27

ENDODONTICS AND PERIODONTOLOGY

- What is the relationship between pulp and periodontal diseases?
- Where may endodontic failure affect the periodontium?
- Which requires priority – to treat pulp or periodontium?

The pulp and the periodontium are the two living organs of teeth. Both are subject to all the variety of disease that affects the body. Furthermore, they have potential communicating channels: some are anatomically regular such as the tooth apex, and some are variants such as accessory and lateral canals.

When inflammation affects the pulp, usually to combat microorganisms from caries, it is subject to all the possible variations that occur in other living tissues, from mere hyperaemia to necrosis and gangrene, but with one important constraint. The pulp is enclosed in the rigid pulp chamber and inflammation greatly increases pressure in the tissues, which is why infection frequently kills the pulp and why it can be so painful.

In the treatment of periodontal diseases, we are often mindful of the behaviour of the patient and his or her susceptibility to disease. In treating pulpal diseases, our concern is frequently for a high level of technical skill in removing bacterial debris and obturating canals.

Although periodontal treatment also requires skill, successful endodontic treatment depends far more on operating skill than on the patient behaviour that is central in controlling bacterial plaque. Recent advances in endodontic knowledge also have helped to elucidate some previously hidden problems.

ROOT CANAL MORPHOLOGICAL VARIATION

We have already mentioned lower molars that can have three roots (Chapter 22). It is good to be aware of the possible variations in root anatomy, both for periodontics and endodontics. But what about the problem of a periodontal-endodontal lesion on a lower incisor? Root filling such a tooth seems relatively straightforward and yet, if we treat

Abstract 27,1 *Root canal morphology of mandibular incisors*

Kartel N, Yanikoğlu FÇ, *Journal of Endodontics* 1992; **18**: 562–564

Root canals were identified in 100 freshly-extracted lower incisors: single canals with one apical foramen were present in 55; multiple canals with one final apical opening were present on 37; and in 8 there were varieties of multiple canal morphology with more than one apical opening. Lateral canals were present in the middle third of the root in 5 teeth and in the apical third in 18 teeth. In addition, 72 apical foramina were laterally positioned. The authors compare their figure of 45% for the presence of a second canal with figures of 41%, 26%, 20% and 12% in previous studies.

Comment: Root treating a lower incisor is clearly not straightforward in many cases. The only question of bias that may be raised over such studies is: did the root canal morphology contribute to the need for the tooth to be extracted, thereby yielding a non-representative sample for analysis?

the pocket on a tooth that seems to have a well-obturated canal, we may be doomed to disappointment.

The problem is that lower incisors quite frequently have aberrant pulp canal anatomy. One well-conducted study is shown in Abstract 27,1. The moral is clear: in treating periodontal diseases, we need to understand what is happening on the other side of the dentine.

APICAL PLAQUE

Persistent apical areas after root filling are often an irritation to the clinician, even when they do not cause discomfort to the patient. Such radiolucencies, if unchanged and symptomless over a long period of time, may indicate that a balance has been reached between contained infection and the body's defences. These areas are not cut off from the rest of the body and may often contain a layer of bacterial plaque (Abstract 27,2).

Abstract 27,2 *Periapical bacterial plaque in teeth refractory to endodontic treatment*

Tronstat L, Barnett F, Cervone F, *Endodontics and Dental Traumatology* 1990; **6**: 73–77

Under strict conditions of asepsis, 10 persistent periapical lesions were surgically exposed and bacterial sampling was performed. Periapical lesions were enucleated and 2–3 mm of apical root was resected. The bacterial samples revealed a predominantly anaerobic flora, and on nine apical root specimens a continuous microscopic layer of microbial plaque was identified. The tenth specimen had small patches of plaque. The authors considered that the microbes could have come from endodontic lesions, but point out the possibility of haematogenous spread from elsewhere in the body.

Comment: If microorganisms are merely present in the periapical tissues, they can be dealt with by the host response. If the apical root surface is colonized by plaque, this is likely to persist unless the biofilm is removed.

Apical plaque is a biofilm, and has the same sophisticated defences as periodontal plaques. In the peculiar, enclosed environment of an apical lesion, other features are worthy of note. The organisms, of relatively few species when compared with periodontal plaque, may not always come from the mouth. *Bacteroides fragilis* is an intestinal organism, and has been identified in an apical plaque.

When discomfort is treated by apical surgery, the removal of the cause is the aim. In the case featured in Figs 27,1–27,3 there were two possible causes: the apex and the root perforation. As far as can be seen in the 8-month post-operative radiograph, the bone has healed around the apex but the area adjacent to the cast post has not. However, symptoms were eliminated completely by the procedure, leading to the conclusion that the

Abstract 27,3 *Factors influencing the success of conventional root canal therapy – a five-year retrospective study*

Smith CS, Setchell DJ, Harty FJ, *International Endodontic Journal* 1993; **26**: 321–333

In a postgraduate clinic in London, 1518 teeth were root treated over a 12-year period. Of these, 821 had been followed up for 5 to 13 years. The overall success rate at 5 years was 84.3%. When examined for relevant factors, there were significantly higher success rates associated with: male gender, full obturation as opposed to short fillings, pre-operative vital pulp and pre-operative normal radiographic appearance. A cumulative graph of failures suggested a tendency to level out at 6–10 years, with a low risk of later occurrence. The overall annual failure rate was 1.7%. Comparing their results with other studies, the authors comment that case selection is of importance, because heroic treatment carries a high risk of failure.

Comment: Clearly, a lot of information is lost in long-term studies, but this is the best sort of information we have. When planning periodontal treatment and discussing it with the patient, one important factor is the success rate of other forms of treatment involved in the plan. Risks must be explained clearly if the patient is to give informed consent.

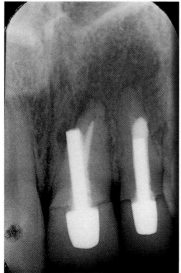 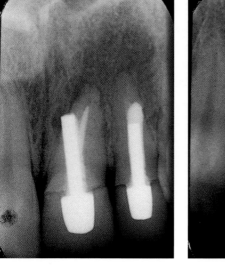 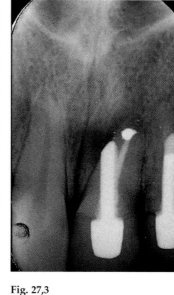

Fig. 27,1

A badly-placed cast post with a root perforation in tooth 21. The patient was experiencing regular moderate discomfort. Note the apical condition of the tooth.

Fig. 27,2

Apical surgery has been performed, and the post trimmed. A small amount of associated cement was removed as well.

Fig. 27,3

Although healing is apparently incomplete next to the post, there is apical regeneration of bone 8 months later, and the tooth is symptomless.

assumed cause (root perforation) may not have been the actual cause. Removal of an apical plaque may have been the solution that worked.

In the case shown in Figs 27,4 and 27,5, surgery was performed in an attempt to tidy up an apical junkyard. Although this was not wholly successful, the bone regeneration was an indication that any apical plaque was removed, allowing inflammation to resolve.

ENDODONTIC SUCCESS AND PERIODONTAL PLANS

Eminent endodontic scientists have pointed out that the enclosed, anaerobic bacterial organization of a necrotic pulp or a periapical area is a relatively static ecosystem that exposure to air may greatly alter. The best endodontic treatment carries a success rate well below 100% (Abstract 27,3). Therefore, before re-opening a quiescent periapical lesion, it may be wise to wait for some indication that it is necessary, and not to assume more than an 80% likelihood of success in root fillings.

These matters all affect periodontal treatment and treatment planning. If faced with a difficult endodontic problem, it may be as well to have more than one plan for dealing with the situation. If teeth have been apparently well root filled and are periodontally healthy but have persistent apical areas, it is acceptable not to re-treat them unless they are likely to be abutments. On multi-rooted teeth, resection of such a root may be an acceptable option.

PERIODONTAL-ENDODONTAL (PERIO-ENDO) LESIONS

Traditional wisdom has said that there are three types of perio-endo lesion: those primarily pulpal in origin, those primarily periodontal in origin, and those resulting from the

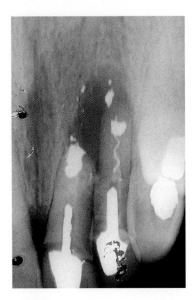

Fig. 27,4

An apical mess with treatment debris scattered around
two apices.

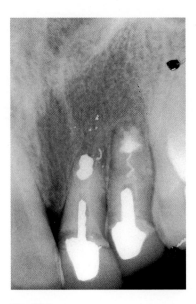

Fig. 27,5

Following apical surgery, despite incomplete debridement, there is bone regeneration 1 year later. This may
relate to removal of associated apical plaque.

meeting of separate pulpal and periodontal
lesions. Then we are told that we should first
treat the presumed origin of the lesion. The
present author has never been able to see the
wisdom in this.

If the pulp is involved, whether primarily
or secondarily, it needs treating because it will
die, or already has died. Furthermore, it can
have painful lesions much more often than
inflammation in the periodontium. Although
a pulpal lesion may drain through the
periodontium, the killing of the pulp by an
apical periodontal lesion seems rare, if not
non-existent. In the case shown in Figs 19,74
and 19,75 there is an extreme example of an
apical periodontal lesion without pulpal
effect.

The pulp has priority in treatment for these
reasons: first, it is likely to cause painful
problems; secondly, it may be the source of
the periodontal lesion, which can resolve in
some circumstances; thirdly, there will be no
healing of the periodontium with an infected,
necrotic pulp connected to it.

Figs 27,6–27,8 show a typical perio-endo
lesion treated with pulpal priority. This was
probably a true combined lesion, because
there were pockets on other teeth also (an
isolated perio-endo lesion with no other
pockets suggests that the patient is not susceptible to periodontitis), and it did not respond
fully until periodontal surgery was performed.

DOES THE PERIODONTAL
CONDITION AFFECT THE PULP?

Apart from perio-endo lesions, there are two
other questions that have been asked about
pulpal-periodontal relations. The first is
whether disease of the periodontium affects
the pulp when the latter is alive and normal,
and the second is whether periodontal treatment may affect the pulp.

Abstract 27,4 is of a time-honoured and
well-designed research study that concludes
that the pulp is largely unaffected by periodontal disease, even when the latter is severe.
This is in agreement with the opinion stated
above, that periodontitis is unlikely to be the
cause of a perio-endo lesion.

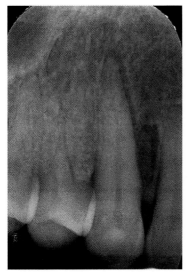

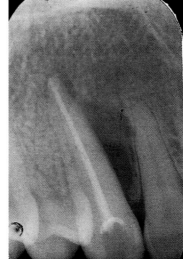

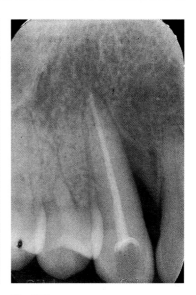

Fig. 27,6

A perio-endo lesion on tooth 13. The tooth is non-vital, and the angular defect is one of several indications of marginal periodontitis in the mouth. The mesial pocket is 12 mm deep, compared with 2 mm on the distal of tooth 12.

Fig. 27,7

The root has been filled, but a deep pocket (10 mm) is still present on the mesial of tooth surface 13.

Fig. 27,8

One year after flap surgery, there is evidence of bone regeneration on the mesial surface of tooth 13 and the PD is 4 mm without BOP. Full treatment was necessary to resolve this true combined perio-endo lesion. The distal PD of tooth 12 is still 2 mm.

Abstract 27,4   *Influence of periodontal disease on the dental pulp*

Mazur B, Massler M, *Oral Surgery, Oral Medicine and Oral Pathology* 1964; **17**: 592–603

In 26 patients, 106 caries-free teeth graded with mild, moderate, severe and very severe periodontitis were removed and histologically examined. In four other patients, pulpal changes were compared in 15 teeth with mild to very severe periodontitis and in 7 control teeth without it; all teeth were caries-free. Pulpal changes were also graded in the same four categories. There were no correlations between the periodontal and pulpal changes. All four pulpal categories were represented in all four periodontal groupings. In the group of patients with normal control teeth, there were no differences in pulpal pathology between these and the periodontitis-affected teeth.

Comment: A classic, well-performed study that is a strong indication that pulpal changes are independent of periodontal disease.

Abstract 27,5   *Endodontic effects of root planing in humans*

Wong R, Hirsch RS, Clarke NG, *Endodontics and Dental Traumatology* 1989; **5**: 193–196

In six patients, 10 teeth with advanced periodontitis had one proximal surface thoroughly root planed (30 strokes with a new curette) and the other was left unplaned as a control. Citric acid at pH 1 was administered to both surfaces to remove the smear layer left by instrumentation. The teeth were carefully extracted 10–14 days later. Examination by light and scanning electron microscopy showed that cementum had not been removed completely from three planed surfaces; of the remaining seven, bacteria were found within tubules of three teeth. In these teeth, the pulp adjacent to the planed areas showed low-grade inflammatory changes. Control areas showed none of these changes.

Comment: This study reminds us not to overdo root planing, but it is probable that the smear layer provides some protection.

Regarding the second question, Abstract 27,5 provides evidence that root planing certainly may have pulpal effects. This is not surprising, because it can cause dentinal hypersensitivity. These effects appear mild and within the coping ability of an intact pulp. However, in the patients selected no oral hygiene measures had been instituted, as this might reduce the colonization of tubules. In addition, the use of citric acid to remove the smear layer might take away one of the obstacles to colonization.

DENTINE AFTER ROOT TREATMENT

There is a possibility of fracture after root treatment of teeth with reduced periodontal support. When the pulp has been removed, so have the live odontoblasts, and the tooth becomes more brittle as a result. When a root has been deducted from the available support, fracture becomes even more likely. Root resections require careful planning to avoid such embarrassment.

CONCLUSIONS

The relationship of the pulp and periodontium suggests that the pulp is the dominant partner, as far as perio-endo lesions and their treatment are concerned. It is also important to be aware that plaque may form apically, and that routine periodontal treatment is unlikely to harm the pulp.

28 FIXED AND REMOVABLE PROSTHODONTICS AND PERIODONTOLOGY

- How do fixed bridges relate to the periodontium?
- How should removable appliances be designed for the reduced periodontium?
- Where there is untreated periodontal disease, what is a suitable approach?

The provision of tooth replacements in the periodontally normal dentition is a well-established art and science. Studies have shown that there is virtually no effect on the periodontium, provided that its healthy state is maintained. A long-term study of patients with removable prostheses indicated that these appliances had no adverse effects, provided that the patients were given good maintenance support and encouraged in preventive dental behaviour (Abstract 28,1). Similarly, fixed prostheses do not cause periodontal damage even in the extreme conditions of cross-arch bridges (Abstract 28,2).

The presence of periodontal disease is a warning that it may be necessary to modify the prosthodontic treatment plan. We may note also that a good periodontal condition contributes to prosthodontic practice in two ways: first, it makes impression-taking easier where there is no bleeding; secondly, there will be less likelihood of recession after placing a crown if there is no pre-existing inflammation.

PERIODONTALLY ALTERED PROSTHODONTIC SITUATIONS

There are two circumstances that require comment. The first is where there is untreated periodontal disease. It is facile to say that the disease must be treated before any tooth replacement; in practice a less than perfect situation is sometimes forced upon us. This comes in two forms: patients may require interim tooth replacement before thorough

Abstract 28,1 *Caries, periodontal and prosthetic findings in patients with removable partial dentures: a ten-year longitudinal study*

Bergman B, Hugoson A, Olsson C-O, *Journal of Prosthetic Dentistry* 1982; **48**: 506–514

In a Swedish dental school clinic, all patients provided with removable partial dentures over a 3 month period in 1968–9 were followed up for 10 years. Thirty patients aged 24–80 years received 33 dentures and the three drop-outs were due to death. Prior to removable partial denture provision, and annually thereafter, hygiene and other support was given. Up to 6 years, a control group of 10 subjects was examined, but after this only four were available. Because there had been no apparent change in this group, it was examined no further. There were no significant changes over the 10 years in plaque, gingivitis, pocket depth and tooth mobility scores. Apart from replacement or adjustment of restorations and dentures where indicated, approximately one new carious surface required treatment in each patient over the whole time. During the 10 years, more than half of the total restorative treatment occurred in five patients, and more than half of the patients required two or fewer restorations only.

Comment: This thorough study indicates that properly constructed removable partial dentures are unlikely to cause caries or periodontal problems. As in long-term periodontal studies, a few patients seem to account for most of the disease.

Abstract 28,2 *A longitudinal study of combined periodontal and prosthetic treatment of patients with advanced periodontal disease*

Nyman S, Lindhe J, *Journal of Periodontology* 1979; **50**: 163–169

From 1969 to 1973, 299 patients who had lost 50% or more of periodontal support were referred to a Swedish university for periodontal treatment and were included in this 5–8 year study. In 48 patients no prosthodontic treatment was required, and these were the control group for the study. The other 251 patients required tooth replacement, and every fifth patient was selected for comparison with the control group. This selected treatment group of 50 patients had 74 bridges: 21 cross-arch with distal abutments; 39 cross-arch with distal cantilevers; and 14 unilateral bridges. In the patients compared there were no differences with respect to plaque, gingivitis, PD, PAL, and bone support over a 5–8 year maintenance period. In the whole group of 251 patients, 332 bridges had been made (respectively, 139, 159 and 34 in the three subgroups). Over the 5–8 year follow-up period, there were 26 failures, none for periodontal reasons. Retainer de-bonding accounted for 11 failures, fractured bridges for 7 and fractured abutments for 8.

Comment: The reason for this outstanding periodontal success was the thorough 3–6 month maintenance programme. The authors also considered that the mechanical failures could have been prevented if known principles had always been followed.

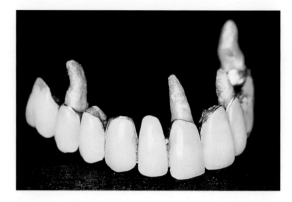

Fig. 28,1

A cross-arch bridge lost through the progression of untreated periodontitis. (Photograph courtesy of Mr B J Smith.)

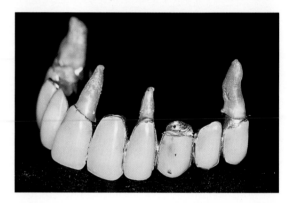

Fig. 28,2

The one abutment that needed to be sectioned was tooth 23. (Photograph courtesy of Mr B J Smith.)

and definitive periodontal treatment; or, in some cases, the response to treatment may be insufficient to guarantee periodontal stability and yet teeth may need replacing.

The second circumstance is where tooth replacement is required in the dentition with healthy but reduced periodontal support. The outstanding study of this condition was published in 1979 (Abstract 28,2), and showed that reduced periodontal support, given sufficient healthy abutments, was no barrier to successful bridgework. Indeed, it is widely believed that these large bridges were successful *because* of the reduced support. Figs 28,1–28,3 show the result of unsatisfactory maintenance support.

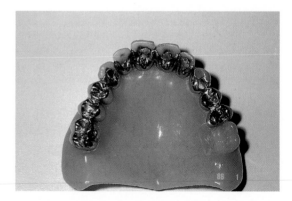

Fig. 28,3

Within 2 days, the bridge became the dentition of a complete denture. (Photograph courtesy of Mr B J Smith.)

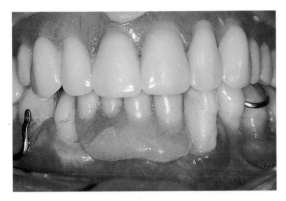

Fig. 28,4

Lower removable partial denture in dentition with progressing periodontitis.

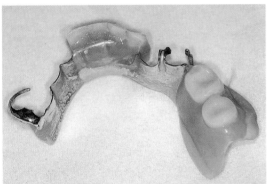

Fig. 28,5

The denture.

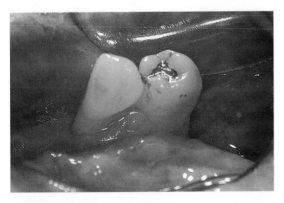

Fig. 28,6

Teeth on the right, lingual view.

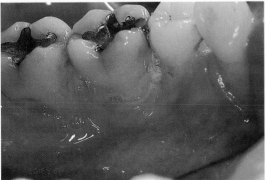

Fig. 28,7

Teeth on the left, lingual view.

On top of these considerations, there is one more: does a missing tooth need replacement? All these questions are more appropriately given detailed attention in texts devoted to prosthodontics but we shall consider also the special situation of the shortened dental arch.

INDICATIONS FOR TOOTH REPLACEMENT IN THE PERIODONTALLY INVOLVED DENTITION

Why do dentists replace teeth? The patient has two significant objectives in restoring appearance and function. The dentist has an additional objective that is of even more significance in the reduced support dentition – a prosthesis is a space maintainer that contributes to the overall effectiveness of the dentition by preventing tooth movement.

This means that when providing any prosthesis we must consider its relationship to the dentition as a whole. Not only do abutments provide support for a prosthesis, but they also are affected by its presence: the prosthesis transmits increased forces to the abutments.

REMOVABLE PARTIAL DENTURES IN THE PERIODONTALLY REDUCED DENTITION

Figs 28,4–28,7 show a failing situation with a removable partial denture. In addition to progressing, unsatisfactorily-treated periodontitis on all teeth, the abutment teeth showed marked hypermobility. Even if they were not hypermobile when the denture was made, the situation was not predictably suited to this sort of prosthesis.

Because of the very limited support on the right, teeth 43 and 44 were particularly at risk of strong lateral force disturbance. A design was required that would enhance stability of the whole arch. Given favourable initial periodontal circumstances, this would need to make use of all the limited support available,

and in such a way that abutments provided maximum resistance to displacement.

Such resistance is least forthcoming when the forces tend to tilt these teeth and most forthcoming when bodily tooth movement is required for displacement, a fact that is well understood in orthodontic practice. Whatever type of prosthesis was to be made, therefore, the situation required as many teeth as possible to be used as abutments, and for them all to be held as rigidly as possible by the prosthesis. In other words, the prosthesis should act as a splint for the remaining teeth.

Guide planes resist displacement (a feature of this prosthesis). Other partial denture features favourable to reduced periodontal support might include: intracoronal attachments sufficiently extensive to resist the tendency for teeth to tilt; rests extended across the vertical axes of abutment teeth or continued mesiodistally across abutments; and perhaps no clasps. In order to reach undercuts, retentive arms tend to displace the tooth each time the prosthesis is inserted or removed. Where teeth have reduced support, such a jiggling force can increase abutment mobility. However, if the guide planes can be so designed as to reciprocate retentive clasp forces during insertion, jiggling will be prevented.

DESIGN OF FIXED PROSTHESES

The needs for rigid linking of abutments and maximum resistance to lateral forces of displacement make a fixed bridge the most suitable prosthesis in the dentition with periodontally reduced support. Because of the proven susceptibility of such a patient to periodontitis, special care is needed to provide access for thorough plaque control and to keep margins supragingival. Figs 28,1–28,3 should be a permanent reminder of the need for periodontal maintenance in all such cases.

It is also useful if the bridge can be provided with contingency features against failure of any questionable abutments. In the case shown in Figs 28,8 and 28,9, subsequent caries in abutment tooth 24 was dealt with by removal of the tooth and retention of a distal cantilever pontic. Another example of abutment removal, this time for periodontal reasons, is shown in Figs 28,10–28,12.

When there are gaps or moderate misalignment of teeth, there may be a simpler option than orthodontics and fixed splinting. Figs 28,13–28,16 show such a case where no orthodontic treatment was performed but bridgework was used to camouflage the appearance. Such work requires careful planning to give space for periodontal maintenance.

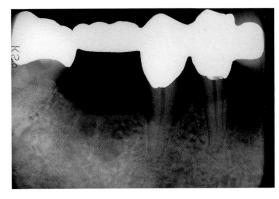

Fig. 28,10

Abutment tooth 45 is periodontally adequate. (Photograph courtesy of Mr B J Smith.)

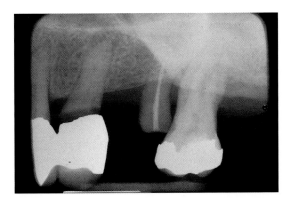

Fig. 28,8

Abutment tooth 24 on a cross-arch bridge has caries. This root was resected and the prosthesis was maintained. (Photograph courtesy of Mr B J Smith.)

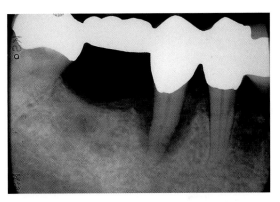

Fig. 28,11

Significant progression of periodontitis 3 years later. (Photograph courtesy of Mr B J Smith.)

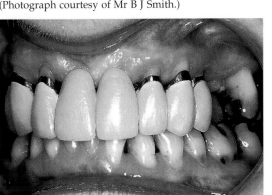

Fig. 28,9

The maintained cross-arch bridge. (Photograph courtesy of Mr B J Smith.)

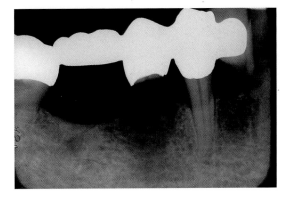

Fig. 28,12

The root was resected and the prosthesis maintained. (Photograph courtesy of Mr B J Smith.)

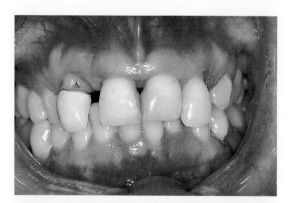

Fig. 28,13

Unsatisfactory appearance, with gaps mesial to tooth 12 and distal to tooth 22, which is overerupted, but periodontal treatment is progressing favourably.

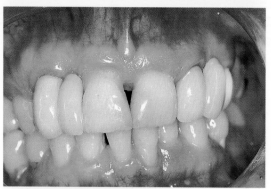

Fig. 28,14

Following periodontal treatment, the gaps have been camouflaged with skilful bridgework.

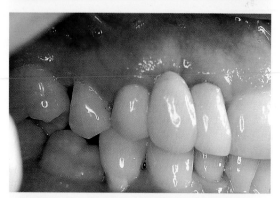

Fig. 28,15

Right bridge.

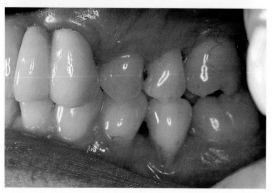

Fig. 28,16

Left bridge.

PROSTHESES IN THE PATIENT WITH UNTREATED PERIODONTAL DISEASE

At the outset of periodontal treatment, when unsavable teeth are to be removed, there may be a requirement for their immediate replacement on the grounds of appearance or maintenance of arch integrity.

If there is a suitable abutment, a single anterior tooth may be replaced with a cantilevered adhesive bridge. The abutment should have no significant attachment loss or pocketing and should be free of other restorative problems.

In other situations, a provisional solution is found in a simple mucosa-borne removable partial denture. When patients already have prostheses, these may be retained during treatment (with modification if necessary) until a more favourable periodontal condition is established. There is no evidence that 'gum-strippers' really do what their nickname suggests. In the presence of good plaque control, they may function satisfactorily until a better-designed solution is possible.

The Every pattern of upper partial denture is sometimes of use, and follows the usual design rules for this appliance: maintenance of proximal contact round the arch, and avoidance of gingival margin areas.

There is one further situation that needs comment. Where a patient is not responding to treatment, either through failure of plaque control or because of other factors, the approach in Case History 1 (Chapter 1) may be followed. Partial dentures may be made with gradual addition of further teeth as it becomes necessary.

The patient should be given particularly sympathetic attention and, as far as possible, should decide when teeth need extraction. To manifest unfeeling rigidity, e.g. by insisting on a clearance, is unnecessary, rejecting behaviour. Our duty as dentists is to advise and to provide what help we can to patients who, in some cases, may desperately need friendship and kindness. This is not to rule out a serious medical condition, such as endocarditis, as a reason for losing teeth.

SHORTENED DENTAL ARCHES

In some patients the pattern of periodontitis is limited to severe loss of molar support, with little or no attachment loss elsewhere. In other patients, molar teeth may be lost for other reasons such as caries. In addition, molar teeth are harder to treat and they respond less well to periodontal therapy.

It is therefore natural to ask whether the molar teeth are essential to the well-being of the whole dentition. Furthermore, if they are lost, need they be replaced?

The answers to these questions are essentially given in the welcome study in Abstract 28,3. Provided that the premolar condition is well maintained, such arches may last a very long time.

Abstract 28,3 *Shortened dental arches and periodontal support*

Witter DJ, De Haan AFJ, Käyser AF et al., *Journal of Oral Rehabilitation* 1991; **18**: 203–212

Periodontal support was compared in 74 patients with shortened dental arches (SDA), 25 with similar arches and distal extension base removable partial dentures (SDA+RPD), and 72 with complete dental arches. Three-quarters of SDA subjects had been in this condition for 5 years or more and 25% for over 15 years. Particular attention was paid to the condition of the most distal premolars. When the three groups were considered together, 28% of SDA+RPD subjects, 19% of SDA subjects and 7% of controls had mobile teeth, a statistically significant difference. There were similar differences in distal premolar bone height. During a 5-year follow-up of the SDA and SDA+RPD groups, 14 teeth were lost, 13 of them premolars and half for periodontal reasons. The authors stress the need for the best possible periodontal maintenance in SDA patients, and suggest that subjects with SDA are probably in a high-risk group for dental diseases.

Comment: A shortened dental arch seems a satisfactory and stable situation on the basis of this and other studies.

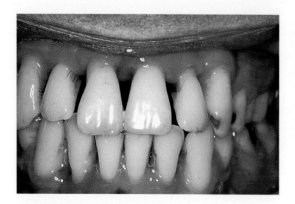

Fig. 28,17

Significant post-surgical gingival recession in a treated patient. (Photograph courtesy of Dr Ravi Saravanamuttu.)

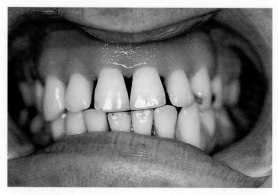

Fig. 28,18

Acrylic gingival veneer in place. Thorough hygiene is essential in this situation. (Photograph courtesy of Dr Ravi Saravanamuttu.)

GINGIVAL VENEERS

Although these may be offered to patients with gingival recession (Figs 28,17 and 28,18), they have been requested from the present author only twice in over 30 years. When they see the result of thorough periodontal treatment, many patients are satisfied with the appearance and some are also wary of any device that they feel might compromise their plaque control.

CONCLUSION

Although judicious provision of tooth replacement may assist in the treatment of patients with periodontal problems, it is as well to be wary of the many possible pitfalls. Simple treatment is often the best approach until the future of the dentition is predictable.

29 ASPECTS OF IMPLANT DENTISTRY

- What are the similarities and differences between implants and teeth?
- What are the main factors affecting implant success?
- How are implants maintained?

This book stops short of any detailed consideration of modern osseointegrated implants, for which the reader should consult other texts. However, everyone interested in the practice of periodontology requires an understanding of this field, with which periodontics is so inextricably linked. For instance, calculus may be a problem around implants (Figs 29,1 and 29,2), and requires special attention. In addition, the practice of implant dentistry often requires more than a passing acquaintance with periodontology and prosthodontics.

Among the first serious attempts to deal with patients who were unable to manage lower complete dentures was the development of subperiosteal implants. An incision was made along the crest of an edentulous ridge, flaps were elevated and the outline of a framework was made in the bone with a large bur over the whole denture-bearing area.

Next, an impression was taken, and a framework was cast, with four projecting abutments (two molar, two anterior) to support a denture. Following the fitting of the cast framework, a denture was made and inserted. Success rates are not known.

Variations on the theme included smaller implants to provide distal abutments for fixed bridges that were attached to natural teeth. Such early attempts at implants were well established by the late 1950s but were practised by very few operators.

One of the defects of these early implants was epithelialization. The whole implant structure was externalized and retained within a

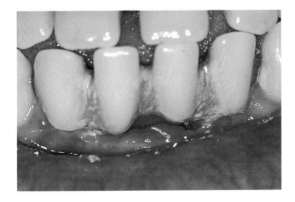

Fig. 29,1

A fixed prosthesis on two implants.

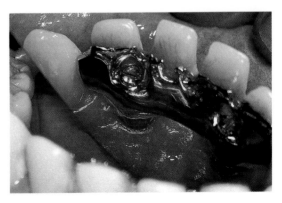

Fig. 29,2

Mirror view shows that there is calculus lingual to the left implant.

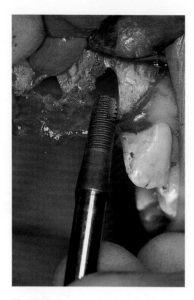

Fig. 29,3

Site prepared with implant about to be inserted. (Photograph courtesy of Dr Paul Palmer.)

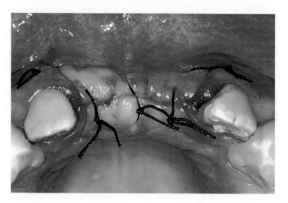

Fig. 29,4

Flap closure after implant insertion. (Photograph courtesy of Dr Paul Palmer.)

close-fitting epithelium-lined tissue. This could lead to good conditions for abscesses in some patients. Consequently, clinicians with an interest in implants sought the elusive goal of osseointegration.

OSSEOINTEGRATION

Following studies in the 1960s and 1970s, the advent of reliable implant dentistry resulted from the work of Per-Ingvar Brånemark, a Swedish orthopaedic surgeon. If the implant was buried in close-fitting bone and covered with mucoperiosteum (Figs 29,3 and 29,4), over the next 3–6 months it would become osseointegrated by the formation of bone around it, and when uncovered could become the base for an abutment around which a tight gingival cuff could form.

To be close to bone, and to provide for stability, a cylindrical form with a screw thread was designed. The implant itself had to be of a biologically compatible material: high-grade titanium was generally used, although

other materials followed in other implant systems. To avoid surface contamination, everything that contacted the implant had to be made of the same high-quality metal.

It is greatly to the credit of the developers of the Brånemark system that they did not rush into commercial production but waited for evidence of long-term reliability. Given the spectacular failure of some previous implant work, the establishment of such credibility was necessary.

In marked contrast to some earlier procedures, operators today are taught to be gentle with the bone. Overheating would cause necrosis, and must be avoided as the osteotomy site is shaped. An implant is seated in the carefully-prepared site with a delicate hand operation method and is never forced.

FACTORS AFFECTING SUCCESS

As a result of the new system with its biologically compatible materials and methods, and operators who understood essential matters of prosthodontic treatment planning, a very high rate of success followed. One large meta-analysis based on many published studies is shown in Abstract 29,1.

Abstract 29,1 *Biological factors contributing to failures of osseointegrated oral implants. (1) Success criteria and epidemiology*

Esposito M, Hirsch J-M, Lekholm U, et al., *European Journal of Oral Science* 1998; **106**: 527–551

This is an analysis of 159 follow-up studies of Brånemark implants up to February 1997. Studies with inadequate data or relating to extreme situations were excluded (totalling 86). This review therefore included 73 published papers. The 5-year biological failure rate is estimated at 7.7%. For the edentulous patient, fixed prostheses had a 5.8% implant failure rate, compared with 12.8% for overdentures. Implants partially supporting bridges failed in 4% of cases, and single tooth implants in 2.4%. Where bone grafts were involved, 14.9% of implants failed, and with other types of adjunctive oral surgery, 7.3% of implants failed. There was a higher maxillary failure rate. The authors attributed about 10% of peri-implantitis to plaque and the rest to overloading.

Comment: This is an extensive summary of many relevant studies. The literature clearly points to occlusal forces as the main cause of peri-implantitis.

The overall long-term success rates for individual implants in the maxilla and the mandible are around 85–90% and 95% upwards, respectively. The main factors that increase failure are tobacco smoking, sparsely trabeculated bone and removable rather than fixed appliances. Although proper treatment for implant patients includes a thorough hygiene programme, there is little evidence that plaque has any major effect. Perhaps this is because it has never been allowed to exist for long in implant patients, but it may also relate to fundamental differences between osseointegrated implants and teeth.

OSSEOINTEGRATED IMPLANTS AND TEETH COMPARED

Whereas the implant is rigidly fixed in bone, the tooth is not. All the complex details of the periodontal attachment apparatus permit the tooth to erupt, take up its position in the arch and move with the gradual remodelling of adjacent tissues. In contrast, the implant is analogous to an ankylosed tooth.

This simile is more readily understood when we consider the special case of an implant placed in a young patient whose alveolar bone has not reached its full adult formation. In this case, the teeth move with bone development, whereas the implant is gradually submerged and requires operative intervention.

In eruption and remodelling of the jaws, therefore, the tooth has a definite advantage over the implant. However, the susceptibility of the periodontium to plaque-induced disease is perhaps a significant disadvantage for the tooth. This is perhaps surprising, for without the benefit of evidence we might expect the implant to be far more vulnerable to ordinary inflammation.

For instance, we could postulate that bone loss following the spread of inflammation could lead to rapid failure of the implant. In fact this event – a plaque-induced peri-implantitis – seems relatively rare. Bacterial plaque is apparently more of a threat to teeth than to implants.

OCCLUSAL STRESSES ON IMPLANTS

However, there is another factor that is more threatening to implants than to teeth, and there is a clue to this in the determinants of increased implant failure. When a tooth is jiggled (as we saw in Chapter 25) then, provided that the plaque is controlled, no attachment loss occurs but bone is invariably lost. In contrast, all the support that the implant has comes from bone, and if the equivalent of occlusal trauma is applied then there may be severe consequences.

Such trauma appears to be a significant factor in implant failure. Forces on the tooth are partly absorbed by the resilient structure of the periodontal ligament, which may adapt to repetitive stress. Where an implant is successfully osseointegrated, these forces are

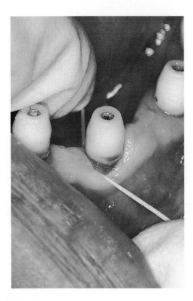

Fig. 29,5

Dental floss applied to an implant awaiting a removable prosthesis.

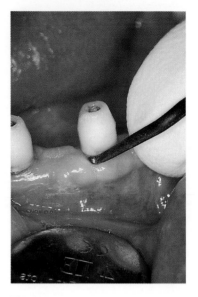

Fig. 29,6

Carbon-fibre scaling instrument for use on implants.

transmitted directly to bone, with no such adaptable cushion to maintain attachment and mitigate injury.

This may help to explain the higher failure rates when implants are used to support removable prostheses, because lateral movements necessarily involve forces not present when the implants are rigidly connected with a fixed bridge. Where bone is sparsely formed, or affected by the myriad of damaging factors in tobacco smoke, it may also be more susceptible to such damage.

The occlusal relations of implant-supported prostheses are an important consideration in implant dentistry, and every effort is made to minimize undesirable stresses on implant-supporting bone.

PERIODONTAL RELATIONS WITH IMPLANTS

There are several situations where implant dentistry is associated with matters of perio-

Abstract 29,2   *Failure rates of restorations for single-tooth replacement*

Priest DF, *International Journal of Prosthodontics* 1996; **9**: 38–45

This paper compared failure rates in different methods of single-tooth replacement. Eleven studies of conventional fixed bridges, 18 of resin-bonded adhesive bridges and 7 of implants were examined. The major causes of failure in conventional bridges were caries and endodontic or periodontal complications. Rates varied from 3% over 23 years to 20% over 3 years. Failure of resin-bonded bridges was usually by debonding and the rates varied from 10% over 11 years to 54% over 11 months. Single-tooth implant failure varied from 9% over 3 years to 0% over 6.6 years.

Comment: There was a wide variation in the results of bridge follow-up studies. If implants show good long-term retention, they may become preferable on the grounds of cost and convenience for restoration, repair or replacement.

dontal health. The most obvious implication is of regular maintenance. The patient is taught to use careful plaque control without damaging the surface of implants (Fig. 29,5). Likewise, special instruments are used by the hygienist or dentist for scaling (Fig. 29,6).

Implants may be used to replace a single tooth, to support other teeth as abutments or to replace an entire arch or dentition. They should be considered seriously when only one anterior tooth is missing and the prognosis for all others is favourable: Abstract 29,2 shows a rare cost-benefit estimation that suggests that an implant is the best option.

In reviewing the periodontal health of a patient who has received implant treatment, the dentist will be able to monitor the healthy support of fixtures. Mobility and marked radiographic bone loss are the principal signs of failure.

CLINICAL ASSESSMENT, DIAGNOSIS AND TREATMENT PLANNING

- How should the patient be involved in decision making?
- How does individual tooth diagnosis assist treatment planning?
- How should prognostic uncertainty be managed?

Periodontal treatment procedures require clear objectives at each stage of the treatment plan. Some patients with periodontal disease are given what is in effect a repeated course of maintenance care of indefinite length.

This may be appropriate after a treatment plan has been formulated and executed with limited success because either the patient was unable to comply with hygiene requirements or the dentist was unable to produce the desired results. However, at the outset, following initial assessment a careful treatment plan is needed, with suitable points for reassessment and further decisions.

The aim of a diagnosis is to formulate a treatment plan, and the aim of a treatment plan is to increase the certainty of future stability. In a state of untreated disease, there is little that is certain except for the possibility that disease will progress further, given time.

However, it is often not possible to make a full periodontal treatment plan at the outset. There may be uncertainties over the condition of individual teeth, or their likely response to treatment. Complete treatment therefore may depend on further information and the whole procedure may take several stages. This is acceptable provided that treatment objectives can be identified at each stage.

DECISION MAKING

The principles of periodontal decision making are outlined in Table 30,1. At each decision point, adequate information is gathered for a decision about appropriate treatment and

Table 30,1: *Periodontal treatment decisions – principles*

Stage of treatment	Information required	Information sources	Periodontal treatment options
Initial assessment	Dental and medical history to date; prognosis for individual teeth; patient's objectives	Patient history and examination; diagnosis of relevant conditions	Hygiene; non-surgical treatment; extractions
Reassessment after non-surgical treatment	Response to defined treatment; results achieved	Initial examination, plaque control records and re-examination	Hygiene; non-surgical treatment; surgical treatment; extractions
Reassessment after further treatment	Results achieved	Previous and current examinations	Hygiene; non-surgical treatment; surgical treatment; extractions

management. It is important to document examination details well (Chapter 5). Depending on the probing assessment, the radiographic examination may involve a detailed set of long-cone paralleling technique periapical views for an advanced problem or a panoramic tomograph for some limited problems. The latter view has improved considerably in quality since tomograms entered dentistry three decades ago.

Diagnosis is often uncertain, particularly with forms of periodontitis. A frequent question to which we would like to know the answer is whether a patient, perhaps aged 30–40 years, has a slow, long-active disease or has recently undergone rapid attachment loss. This may have implications for our treatment and is occasionally of medico-legal significance.

The initial assessment is usually incapable of providing one of the most important pieces of information for periodontal management, namely the response to treatment. Although we know a considerable amount about the reponse of groups of patients to treatment, there is no way of knowing that of the individual patient who attends for the first time.

It is therefore wise to be cautious in treatment planning at the initial stage, because there is one major unknown factor in the degree of the patient's response. Although some teeth may appear to have very good reasons for extraction, for instance, there are many other teeth for which the prognosis may be less clear.

Once the result of an initial course of treatment has been properly assessed, the future may be planned with a greater degree of confidence. Where relevant, decisions on surgery may be made in the knowledge that there has been a suitable improvement following thorough control of subgingival plaque.

CASE MANAGEMENT: A COMMENT ON PROBING CHARTS

For elegant presentation of results, various anatomical charts have been devised. However, these charts have disadvantages when speedy review of a patient's progress is required. One drawback is that it is harder to

put together the buccal and lingual aspects of the same teeth; another is that sequential charting is not easy to follow over a period of time involving several repeated assessments, each of which requires a separate page.

Another form of chart that has been used successfully for many years is shown in the cases presented in this chapter and earlier in this book. Using the charting customs given in Conventions and Abbreviations at the start of this book, it is possible to record measurements in a way that shows six probing points together for each tooth. Bleeding is noted as a dot by the probing measurement, and pus as a 'P'.

For management of periodontitis, up to three PD charts may be placed on one page. The recession also may be recorded as a separate chart if desired, but for all practical purposes, PD is the central treatment management tool.

SHARING DECISIONS WITH THE PATIENT

Frequently there are alternative ways of treating the same periodontal problem, and these will need discussion. It is important to involve the patient from the outset, however, because the objectives of treatment require consideration at the earliest stage. Furthermore, they depend on the patient's compliance. Sometimes the patient has conflicting objectives: for instance, it may not be possible to retain all teeth and improve appearance at the same time.

Loss of teeth is one of the permanent changes that may result from periodontal diseases. Because this is a final event, any recommendation for extraction should be discussed clearly. It may be helpful to take the patient through the reasoning that leads the clinician to give such advice. The patient will probably want to know the likely status of what remains, and what sort of replacement, if any, is indicated.

EXTRACTION DECISIONS

Table 30,2 lists a number of reasons suggesting why a tooth should be removed. In each

Table 30,2: *Reasons why extraction may be indicated*

Tooth-based: periodontal	Advanced attachment loss; minimal remaining radiographic bone support; severe or untreatable furcation involvement
Tooth-based: caries or pulp-related	Advanced caries of crown or root; severe pulpal or periapical lesion; untreatable periodontal-endodontal lesion
Dentition-based	Overeruption; drifting; untreatable position in mouth; too few remaining teeth in arch
Patient-based	Significant medical reason; physical or behavioural disability; patient objectives

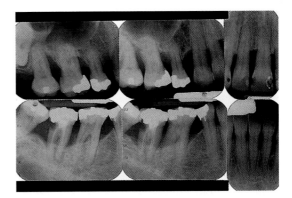

Fig. 30,1

Right-side radiographs of 45-year-old female patient with advanced periodontitis. Note that tooth 47 has significant distal caries, possibly fused roots and under 50% bone support.

case, the indication is not absolute, but relative. There may be an appropriate alternative treatment or even lack of treatment. In some cases, for instance, teeth with markedly reduced support may be retained as the abutments for a cross-arch bridge, but such a case requires very careful selection. Some overerupted teeth may be orthodontically intruded, although this is less likely for a lone molar.

The patient's objectives are also very important. If extraction is either desired or abhorred, such views may have quite an effect on our approach to treatment. The four levels of consideration given in the table are typical of the multi-level approach to treatment decisions that technical dental achievement requires at the present time.

An example of contrasting extraction decisions is apparent in the case outlined in Figs 30,1–30,9. The patient presented with two lower molar roots affected by distal caries and significant periodontitis. On tooth 47 the roots were close together (in fact, fused) with an unmanageable furcation; the decision was to extract this tooth. However, on tooth 36 the root morphology permitted a distal root resection. In the same patient, tooth 22 presented a problem because of significant attachment

		3 4 2	3 2 8	4 2 3		7 2 7	6 2 8	10 2 7
		3 8 2	5 2 8	5 2 3		6 5 6	7 5 8	8 5 7
8	**7**	**6**	**5**	**4**	**3**	**2**	**1**
8	**7**	**6**	**5**	**4**	**3**	**2**	**1**
5 7 8	9 4 8	5 3 8		4 2 3	3 2 2	2 2 2	2 2 6
4 2 8	9 3 10	8 2 9		4 2 3	4 2 3	3 3 3	3 3 6

Fig. 30,2

Probing chart shows advanced disease for tooth 47. This tooth was extracted.

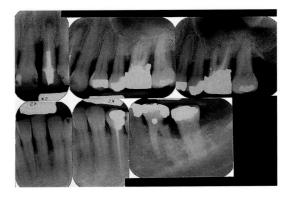

Fig. 30,3

On the left side, tooth 36 has significant distal caries, but support is better and root morphology is more favourable.

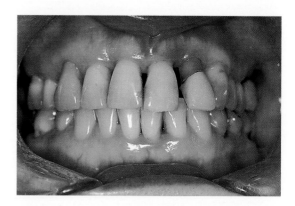

7 7 9	9 7 8	9 2 5	7 2 7	8 2 7	6 3 10	9 3 10
8 6 10	9 7 7	8 6 3	7 2 5	7 5 6	8 3 7	7 7 12
1	2	3	4	5	6	7
1	2	3	4	5	6	7
5 2 5	3 2 2	3 2 2	3 2 3	3 2 2	4 6 6	8 4 5
3 2 7	4 2 3	3 2 2	3 2 2	3 2 3	3 2 4	10 3 3

Fig. 30,4

Chart shows less pocketing for tooth 36 than for tooth 47.

Fig. 30,7

The same patient showing tooth 22.

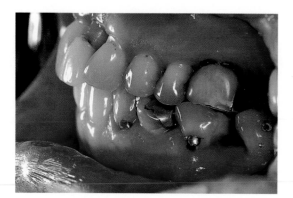

Fig. 30,5

Tooth 36, showing caries.

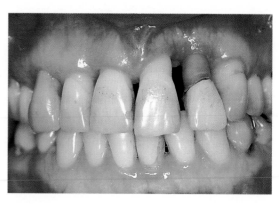

Fig. 30,8

Following root planing and surgery tooth 22 has more reduced support.

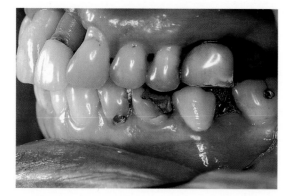

Fig. 30,6

Following distal root resection, tooth 36 is restored with a crown.

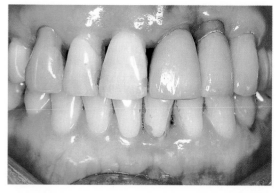

Fig. 30,9

To maintain tooth 22 in the arch, a three-unit splint was fitted.

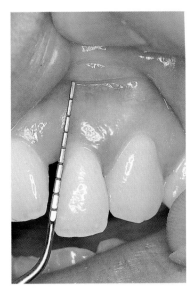

Fig. 30,10

LJP lesion on the mesial surface of tooth 22 in a 21-year-old female.

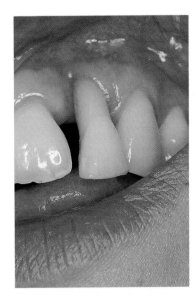

Fig. 30,12

Tooth 22, after incisal reduction.

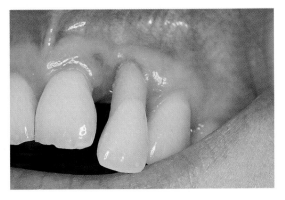

Fig. 30,11

Tooth 22, following surgery.

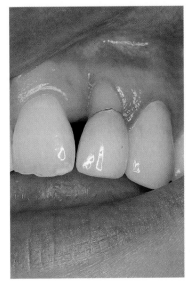

Fig. 30,13

22 splinted to 23.

loss and an apical area with a cast post and crown present. If this tooth was to be retained, which the patient strongly desired, the decision would have to include flap surgery and apical curettage at least. In the event, this was performed, but because of the limited remaining support a full-coverage splint was provided rather than a crown. Teeth 21 and 23 provided stability for the mobile tooth 22. A bridge would have been a reasonable alternative.

Where there are such alternatives, patients' objectives (such as retaining teeth subject to the limitations of actual treatment success) may play a part in deciding the course to be taken. In Figs 30,10–30,13 we see the result of retaining tooth 22 shown at surgery in Fig. 4,2. The overeruption meant that the tooth had to be reduced, but the appearance was still unaesthetic and a crown was required.

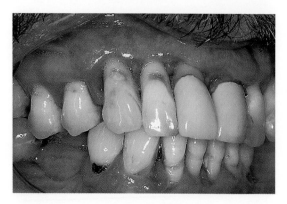

Fig. 30,14

Advanced periodontitis in a 50-year-old male: right side.

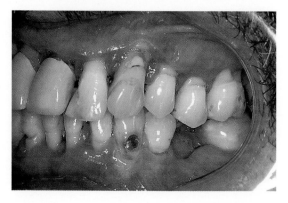

Fig. 30,16

Left-side view.

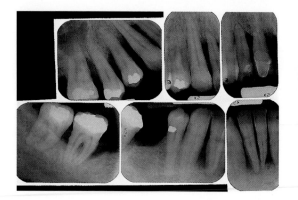

Fig. 30,15

Radiographs show very advanced bone loss on most of the teeth.

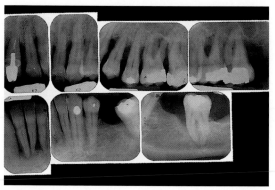

Fig. 30,17

Similar advanced bone loss.

Because of reduced support, the crown was provided as part of a full-coverage splint linked to tooth 23. The outcome was satisfactory and the gain was retention of tooth 22; however, tooth 23 required a significant loss of sound enamel. An alternative simpler treatment might have used an adhesive bridge cantilevered off tooth 23 to replace tooth 22.

CONTINGENT TREATMENT PLANNING

We have seen that a complete periodontal treatment plan may not be possible at the outset of treatment, because there is uncer-

tainty over aspects of the response to therapy, both in the patient's plaque control and in the operator's part of treatment.

In Figs 30,14–30,20 we see what happened to a 50-year-old man with advanced periodontitis whose dentist advised clearance and complete dentures. A full periodontal examination showed that there were three teeth with a definite prognosis of 'savable'; the others had either 'unsavable' or 'doubtful' predictions. The upper arch was heading for a complete denture. In the lower arch, a partial denture might have been an appropriate treatment outcome.

The patient was extremely keen to keep all teeth if this was possible, and a simple contin-

Fig. 30,18

PD charts before and after one course of OHI and root planing, with adjunctive systemic metronidazole. The probing reductions are profound, and mostly by shrinkage.

Fig. 30,19

PD charts for left side show similar reductions.

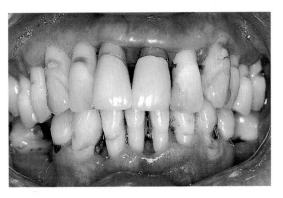

Fig. 30,20

6 months after root planing: note the recession.

gency plan was therefore designed: if a thorough course of oral hygiene and root planing improved the condition, more teeth might be retained as supports for the inevitable dentures. Because frequent pus on probing suggested multiple abscesses caused by anaerobic organisms, metronidazole would accompany the root planing. No teeth would be removed until their future had been put to the test by non-surgical treatment.

The outcome was a surprise to both periodontist and patient. Much of the effect was through recession but there was also a considerable gain of clinical attachment presumably through resolution of inflammation at the base of pockets. An apparently untreatable patient with a need for extraction of most teeth became a treated patient who had lost no teeth and was on a maintenance programme. Five years later, the condition was the same and no teeth had been lost.

In this case, the patient wished to avoid the need for any prosthesis. This was in agreement with clinical objectives because, in the event of all or most teeth being retained, partial dentures might produce large unavoidable lateral stresses in mastication. In passing, we should note that this was one response in one patient, that it was extreme and is by no means an indication that all patients will respond similarly. However, it illustrates the principle of contingent treatment and the need for assessment of treatment response before extracting teeth, unless the indication for their removal is very definite.

AESTHETIC ASPECTS OF TREATMENT PLANNING

In the patient shown in Figs 30,21–30,34 the presenting complaint was the unpleasant

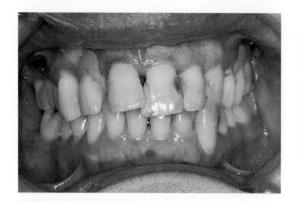

Fig. 30,21

A 57-year-old female who was unhappy with aesthetics and desired a bridge. The drifting of anterior teeth is a clear warning that there is underlying periodontitis.

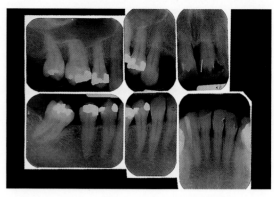

Fig. 30,24

Radiographs of right side.

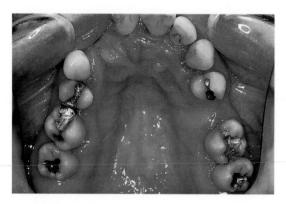

Fig. 30,22

Upper occlusal view.

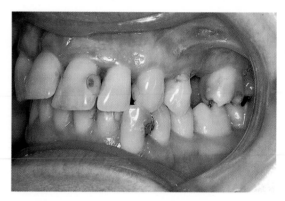

Fig. 30,25

Left side.

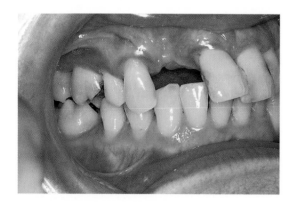

Fig. 30,23

Right side without denture.

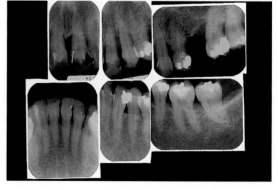

Fig. 30,26

Radiographs of left side.

2			3|2|4	5|2|3				3|2|3	2|2|2				3|2|3
			4|3|5	6|2|3	X			3|3|3	3|3|3	X			3|3|3
1			5|3|3	3|3|3				3|3|4	3|2|3				3|2|5
			5|3|5	5|4|5				4|3|5	7|6|6				5|5|3
8			**7**	**6**		**5**		**4**	**3**		**2**		**1**
8			**7**	**6**		**5**		**4**	**3**		**2**		**1**
1			3|4|4			3|3|4	3|2|3	3|2|2	3|1|2	2|1|2			
			3|2|3			3|1|13	2|1|13	2|1||2	2|1|12	2|1|13			
2			3|4|3			3|2|3	3|1|12	2|2|13	3|1|13	3|2|3			
			2|1|13			2|1|13	2|1|13	2|1|13	3|1|12	3|2|12			

Fig. 30,27

PD charts of right side: chart 1 shows condition 3 months after root planing (BOP affected all pockets over 4 mm); chart 2 is 3 months after surgery. Note that teeth 16 and 17 have not reduced further.

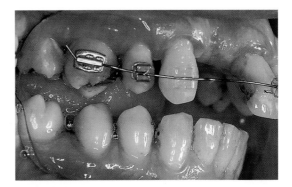

Fig. 30,29

Orthodontics in progress on right side. Periodontal maintenance proved difficult throughout. The appliance added a negative factor in a patient who already found hygiene a struggle.

3|2|2	3|2|2	2|1||5	3|1|13				2|2|3	4|2|3			
3|3|2	2|1|2	2|2|4	3|3|3	X			5|3|3	4|2|5			
6|2|5	5|3|2	2|2|3	3|2|2				5|3|5	5|6|8			
6|6|3	4|3|4	9|8|8	6|4|4				8|4|7	6|4|5			
1	**2**	**3**	**4**		**5**		**6**	**7**		**8**	
1	**2**	**3**	**4**		**5**		**6**	**7**		**8**	
2|1|12	2|1|2	2|2|3	3|2|13	4|2|14	5|3|15	4|4|5			
3|1|13	3|1|13	3|1|13	3|1|14	5|1|14	3|3|3	3|2|5			
2|1|12	2|1|12	2|2|13	3|1|13	3|1|13	5|1|14	5|3|6			
2|1|12	3|2|2	3|1|13	2|2|1	3|3|1	3|3|2	4|2|3			

Fig. 30,28

PD charts of left side show reductions in all areas following surgery. Surgery was not done for teeth 36 and 37.

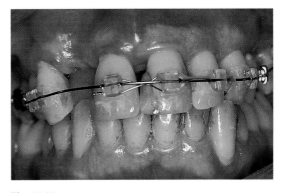

Fig. 30,30

Central view of appliance.

appearance of a mucosal-borne partial denture. The patient was intent upon a fixed bridge to improve aesthetics, but her dentist had rightly insisted on priority for the periodontal problems.

The periodontitis had resulted in drifting and slight overeruption of upper incisors, and therefore the overall plan would include orthodontic treatment. A suitable bridge also would be able to provide permanent ortho-dontic retention. Thus, the overall plan was clear, given a satisfactory periodontal outcome.

Initial non-surgical treatment was carried out mainly by a hygienist and produced a favourable response. Subsequent flap surgery was performed for all pockets, with resection of a wide margin in the posterior lingual and palatal regions. During this phase of treatment the patient did not maintain consistently

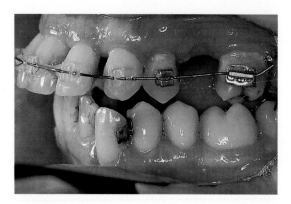

Fig. 30,31

Appliance on left side.

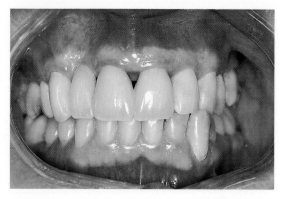

Fig. 30,33

Central view of bridge.

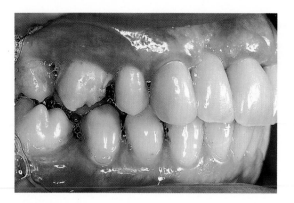

Fig 30,32

As a permanent orthodontic retainer and aesthetic fixed prosthesis, a bridge was fitted with teeth 21, 11 and 13 as abutments, and a pontic at tooth 12. Right-side view.

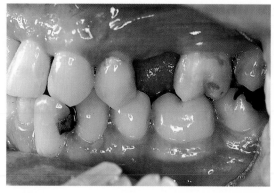

Fig. 30,34

Left view. There is plaque on the mesial surface of tooth 27. This patient requires permanent 3-monthly maintenance.

excellent plaque control, but the response to surgery was surprisingly good e.g. on teeth 13 and 23.

Orthodontics took nearly 1 year, reflecting the relatively good support of the teeth that were realigned and intruded. The bridge included both of the upper central incisors as abutments, to maintain the colour match. The patient was pleased with the result.

Throughout the 2 years of treatment, plaque control first reached a high level in the initial hygiene treatment, but subsequently was variable. At the 5-year reassessment there were still problems in the upper molar regions, with residual pockets. The pattern of erratic plaque control was largely related to accessibility: anterior teeth and premolars were acceptably maintained but molars were maintained less satisfactorily.

The initial periodontal objective of this patient was her appearance. She may not have had the commitment to plaque control that sometimes comes with a desire to keep teeth at all costs. Patients like this will always need a permanent programme of maintenance, with subgingival debridement every 3–6 months.

DECISIONS AT THE REASSESSMENT AFTER NON-SURGICAL TREATMENT

How do we make use of the further knowledge that we are given by reassessment – the knowledge of response to treatment? This needs to be interpreted in the light of the main behavioural factors that condition treatment: plaque control and smoking. It is a principle of ethical treatment that the patient should be given appropriate attention that is likely to improve health. First, let us look at the question of plaque control.

If plaque has been well controlled by the patient with excellent compliance from the time of initial instruction, and scores of below 10% have been recorded regularly at each root planing and scaling appointment, then there is little that remains to be achieved in most patients. A score of below 5% is even better, of course, as is the rarely-attained level of zero. But for all practical purposes, the 10% threshold indicates good compliance.

Compliance, or adherence to instructions, is not solely to be measured by the plaque score. If there is marginal gingival inflammation where plaque has been removed, and if the inflammation is more generally present, then the implication is that the patient has recently cleaned the teeth thoroughly but has not done this habitually. It signals a person who either finds plaque control too difficult or too time consuming, but also a patient who has not understood the need and importance of this behaviour.

If, for any reason, plaque control does not appear adequate, then this should be explained in a way that is not likely to alienate the patient. Credit may be given for anything that has been achieved and the patient's attention should be directed to problem areas with actual oral hygiene practice. The clinician must indicate that few clinical procedures can produce lasting results in the absence of good plaque control.

If repeated instruction and help does not produce the desired result, then a maintenance programme is instituted, with regular encouragement in oral hygiene and subgingival debridement at 3–6 month intervals; during such a programme the patient can be reassessed every 1–2 years, and if better compliance is forthcoming, a decision may be taken to return to a definite treatment plan.

Fig. 30,35

Excellent right-side response to OHI and root planing in female smoker, aged 46 years, who smoked 15 cigarettes per day for 25 years.

Fig. 30,36

Left-side response is similarly good. The plaque control is virtually total, and surgery is appropriate for the next stage of treatment.

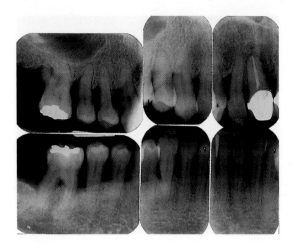

Fig. 30,37

Right-side radiographs show the advanced bone loss that is the background for the excellent response to non-surgical treatment.

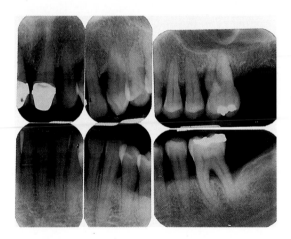

Fig. 30,38

Similar advanced disease on the left side.

EFFECT OF SMOKING ON THE TREATMENT PLAN

Although smoking is probably the most significant environmental factor in periodontitis, it is as well to put it in perspective. Smoking exacerbates the disease, and also reduces the treatment effect. It does not produce disease where there is no plaque. For

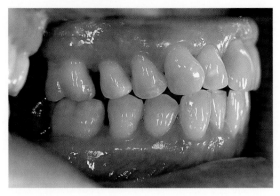

Fig. 30,39

At 3 months post-root planing, reassessment shows excellent plaque control and an absence of gingival inflammation are apparent. Right view.

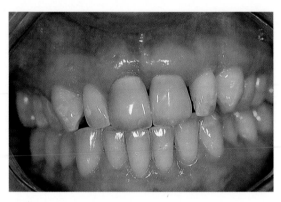

Fig. 30,40

Central view.

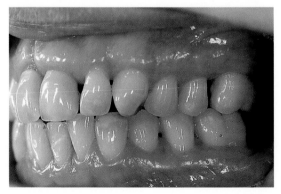

Fig. 30,41

Left view.

these reasons, all types of periodontal treatment may be considered, but with two provisos: first, plaque control needs to be near-perfect; secondly, the prognosis in a smoker should be viewed as less satisfactory than in a non-smoker with a similar condition.

When apprised of the situation, some smokers are able to produce outstanding plaque control but unable to quit the habit. An example of the response to initial treatment in such a patient is shown in Figs 30,35–30,41. Subsequently, surgery was planned and performed uneventfully with satisfactory results.

MANAGEMENT STRATEGY IN ACTION

To illustrate the decisions made at each stage of management, we will consider two typical case histories of patients with advanced periodontitis: a 37-year-old man whose response to treatment was very satisfactory, and a 38-year-old female whose response was satisfactory but who needed a long-term follow-up.

In Figs 30,42–30,50, the initial radiographs, final photographs and sequential PD charts are given for a patient treated for advanced periodontitis affecting most of the teeth. Only teeth 11, 21, 31–33, 41 and 42 appeared largely unaffected. There were no furca involvements greater than grade 1, and there was recession of 1–3 mm only on the palatal aspects of teeth 16, 17, 26 and 27. On the basis of attachment loss, position in the dental arch and radiographic support, the individual tooth prognoses were assessed as: teeth 28, 38, 48 unsavable; teeth 14–18, 25–27, 37 and 46 doubtful; all remaining teeth savable or unaffected.

Because of the status of the third molars, the patient was advised to have them removed at the outset of treatment, and agreed. This also made treatment access easier for the four second molars.

The response to non-surgical treatment was excellent (probing chart 2). Plaque control was maintained throughout treatment at a level where less than 5% of surfaces were affected. At the reassessment, the following treatment

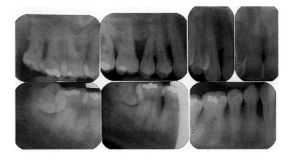

Fig. 30,42

Advanced periodontitis in a 37-year-old male: right-side radiographs.

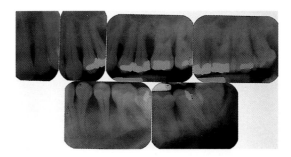

Fig. 30,43

Left side.

3		3 3 4	4 2 4	5 3 2	2 2 7	6 2 4	3 2 2	2 2 2
		2 2 3	3 2 3	4 2 3	3 3 7	3 3 3	5 6 2	2 2 2
2		5 3 6	7 3 7	8 2 3	2 2 5	3 1 4	3 2 2	2 2 2
		6 4 6	5 2 5	7 3 3	3 3 8	5 6 4	5 6 2	2 2 3
1	6 7 9	7 5 9	10 3 10	11 9 3	3 3 9	7 3 5	7 2 3	3 1 2
	3 5 7	8 5 8	8 2 5	7 9 2	2 2 9	9 5 4	8 6 2	2 2 2
	8	**7**	**6**	**5**	**4**	**3**	**2**	**1**
	8	**7**	**6**	**5**	**4**	**3**	**2**	**1**
1	5 5 7	5 2 3	9 2 2	2 2 4	1 1 3	2 1 2	2 1 1	1 1 1
	7 8 8	9 5 2	10 8 2	4 1 2	1 1 5	8 2 2	2 2 2	3 1 2
2		3 2 3	4 2 3	3 2 5	2 2 3	5 1 2	2 1 1	2 2 1 2
		5 3 2	3 2 2	2 1 1 3	3 1 1 2	5 1 2 3	3 3 1 2	2 1 1 2
3		2 1 3	3 2 2	2 2 3	2 1 1 2	5 2 2	1 1 1	1 1 1
		2 1 2	5 2 3	3 2 3	2 2 2	4 1 1 2	2 1 1	2 1 2

Fig 30,44

First 3 probing charts of the right side (see text).

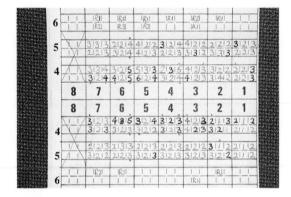

Fig. 30,45

First 3 probing charts of the left side (see text).

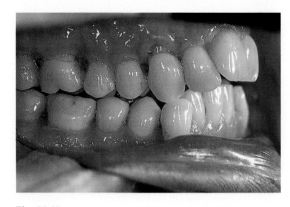

Fig. 30,48

Right view 5 years after surgery.

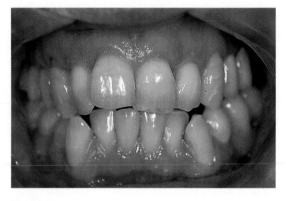

Fig. 30,46

Probing charts 4 and 5 of the right side with final recession chart (see text).

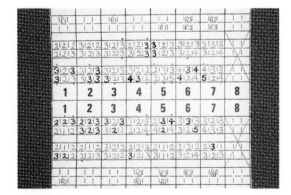

Fig. 30,49

Central view.

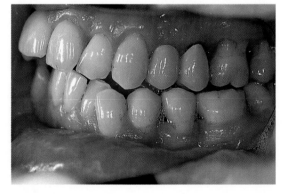

Fig. 30,47

Probing charts 4 and 5 of the left side (see text).

Fig. 30,50

Left view.

was planned and subsequently performed: further root planing for teeth 22–24, 43, 45 and 47; flap surgery for teeth 12–17, 25–27 (with distal wedge resection), and 35–37.

Three months after completion of this treatment, further improvements had occurred (probing chart 3). However, the result at this stage was less than adequate in teeth 13–15, 25, 34 and 46, which all had a PD of 5 mm. These were all planed again and after 2 years (probing chart 4) the condition was improved in the worst-affected teeth (teeth 13 and 14), but with slight recurrences in several places (teeth 15, 16, 26 and 27).

By this time maintenance was every 3 months, and 5 years after surgery (6 years after initial assessment: probing chart 5) there were minimal bleeding points and maximum PD of 4 mm only on seven teeth. At this stage, the disease was considered controlled, but maintenance continued on a permanent basis.

To give a fuller picture of the changes from start to finish, the presence of recession is marked in the midsurface spaces on the final chart. In progressing from the initial presentation of disease to the result 6 years later, considerable inflammation was resolved and recession contributed to the reduction of pockets.

AN ILLUSTRATION OF THE NEED FOR PERMANENT MAINTENANCE

In the next case, shown in Figs 30,51–30,60, a severe problem was treated first with root planing and adjunctive metronidazole. This was a few years ago, but I would still use metronidazole today in such a case because of the presence of suppuration in deep pockets. The response was again excellent (the second chart is 6 months later) and the patient was put on a maintenance programme.

However, at 18 months (chart 3) there was sufficient recurrence of disease, despite good oral hygiene and repeated root planing, to suggest a need for further treatment. Access flap surgery was performed for teeth 11–16, 21–26, 37 and 45. At this stage, it was confirmed that the problem on the buccal surface of tooth 37 was linked to unfavourable

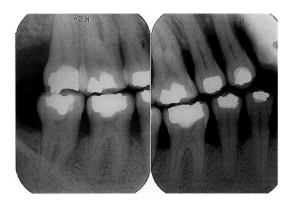

Fig. 30,51

38-year-old female with advanced periodontitis: right posterior radiographs.

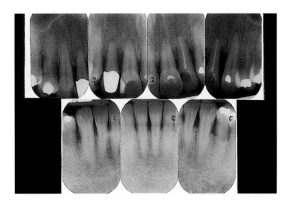

Fig. 30,52

Anterior radiographs.

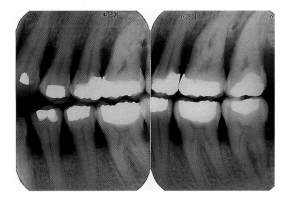

Fig. 30,53

Left posterior radiographs. Tooth 37 has furca involvement with unfavourable morphology.

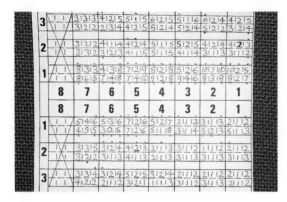

Fig. 30,54

First three probing charts of right side (see text).

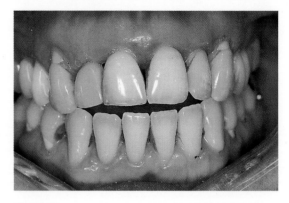

Fig. 30,57

Central view.

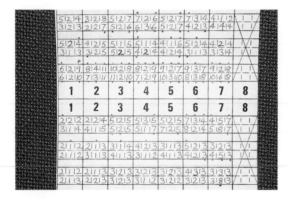

Fig. 30,55

First three probing charts of left side (see text).

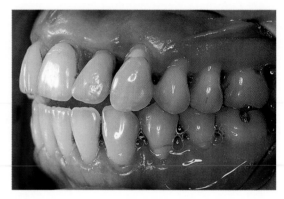

Fig. 30,58

Left side.

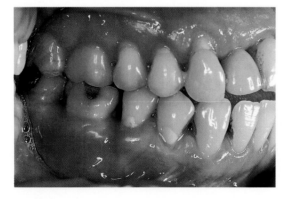

Fig. 30,56

Appearance of right side at this stage.

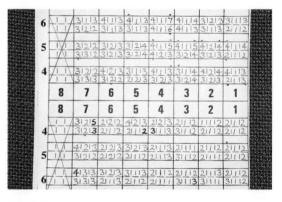

Fig. 30,59

Probing charts 4–6 of the right side (see text).

```
5|1|3  2|1|4  2|1|3  5|1|5  3|1|5  3|2|4  3|1|3  |  |
1|1|2  2|1|1  2|2|3  2|1|2  2|1|2  3|1|3  2|2|2  |  |

4|2|4  3|2|5  5|1|4  5|1|5  4|1|5  3|2|3  4|2|4  |  |
2|1|2  2|1|3  5|2|3  4|3|3  4|2|3  2|3|4  3|3|4  |  |

4|1|4  3|3|5  4|2|4  5|1|4  4|1|4  4|2|5  5|2|4  |  |
2|1|2  2|1|4  3|2|3  3|2|3  3|2|3  3|2|4  4|3|3  |  |

   1      2      3      4      5      6      7      8

   1      2      3      4      5      6      7      8

2|1|1  1|1|2  2|1|2  3|2|3  3|2|2  3|2|3  3|2|3  |  |
2|1|2  2|1|2  2|1|2  3|1|2  3|1|2  3|1|3  3|7|3  |  |

2|1|1  2|1|2  2|1|3  3|2|3  3|1|3  3|2|2  2|1|3  |  |
2|1|2  2|1|2  3|1|2  3|1|3  3|1|2  3|1|3  3|8|2  |  |

2|1|2  2|1|3  2|1|2  2|1|2  1|1|2  1|2|1       |  |
2|1|2  2|1|1  2|1|4  5|1|3  3|1|4  2|1|3       |  |
```

Fig. 30,60

Probing charts 4–6 of the left side (see text).

furcation morphology, and the patient was advised that the tooth could not be guaranteed.

One and two years after surgery, the majority of problems were kept in check with the maintenance programme (charts 4 and 5). By the sixth year after surgery (chart 6), however, although bleeding was minimal there was a clear tendency for one pocket to increase in depth on the mesial surface of tooth 14. When 2 mm of recession was taken into account it had regressed to, or even beyond, the state at initial assessment 8 years previously. This is an example of the need for permanent maintenance and occasional retreatment, which in this case was performed surgically because the pocket had recurred despite regular maintenance scaling and planing.

It is also apparent that tooth 37 was lost between the second and sixth years after surgery (actually about 4 years later). The patient wanted to retain this tooth as long as possible despite the unfavourable prognosis, and there was no reason other than the possibility of discomfort to do otherwise. When it eventually developed a small abscess, the patient accepted its extraction.

CONCLUSION: THE HUMAN FACE OF PERIODONTICS

We have come full circle in this book, which started with the human environment of the periodontium. We then considered the essential scientific and other questions that are of importance in understanding disease and treatment, and ended with the application of periodontal knowledge in the management of patients.

Although scientific knowledge is the foundation of any clinical discipline, the way in which it is applied is equally important. In some respects, modern scientific medicine has acquired a tarnished image. On the one hand, the media are so full of excitement about amazing new advances that some patients expect there to be a miracle cure for every problem. On the other hand, we frequently read of the anger of those who rightly or wrongly feel that they have suffered because of clinical incompetence or arrogance.

The answer is to practise scientifically but with sensitivity and gentleness. Patients need scientific advice, but they also have their own objectives and feelings, however these may appear to the clinician. If patients wish to go against our advice, then as long as they understand our reasons for offering it, we have a duty to support them as far as it is possible. Clearly, discussions and disagreements must be recorded in the notes to avoid problems.

One final caveat: we do not know all the patient's other problems. One of the author's long-term patients is a lady who worked very hard at plaque control and then disappeared for a long period in the middle of her treatment, failing to keep appointments. It transpired that she had two major concerns: possible recurrence of a malignancy that had been treated some years before, and a severe illness affecting her daughter, who nearly died as a result.

We cannot know the burdens which our patients face in other aspects of life, unless they confide in us. It is therefore a good strategy to cultivate humility and friendliness, rather than the detachment and lack of feeling that is sometimes described by unhappy patients in the media. Kindness and sympathy must be the first rule in clinical periodontics.

REFERENCES

Budnick LD (1984) Toothpick-related injuries in the United States, 1979 through 1982. *Journal of the American Medical Association* **252**: 796–797.

Dean HT, Arnold FA, Elvove E (1942) Domestic water and dental caries. *Public Health Reports* **57**: 1155–1179.

Ericsson I, Lindhe J (1977) Lack of effect of trauma from occlusion on the recurrence of experimental periodontitis. *Journal of Clinical Periodontology* **4**: 115–127.

Ericsson I, Lindhe J (1982) Effect of longstanding jiggling on experimental marginal periodontitis in the beagle dog. *Journal of Clinical Periodontology* **9**: 497–503.

Hancock EB (1981) Determination of periodontal disease activity. *Journal of Periodontology* **52**: 492–499.

Kantor M, Polson AM, Zander HA (1976) Alveolar bone regeneration after removal of inflammatory and traumatic factors. *Journal of Periodontology* **47:** 687–695.

Kennedy JE, Polson AM (1973) Experimental marginal periodontitis in squirrel monkeys. *Journal of Periodontology* **44**: 140–144.

Kieser JB (1974) An approach to periodontal pocket elimination. *British Journal of Oral Surgery* **12**: 177–195.

Kinane DF, Cullen CF, Johnston FA, et al (1989) Neutrophil chemotactic behaviour in patients with early-onset forms of periodontitis (II). Assessment using the under agarose technique. *Journal of Clinical Periodontology* **16**: 247–251.

Lindhe J, Hamp S, Löe H (1973) Experimental periodontitis in the beagle dog. *Journal of Periodontal Research* **8**: 1–10.

Lindhe J, Ericsson I (1976) The influence of trauma from occlusion on reduced but healthy periodontal tissues in dogs. *Journal of Clinical Periodontology* **3**: 110–122.

Lindhe J, Ericsson I (1982) The effect of elimination of jiggling forces on periodontally exposed teeth in the dog. *Journal of Periodontology* **53**: 562–567.

Löe H, Silness J (1963) Periodontal disease in pregnancy. I. Prevalence and severity. *Acta Odontologica Scandinavica* **21**: 533–551.

Loesche WJ (1976) Chemotherapy of dental plaque infections. *Oral Sciences Reviews* **9**: 65–107.

Lundqvist C (1952) Oral sugar clearance, its influence on dental caries activity. *Odontologisk Revy* **3**: Suppl. 1.

McCormick J (1993) Olfaction. In praise of stinks. *Lancet* **341**: 1126–1127.

O'Leary TJ, Drake RB, Naylor JE (1972) The plaque control record. *Journal of Periodontology* **43**: 38.

O'Mullane DM (1976) Efficiency in clinical trials of caries preventive agents and methods. *Community Dentistry and Oral Epidemiology* **4**: 190–194.

Page RC, Baab DA (1985) A new look at the etiology and pathogenesis of early-onset periodontitis. Cementopathia revisited. *Journal of Periodontology* **56**: 748–751.

Page RC, Schroeder HE (1976) Pathogenesis of inflammatory periodontal disease. A summary of current work. *Laboratory Investigation* **34**: 235–249.

Page RC, Schroeder HE (1982) *Periodontitis in Man and Animals. A comparative review* (Basel: Karger).

Parakkal PF (1979) Proceedings of the workshop on quantitative evaluation of periodontal diseases by physical measurement techniques. *Journal of Dental Research* **58**: 547–553.

Polson AM, Zander HA (1983) Effect of periodontal trauma upon intrabony pockets. *Journal of Periodontology* **54**: 586–591.

Polson AM, Meitner SW, Zander HA (1976a) Trauma and progression of marginal periodontitis in squirrel monkeys. III. Adaptation of interproximal alveolar bone to repetitive injury. *Journal of Periodontal Research* **11**: 279–289.

Polson AM, Meitner SW, Zander HA (1976b) Trauma and progression of marginal periodontitis in squirrel monkeys. IV. Reversibility of bone loss due to trauma alone and trauma superimposed upon periodontitis. *Journal of Periodontal Research* **11**: 290–298.

Polson AM, Adams RA, Zander HA (1983) Osseous repair in the presence of active tooth hypermobility. *Journal of Clinical Periodontology* **10**: 370–379.

Ramfjord SP, Nissle RR (1974) The modified Widman flap. *Journal of Periodontology* **45**: 601–607.

Schroeder HE, de Boever J (1970) The structure of microbial dental plaque. In: McHugh WD, ed, *Dental Plaque, a symposium* (E, S Livingstone: Edinburgh), pp 49–74.

Socransky SS (1979) Criteria for the infectious agents in dental caries and periodontal disease. *Journal of Clinical Periodontology* **6**: 16–21.

Watts TLP (1995). Coenzyme Q10 and periodontal treatment: is there any beneficial effect? *British Dental Journal* **178**: 209–213.

INDEX

Note: page references in *italics* are to figures; those in **bold** are to tables.